T0192776

Nutrition and HIV

Epidemiological Evidence
to Public Health

Nutrition and HIV

Epidemiological Evidence
to Public Health

Edited by

Saurabh Mehta

and

Julia L. Finkelstein

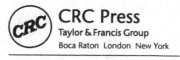

CRC Press
Taylor & Francis Group
Boca Raton London New York

CRC Press is an imprint of the
Taylor & Francis Group, an **informa** business

CRC Press
Taylor & Francis Group
6000 Broken Sound Parkway NW, Suite 300
Boca Raton, FL 33487-2742

First issued in paperback 2021

ISBN 13: 978-1-03-209544-8 (pbk)
ISBN 13: 978-1-4665-8581-2 (hbk)

Library of Congress Cataloging-in-Publication Data

Names: Mehta, Saurabh, author. | Finkelstein, Julia L., author.
Title: Nutrition and HIV : epidemiological evidence to public health /
Saurabh Mehta and Julia L. Finkelstein.
Description: Boca Raton : Taylor & Francis, 2018. | "A CRC title, part of the
Taylor & Francis imprint, a member of the Taylor & Francis Group, the
academic division of T&F Informa plc."
Identifiers: LCCN 2017053162 | ISBN 9781466585812 (hardback : alk. paper)
9781351246989 (ebook)
Subjects: LCSH: AIDS (Disease)--Nutritional aspects. | AIDS (Disease)--Diet
therapy. | AIDS (Disease)--Epidemiology.
Classification: LCC RC607.A26 M444 2018 | DDC 616.97/92--dc23
LC record available at http://lccn.loc.gov/2017053162

Visit the Taylor & Francis Web site at
http://www.taylorandfrancis.com

and the CRC Press Web site at
http://www.crcpress.com

Contents

List of Figures

List of Tables

Foreword

Ron:
I thought AZT's supposed to help me.

Dr. Vass:
The only people AZT helps are the people who sell it. (beat) It kills every cell it comes in contact with, good and bad.

Ron:
So medically speakin', I kicked my own ass!

Dr. Vass:
(nods as he writes)
I'm prescribing a regimen of vitamins as well as the mineral zinc to build your immune system back up. You'll also be taking Aloe and essential fatty acids.

Dallas Buyers Club script

The above excerpt from the script for the 2013 American film *Dallas Buyers Club* is from a scene that touched me in both personal and professional ways. This encounter between Ron (Matthew McConaughey) and Dr. Vass (Griffin Dunne) represents a historical turning point in the role of nutrition in the management of the HIV epidemic. I have long reflected on the particular period reflected in the movie. There has been an unprecedented search to understand the impact that nutrition has on the health and wellbeing of individuals living with HIV/AIDS. The almost messianic merits of "alternative" approaches to HIV and AIDS prevention and treatment played an important role during one of the worst moments of the epidemic. We finally reached the point of acknowledging that fighting against HIV also entails dealing with lifestyle modifications. The various definitions of healthy lifestyles are vague, but equally uncertain are the nutritional recommendations regarding HIV and AIDS. Numerous research efforts have produced myriad results that appear to conflict with each other. The concept of *evidence-based medicine* gained visibility at about this same time. Given the existing scientific evidence and experience to date, it would be irresponsible to ignore the importance of nutrition in patient-centered care for those living with HIV.

I lived similar scenes of despair when I lost friends and family members to this disease. During my research at the Latin American Center for Sexually Transmitted Diseases in Puerto Rico, many patients poured through the clinic doors reporting allegedly efficacious nutrition interventions. Like Ron, the main character in *Dallas Buyers Club*, patients in many hospitals were looking for hope in the midst of a terrible health and stigmatizing drama. Because I was witnessing all too often the accelerated deterioration of HIV-affected individuals' health and wellbeing, I felt compelled to dig deeper into nutrition as a determinant of health in this group. What seemed to be an obvious research gap at the time still remains a mix of conflicting certainties and ongoing controversies.

Today, we are able to use many tools to reshape what was once an unavoidable death sentence. We have transformed the challenges of the infection by creating an orchestrated effort to manage what we can gladly consider a chronic condition. Nutrition plays a clear and relevant role in promoting health and preventing and treating this infection and its co-morbidities. We have the evidence necessary to help countries achieve the sustainable development goals by 2030. The retrieval, synthesis, and assessment of evidence on the effects of various aspects of nutrition presented in this book are certainly a welcome contribution to these ongoing efforts.

Juan Pablo Peña-Rosas, MD, PhD, MPH
Coordinator, Evidence and Programme Guidance
Nutrition for Health and Development
World Health Organization

Preface

In 1981, the Centers for Disease Control and Prevention published case studies on an immune dysfunction that was later recognized as the Acquired Immune Deficiency Syndrome (AIDS), and the causal linkage to infection with the human immunodeficiency virus (HIV) was established a few years hence. The world continues to lose more than a million lives every year to this epidemic, and nearly two million were infected with HIV in the last year alone. Though a vaccine or cure is still elusive, considerable progress in terms of a decline in mortality due to AIDS has been achieved through the increasing availability and coverage of antiretroviral treatment (ART).

The new Sustainable Development Goals, adopted by countries of the United Nations in 2015, include a commitment to end the AIDS epidemic by 2030. Considerable emphasis on prevention of new infections and treatment of those living with HIV will be needed to make this goal achievable. With nearly 37 million people now living with HIV, it is a communicable disease that behaves like a noncommunicable disease (NCD). For example, HIV infection is associated with increased risk for type 2 diabetes mellitus, independent of other risk factors such as age, sex, ethnic origin, sexual orientation, family history of NCDs, smoking, illicit drug use, or heavy alcohol use. People living with HIV (PLHIV) may now spend decades of their lives infected and have an increased burden of other complications, including dyslipidemias and cardiometabolic outcomes.

We believe that a comprehensive approach that includes nutritional interventions is likely to maximize the benefit of antiretroviral therapy in preventing HIV disease progression and other adverse outcomes in HIV-infected men and women. Nutrition is a modifiable risk factor that has been acknowledged to be one of the most cost-effective approaches for intervention in a number of health outcomes by forums such as the Copenhagen Consensus; for example, recent analyses in *JAMA* have suggested that nutrition-related issues constitute 50% or more of the risk factors for mortality both in the United States and globally.

This book highlights the evidence base for linking nutrition and HIV and identifies research gaps to inform the development of guidelines and policies that focus on people living with HIV. We are grateful to CRC Press for focusing this volume on such an important topic, as well as to the contributors for making this work possible. We also acknowledge Dr. Juan Pablo Peña-Rosas for kindly writing the foreword for this book. Additionally, we wish to thank Patricia Mason for her attention to detail and tireless work in helping us copyedit the chapters.

About the Editors

Saurabh Mehta, MBBS, ScD, is a physician with expertise in infectious disease, nutrition, epidemiology, and diagnostics. He trained in medicine at the All-India Institute of Medical Sciences in New Delhi, India, and then received his doctoral degree in epidemiology and nutrition from Harvard University in Cambridge, Massachusetts. He is currently an associate professor of global health, epidemiology, and nutrition in the Division of Nutritional Sciences at Cornell University in Ithaca, New York. The overarching focus of his research program is to identify, diagnose, and intervene on modifiable risk factors such as nutrition to improve population health, with advances in technological innovation being an integral component of his approach. His research is accomplished through a combination of active surveillance programs, development of smartphone diagnostics for nutrition and infection, and randomized controlled trials primarily in resource-limited settings in India, sub-Saharan Africa, and Latin America.

Julia L. Finkelstein, MPH, SM, ScD, is the Follett Sesquicentennial Faculty Fellow and assistant professor of epidemiology and nutrition in the Division of Nutritional Sciences, Cornell University. She is also an adjunct associate professor at St. John's Research Institute in Bangalore, India, and a Faculty Fellow at the Center for Geographic Analysis, Harvard University. She received her bachelor of science degree from McGill University, Montreal, Quebec; her master of public health degree from Brown University, Providence, Rhode Island; and master of science and doctor of science degrees in epidemiology and nutrition from Harvard University. Dr. Finkelstein is an epidemiologist with expertise in designing and conducting randomized clinical trials, cohort studies, and surveillance programs in resource-limited settings. Her research focuses on the intersection of micronutrients, infections, and maternal and child health. The goal of the Finkelstein Laboratory is to elucidate the role of micronutrients (i.e., iron, vitamin B_{12}, and folate) in the etiology of infections and adverse pregnancy outcomes with the goal of improving the health of mothers and young children. This approach integrates nutrition, epidemiology, immunology, and biostatistics with an emphasis on the translation of laboratory findings and epidemiologic evidence to inform interventions and public health practice in at-risk populations. Dr. Finkelstein serves as an external expert with the World Health Organization (WHO) Nutrition Guidelines Group; as a core faculty member in the Pan American Health Organization/World Health Organization (PAHO/WHO) Collaborating Centre for Implementation Research in Nutrition and Global Policy; as an expert consultant for the WHO Vitamin and Mineral Information System Database, a global database of anemia and micronutrient biomarkers for all countries; and as an NIH reviewer for the National Institute of Diabetes and Digestive and Kidney Diseases (NIDDK).

About the Contributors

Haritha Aribindi is an M.D. candidate and Harrison Scholar at the Medical College of Georgia in Augusta. She graduated with distinction from Cornell University, Ithaca, New York, majoring in biological sciences with a concentration in human nutrition. As part of the Finkelstein Laboratory, she assisted with systematic literature reviews and fieldwork as part of a periconceptional surveillance program in southern India. Her research focused on the role of micronutrients in the etiology of anemia in women of reproductive age.

Anna Coutsoudis, PhD, is a public health scientist who held the post of professor in the Department of Paediatrics and Child Health, Nelson R. Mandela School of Medicine, University of KwaZulu-Natal, Durban, South Africa. In 2016, she was awarded professor emeritus status. She has done extensive research on HIV and nutrition, especially in breastfeeding, and has published over 120 peer-reviewed journal articles. Her research work has played an important role in shaping World Health Organization (WHO) guidelines on HIV and infant feeding, and she is a member of several WHO committees and guideline groups. She has served as chairperson of the Technical Steering Committee of the WHO Department of Child and Adolescent Health and Development. She is committed to improving maternal and child health in vulnerable communities through strategies that empower communities. In recognition of her contributions, she was recently awarded the Science for Society Gold Medal award by the Academy of Science of South Africa. In 2000, Dr. Coutsoudis established the first community-based breast milk bank in South Africa specifically to provide donor breast milk to AIDS orphans, and she was one of the founding members of the Human Milk Banking Association of South Africa, which she currently chairs. Over the last several years, she has been collaborating with the Department of Health to scale up donor human milk banking in South Africa. She is currently leading research into low-cost, accessible technology for pasteurization of donor human milk and projects to set up human milk banks in several African countries.

Suzanne Filteau, PhD, trained first in chemistry and then completed postgraduate studies in nutrition. Her research focuses on interactions between nutrition and infectious diseases, mainly in women and children in low-income countries and mainly with HIV. Her work in Africa has investigated infant feeding and maternal health in the context of endemic HIV. She has been a principal investigator of two large randomized controlled trials related to HIV in Africa: a trial of multiple micronutrient fortification of complementary foods for Zambian children and a trial of nutritional supplements to decrease the early mortality of HIV-infected Zambian and Tanzanian adults starting antiretroviral therapy. She has also been involved in other micronutrient studies, including those involving vitamin D and child health in India.

Henrik Friis, MD, PhD, is a former associate professor of epidemiology and current professor of international nutrition and health at the Department of Nutrition, Exercise and Sports, University of Copenhagen, Denmark. For the last 30 years, he has done research with collaborators in various low-income countries, mainly in Africa, and has supervised a large number of PhD students. The focus of the research has been the role of nutrition in relation to infections. The main aim has been to develop and test micronutrient interventions for school children and pregnant women, as well as food-based interventions for adults with HIV and tuberculosis and for children with acute malnutrition.

Ameena Goga, MD, MS, PhD, is a chief specialist scientist at the South African Medical Research Council and holds the post of extraordinary professor in the Department of Paediatrics, University of Pretoria. She is a pediatrician with a PhD in pediatrics and master's degree in epidemiology and mother and child health. She has worked at the policy level at the South African National

Department of Health, as a clinician at the implementation level (hospitals, clinics, and households), as a mentor, and as a researcher. Her most recent work included the follow-up of HIV-exposed, uninfected infants to determine 18-month outcomes. Her work has helped shape national infant feeding and PMTCT policies and targets.

Heather S. Herman is a research specialist with the Finkelstein Laboratory at Cornell University, Ithaca, New York. After earning her bachelor of science degree in human biology at Cornell University in 2016, she worked as a senior research analyst and public health advisor at Jacobi Medical Center, Bronx, New York, for Project BRIEF, an HIV testing and research program funded by the Centers for Disease Control and Prevention. At Jacobi, her clinical work included performing rapid HIV screening and diagnosis of and counseling for HIV-infected patients. Her research has focused on assessing the training of healthcare providers with regard to HIV care for a low-income, urban community in Bronx County, New York. As part of the Finkelstein Laboratory, her research has focused on the intersection of nutrition and infectious diseases, and she is particularly interested in zoonotic diseases. She has conducted fieldwork in Guayaquil, Ecuador, and trained on the Cochrane Systematic Review methodology at the Third Annual WHO/Cochrane Summer Institute for Systematic Reviews in Nutrition for Global Policy-Making.

Samantha L. Huey is a doctoral student in the Mehta Research Group. In 2013, Samantha graduated with honors from Cedar Crest College, Allentown, Pennsylvania, with a bachelor of science in biology with minors in nutrition and global diseases. Her graduate research focuses on characterizing the relationships among vitamin D, immune function, and the gut microbiome among children. Currently, she is conducting fieldwork in Mumbai, India, for a large randomized controlled trial focused on efficacy of biofortified crops in improving growth and immune competence.

Nabila R. Khondakar graduated with distinction in biological sciences from Cornell University, Ithaca, New York. As part of the Finkelstein research group, she has conducted systematic literature reviews on anemia, iron, and adverse pregnancy outcomes. Her research interests focus on the role of iron in infection and maternal and child health outcomes. She is currently an MD candidate at SUNY Downstate College of Medicine, Brooklyn, New York.

Alexander J. Layden is an MD–PhD candidate in the Department of Epidemiology at the University of Pittsburgh, Pennsylvania. He earned his bachelor of science degree in biology at Cornell University, graduating with high honors (*magna cum laude*) with distinction in research. He conducted his undergraduate honors thesis with Dr. Finkelstein on vitamin B_{12} transport across the placenta. As part of the Finkelstein research group, Mr. Layden investigated the role of micronutrients in the etiology of adverse maternal and child health outcomes in India and Ecuador. He is currently researching the etiology of placental inflammation and its consequences for perinatal health in domestic and global populations.

Mette Frahm Olsen, PhD, has a background in public health science and is researching global health and nutrition at the University of Copenhagen. Her doctoral thesis investigated the effects and feasibility of nutritional supplementation for HIV patients starting antiretroviral treatment and was based on a randomized trial in Jimma, Ethiopia. Mette is currently involved in studies in Ethiopia, Tanzania, and Uganda, focusing on nutrition among either adults with infectious diseases or children with acute malnutrition. Her fields of interest include malnutrition and infectious diseases, body composition assessment methodology, child development, and long-term consequences of malnutrition. She enjoys working where academic thinking meets real-world challenges and conducting research that can support better healthcare decision making. She has experience with a broad range of research methodologies, including quantitative and qualitative approaches. She has been involved with communicable disease surveillance as an epidemiologist at the WHO Regional

Office for Europe and has worked with various nongovernment organizations, including the Danish Family Planning Association, Amnesty International, and Red Cross Youth.

Amanda L. Wilkinson, PhD, earned her doctorate in nutrition from Cornell University in 2015. She graduated with a concentration in international nutrition and minors in epidemiology and human nutrition. Her graduate research focused on examining the interactions among HIV infection, inflammation, and maternal and child health and how they affect pregnant women and infants in sub-Saharan Africa. Dr. Wilkinson received her bachelor of science degree in nutritional sciences from Pennsylvania State University, State College, Pennsylvania, where she graduated with distinction from the Schreyer Honors College. Her current research interests are in the areas of nutritional epidemiology, infectious diseases, and under-5 child mortality prevention.

Elaine A. Yu, MPH, PhD, currently focuses on metabolic abnormalities and infectious diseases (tuberculosis, human immunodeficiency virus) among clinical populations internationally and in the United States. Her research interests include how diabetes, infectious diseases, and malnutrition intersect, especially in resource-limited contexts. She is a postdoctoral fellow at Cornell University, Ithaca, NY, where she completed her doctorate in nutrition. Previously, she earned her bachelor of arts degree at the University of California, Berkeley, her master of public health degree at Emory University, Atlanta, Georgia.

Abbreviations

3TC	Lamivudine
ABCA1	ATP-binding cassette transporter A1
ACT	α1-Antichymotrypsin
AFASS	Acceptable, feasible, affordable, sustainable, safe
AGP	Alpha-1-acid glycoprotein
AHR	Adjusted hazard ratio
AIDS	Acquired Immune Deficiency Syndrome
ALP	Alkaline phosphatase
AMD	Adjusted mean difference
AMH	Anti-Müllerian hormone
AOR	Adjusted odds ratio
APR	Adjusted prevalence ratio
ARI	Acute respiratory infection
ART	Antiretroviral therapy
ARV	Antiretroviral
ATRA	All-*trans*-retinoic acid
AZT	azidothymidine (zidovudine)
BAN Study	Breastfeeding, Antiretrovirals, and Nutrition Study
BAP	Bone alkaline phosphatase
BDI	Beck Depression Inventory
BF	Breastfeeding
BMD	Bone mineral density
BMI	Body mass index
BSAP	Bone-specific alkaline phosphatase
BSID	Bayley Scales of Infant Development
C	Control group
CAD	Coronary artery disease
CAPRISA	Centre for the AIDS Programme of Research in South Africa
cART	Combination antiretroviral therapy (also HAART)
CBA	Competitive binding assay
CC	Case-control study
CDC	Centers for Disease Control and Prevention
cEVR	Complete early virologic response
CI	Confidence interval
cIMT	Carotid intima–media thickness
CLIA	Chemiluminescence immunoassay
CoDe	Coding Causes of Death in HIV
CpG	Cytosine–phosphate–guanine
CRP	C-reactive protein
CTX	Cotrimoxazole
Cu/Zn	Copper/zinc ratio
CVL	Cervicovaginal lavage
D_2	Ergocalciferol
D_3	Cholecalciferol
DBP	Diastolic blood pressure
DMSO	Dimethyl sulfoxide

DOTS	Directly Observed Treatment Short-Course
DPD	Desoxypyridinoline
EBF	Exclusive breastfeeding
ECLIA	Electrochemiluminescence immunoassay
EFF	Exclusive formula feeding
EFV	Efavirenz
EIA	Enzyme immunoassay
ELISA	Enzyme-linked immunosorbent assay
EMTCT	Elimination of mother-to-child transmission
FAO	Food and Agriculture Organization of the United Nations
Fe	Iron
Ff	*FokI* polymorphism
FF	Formula feeding
FFQ	Food frequency questionnaire
FGF-23	Fibroblast growth factor 23
FMD	Flow-mediated dilatation
FMLP	Formyl peptide
FVB/N	Control mice strain
GABA	Gamma-aminobutyric acid
HAART	Highly active antiretroviral therapy
HAZ	Height-for-age *z*-score
Hb	Hemoglobin
HCV	Hepatitis C virus
HDL	High-density lipoprotein
HERS	HIV Epidemiology Research Study
HIV	Human immunodeficiency virus
HIVAN	HIV-associated nephropathy
HMO	Human milk oligosaccharide
holoTC	Holotranscobalamin
HOMA-IR	Homeostatic model assessment of insulin resistance
HPLC	High-performance liquid chromatography
HR	Hazard ratio
hs-CRP	High-sensitivity C-reactive protein
HSCL-25	Hopkins Symptom Checklist-25
ID	Iron deficiency
IDA	Iron deficiency anemia
IFN-γ	Interferon-gamma
IL	Interleukin
Int	Intervention group
IQR	Interquartile range
IR	Incidence ratio
IRR	Incidence rate ratio
IU	International unit
IUGR	Intrauterine growth restriction
LAZ	Length-for-age *z*-score
LBW	Low birthweight
LC/MS/TS	Liquid chromatography/mass spectroscopy/tandem spectroscopy
LNS	Lipid-based nutrient supplement
LPT	Late postnatal transmission
LRTI	Lower respiratory tract infection
LTR	Long terminal repeat

MAC	*Mycobacterium avium* complex
MACS	Multicenter AIDS Cohort Study
MAF	Macrophage-activating factor
MAPK1/2	Mitogen-activated protein kinase 1 and 2
MBF	Mixed breastfeeding
MBL-2	Mannose-binding lectin 2 gene
MCV	Mean corpuscular volume
MD	Mean difference
MDD	Major depressive disorder
MDI	Mental Development Index
MeSH®	Medical Subject Headings
MKP-1	Mitogen-activated protein kinase phosphatase-1
MMA	Methylmalonic acid
MMN	Multiple micronutrients
MOR	μ-Opioid receptor
MPL	Monophosphoryl lipid A
MPR	Membrane proximal region
MSM	Men who have sex with men
MTCT	Mother-to-child transmission
MUAC	Mid-upper arm circumference
MVA	Modified vaccinia Ankara
NAC	*N*-acetylcysteine
NACO	National AIDS Control Organisation
NBF	Not breastfeeding
NCD	Noncommunicable disease
NFHL	Nutrition for Healthy Living
NIDS	Nutritive immune-enhancing delivery system
NNRTI	Non-nucleoside reverse transcriptase inhibitor
NRTI	Nucleoside reverse transcriptase inhibitor
NUSTART	Nutritional Support for Africans Starting Antiretroviral Therapy
NVP	Nevirapine
OGTT	Oral glucose tolerance test
OR	Odds ratio
PAF	Population attributable fraction
ParBF	Partial breastfeeding
PCP	*Pneumocystis carinii* pneumonia
PCR	Polymerase chain reaction
PDI	Psychomotor Development Index
PEPFAR	President's Emergency Plan for AIDS Relief
PHA	Phytohemagglutinin
PI	Protease inhibitor
PLHIV	People living with HIV
PLP	Pyridoxal 5′-phosphate
PMP	Pyridoxamine 5′-phosphate
PMTCT	Prevention of mother-to-child transmission
PNP	Pyridoxine 5′-phosphate
POC	Prospective observational study
POMS	Profile of Mood States
PR	Prevalence ratio
PredBF	Predominant breastfeeding
PTH	Parathyroid hormone

PTH-rp	Parathyroid hormone-related peptide
PYR	Pyridinoline
QOL	Quality of life
RAR	Retinoic acid receptor
RBP	Retinol-binding protein
RCT	Randomized controlled trial
RDA	Recommended dietary allowance
RE	Retinol equivalent
RF	Replacement feeding
RH	Relative hazard
RIA	Radioimmunoassay
ROS	Reactive oxygen species
RPV	Rilpivirine
RR	Risk ratio or relative risk
RTV	Ritonavir
SAA	Serum amyloid A
SBMC	Spine bone mineral content
SBMD	Spine bone mineral density
SD	Standard deviation
sdNVP	Single-dose nevirapine
SE	Standard error
SEM	Standard error of the mean
SF	Serum ferritin
SGA	Small-for-gestational age
SIV	Simian immunodeficiency virus
SMZ–TMP	Sulfamethoxazole–trimethoprim
SOC	Standard of care
STAI	State–Trait Anxiety Inventory
sTfR	Soluble transferrin receptor
SVR	Sustained virologic response
TB	Tuberculosis
TBBMC	Total body bone mineral content
TBBMD	Total-body bone mineral density
TBI	Total body iron
TDF	Tenofovir
tHcy	Total homocysteine
TLR	Toll-like receptor
TMP–SMZ	Trimethoprim–sulfamethoxazole
TNF-α	Tumor necrosis factor alpha
TOV	Trial of Vitamins
TOV2	Trial of Vitamins 2
TOV3	Trial of Vitamins 3
TRP	Tubular reabsorption of phosphate
UN	United Nations
UNAIDS	Joint United Nations Programme on HIV/AIDS
UNICEF	United Nations Children's Fund
URI	Upper respiratory infection
VDR	Vitamin D receptor
VL	Viral load
WAZ	Weight-for-age z-score

WHO   World Health Organization
WLZ   Weight-for-length z-score
WtVA–   Wild-type, vitamin A-deficient
ZDV   Zidovudine
ZVITAMBO   Zimbabwe Vitamin A for Mothers and Babies

1 Human Immunodeficiency Virus and Vitamin A

Samantha L. Huey and Saurabh Mehta

CONTENTS

INTRODUCTION

Great strides have been made to reduce the number of human immunodeficiency virus (HIV) infections and HIV/acquired immunodeficiency syndrome (AIDS)-related deaths, but the war against HIV is far from over. From 1981 to the present, human immunodeficiency virus, the etiological agent of AIDS, has unwaveringly killed an estimated 39 million individuals (Mehta and Fawzi, 2007; WHO 2014c; UNAIDS, 2013). Antiretroviral therapy (ART) has become more affordable and accessible in recent years, allowing those infected with HIV to obtain this life-saving treatment. Nevertheless, patients still suffer immune dysfunction and are at high risk for opportunistic infections. Nutrition in the form of vitamin supplementation has been shown to improve host immune response and post-treatment status. Additionally, vitamin supplementation enhances the quality of life for those battling HIV-associated morbidities, both physically in terms of improved body mass index (BMI) and immune markers and psychologically by improving symptoms of depression. Nutritional status and micronutrients, particularly vitamin A, as well as B-complex, C, D, and E vitamins, modulate the pathogenesis of HIV infection and AIDS progression in infected adults, pregnant or postpartum women, and children. Including vitamin A as an adjuvant in HIV vaccines for HIV transgenic rat models (Yu and Vajdy, 2011) has also shown promising results. What is yet to be determined is the particular combination of supplement composition and dosage for each target population that will yield the greatest prevention and treatment benefits; evidence from observational studies and randomized controlled trials is contradictory. This chapter presents an overview of recent studies that have focused on nutrition, with an emphasis on vitamin A, in individuals with HIV/AIDS.

METHODS

In 2015, we searched the PubMed database for English-language articles published between the years 2006 and 2015 by using the following terms: *HIV, beta-carotene, vitamin A, HIV-1, HIV infection, retinoid acid*, and *retinol*. Studies were selected by one author (S.L.H.) according to eligibility criteria: experimental, cross-sectional, or intervention studies with exposure of vitamin A or β-carotene status or supplementation and treatment in both humans and animals, and outcome of HIV pathogenesis. Studies conducted before the year 2006 were excluded, as these studies had been discussed in detail in a previous review (Mehta and Fawzi, 2007). Other reviews, commentaries, and non-primary research articles were also excluded. For each article, we abstracted the study location, study design, methods, sample size, exposure, outcome, and main findings, including effect estimates. From the 275 studies found, 28 studies were selected for inclusion in this review (Figure 1.1).

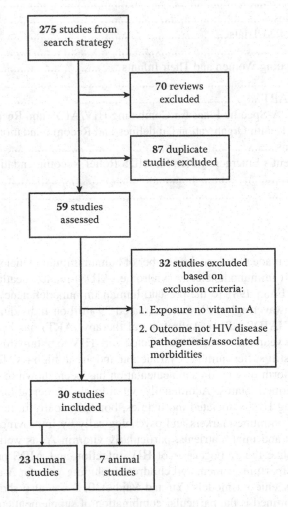

FIGURE 1.1   Study selection. Search terms: "vitamin A AND HIV infection"; "β-carotene HIV"; "β-carotene vitamin A HIV AIDS"; "HIV AND vitamin A"; "prospective cohort study vitamin A HIV"; "mouse study vitamin A HIV"; "animal vitamin A HIV"; "model HIV vitamin A"; "HIV-1 AND vitamin A."

BIOLOGICAL RATIONALE

Nutrients, especially vitamins, have a profound impact on immunity and HIV infection progression and can help support host recovery from side effects of ART. The most studied of the vitamins, vitamin A, impacts HIV disease outcomes and transmission, but supplementation can also be detrimental in certain populations. Vitamin A is a family of retinoid compounds with all-*trans*-retinol biologic activity (Villamor et al., 2005). In the body, vitamin A is important for the maintenance of the integrity of the epithelium in the respiratory and gastrointestinal tracts, as well as in the prevention of night blindness. Night blindness is the world's foremost cause of preventable blindness in children (Villamor and Fawzi, 2005; Katona and Katona-Apte, 2008). Vitamin A has received much attention and focus in the arena of infectious diseases, particularly after Scrimshaw observed that "no nutritional deficiency is more consistently synergistic with infectious disease than that of vitamin A" (Scrimshaw et al., 1968, p. 94). Increased prevalence of measles, diarrheal infections, blindness, and anemia has been linked to low vitamin A status (Semba, 1994; Villamor and Fawzi, 2005; Katona and Katona-Apte, 2008).

Immunologically, vitamin A has been shown to increase natural killer cell function *in vitro* and to stimulate phagocytosis (Kaio et al., 2013). β-Carotene, a precursor of vitamin A, has been shown to maintain the immune response and can also act as an antioxidant (Baeten et al., 2007). The retinoic acid receptor (RAR) supports robust antibody responses by promoting T-helper type 2 cells (Th_2) and Th_{17}, as well as regulatory T-cell (T_{reg}) development and responses (Mora et al., 2008; Reilly et al., 2012). The Th_2 cytokines interleukin-4 (IL-4), IL-5, and IL-10 are associated with strong antibody production, eosinophil activation, and inhibition of several macrophage functions (a phagocyte-independent protective response) (Mora et al., 2008; Reilly et al., 2012). Retinoic acid can also inhibit B-cell apoptosis and modulate antigen presentation on dendritic cells (Mora et al., 2008). Deficiency has been associated with abnormalities in T-cell subsets such as the selective loss of $CD4^+$ helper T cells from lymph nodes, thymus, and spleen (Srinivas and Dias, 2008) and associated decreases in the Th_2 antibodies IgE, IgG1, and IgA (Long et al., 2010). In a mouse model, vitamin A deficiency resulted in a reduction of Th_2 cells; vitamin A supplementation reversed the defect (Mora et al., 2008; Motswagole et al., 2013).

The relationship between nutritional status and infection, particularly HIV, is locked in a vicious cycle (Scrimshaw et al., 1968): HIV/AIDS lowers appetite and impairs the absorption, utilization, and excretion of nutrients; in turn, lowered nutritional status increases infection susceptibility (WHO, 2003; Evans et al., 2013). Co-morbidities—such as increased diarrheal and respiratory diseases in the case of HIV—result in further malnourishment (Katona and Katona-Apte, 2008). Vitamin A, in particular, has been shown to modulate immune function and HIV pathogenesis.

There is evidence in the literature demonstrating that HIV infection impairs nutrient metabolism (Kassu et al., 2007; Katona and Katona-Apte, 2008; Buccigrossi et al., 2011; Evans et al., 2013). HIV infection is initiated on the intestinal mucosal surface and induces infiltration of the gut mucosa, causing the release of T cells, damage to the intestinal wall, and epithelial apoptosis (Epple et al., 2010). The mechanisms of impaired absorption are not well characterized, but increased permeability due to altered intestinal mucosal architecture was seen in human mucosa specimens *in vitro* in a recent study (Buccigrossi et al., 2011). HIV-1 transactivator factor, a viral factor referred to as Tat, induced an enterotoxic effect on intestinal epithelial cells that may explain the diarrhea that often occurs with HIV infection. Tat also caused oxidative stress followed by apoptosis of enterocytes. These effects were prevented by the administration of the antioxidant *N*-acetyl-cysteine. In HIV-positive patients not taking ART, chronic oxidative stress causes perturbations of the antioxidant defense system, which may be explained by the role of Tat in HIV enteropathy.

Nutrient utilization and requirements are altered during HIV infection. Increased inflammation and increased oxidation of retinol, a form of vitamin A, result in increased tissue retinol requirements (Neves et al., 2006). However, with severe protein malnutrition and lower levels of retinol-binding protein (RBP), less retinol is mobilized from hepatic stores (possibly as a result of the acute phase response). Fever, which often occurs in HIV, also increases energy and micronutrient requirements (Katona and Katona-Apte, 2008). Excretion of nutrients is heightened during HIV infection, resulting in poorer nutritional status. Several studies have shown that HIV infection-associated fever diminishes the ability of the proximal tubules of the kidneys to absorb low-molecular-weight proteins such as RBP, leading to its loss—and thus that of retinol—in a 1:1 retinol:RBP ratio in the urine, a condition known as febrile proteinuria (Neves et al., 2006; Kassu et al., 2007; Srinivas and Dias, 2008). This loss further exacerbates nutrient deficiency.

Anorexia, induced by both the HIV infection and ART therapy for it, is a major factor in HIV/AIDS-related wasting and malnutrition. Lack of appetite is caused by multiple factors—including nausea and vomiting, difficulty swallowing (dysphagia) or painful swallowing (odynophagia), as well as esophageal candidiasis, a common opportunistic fungal infection affecting HIV patients (Neves et al., 2006; Mda et al., 2010; Evans et al., 2013). Additionally, mental status can impact dietary intake, as observed among HIV-infected adults with depression (Purnomo et al., 2012). One trial found that micronutrient supplementation improves appetite, indicating that vitamin and/or mineral supplementation may play a role in regulating hunger levels (Mda et al., 2010). In agreement with this finding, another study showed associations between the low ingestion of retinoids and carotenoid precursors with dietary distortion and anorexia (Neves et al., 2006). As a result, wasting, protein depletion, micronutrient deficiencies, and reduction in body cell mass are found in untreated HIV/AIDS patients (Katona and Katona-Apte, 2008). As an adjunct to ART therapy, nutrition interventions can improve appetite and help replenish some of the extra vitamins that are lost, improving quality of life and, potentially, adherence to ART.

Dietary vitamin A may be obtained as retinyl palmitate from animal sources or in the form of pro-vitamin A (including the carotenoids β-carotene, α-carotene, and γ-carotene and the xanthophyll β-cryptoxanthin) from plant sources, such as dark leafy greens and orange-colored vegetables (Solomons, 2012). Because animal-sourced foods are less common in resource-poor regions, and carotenoids are not as effective in boosting vitamin A status (based on an intestinal carotenoid-to-retinol conversion ratio of 12:1), vitamin A deficiency (defined as less than 0.70 µmol/L or less than 20 µg/dL serum retinol) is a major problem in many areas of the world (WHO, 2009), especially in HIV-infected persons (Nunnari et al., 2012). In 122 countries, vitamin A deficiency affects 250 million children, raising the risk of night blindness and infection of HIV (WHO, 2009, 2014a).

It is well established that vitamin A supplementation improves growth and reduces morbidity in HIV-infected children (Villamor et al., 2002; Ndeezi et al., 2010; Kaio et al., 2013). Adults also benefit from supplementation of vitamin A, including decreased mortality in advanced AIDS patients (Austin et al., 2006). However, vitamin A supplementation is *not* recommended for pregnant women or lactating mothers, despite findings from observational studies showing that low vitamin A status increases the risk of mother-to-child transmission (MTCT). Supplementation can also increase the risk of MTCT (Fawzi et al., 2002). One mechanism to explain this counterintuitive finding is that vitamin A supplementation appears to cause increased viral shedding in breast milk and higher prevalence of mastitis, leading to vertical transmission from mother to breastfeeding infant (Baeten et al., 2002; Kantarci et al., 2007; Villamor et al., 2010). Additionally, the HIV genome contains retinoic acid receptors, by which vitamin A may stimulate transcription and replication of the virus. Vitamin A may also increase the expression of CCR5 receptors on monocytes/macrophages, which would increase the susceptibility of cells to HIV infection (Webb et al., 2011). The findings from cross-sectional studies may be explained by the acute phase response, a process that causes the body to blockade nutrients (such as vitamin A and iron) deep in storage tissue to hypothetically prevent the utilization of nutrients by pathogens (Zvandasara et al., 2006). Additionally, inflammatory cytokines such as interleukin-2 (IL-2), IL-6, IL-10, and TNF-α stimulate the movement and storage of iron into macrophages during the acute phase response (WHO and CDC, 2007). The resulting effect is lowered retinol-binding protein levels, and thus lower serum retinol status, which would explain why low vitamin A status is found among HIV patients and also found to increase transmission from mother to child (Mehta and Fawzi, 2007).

In the following sections, laboratory studies, animal studies, observational studies, randomized controlled trials, and vitamin A interactions with ART are discussed. The primary exposure is vitamin A status or an intervention with vitamin A, and the outcomes include various HIV-related symptoms and co-morbidities.

EVIDENCE FROM STUDIES

LABORATORY/EXPERIMENTAL EVIDENCE

Two *in vitro* studies explored the effect of all-*trans*-retinoic acid (ATRA) on HIV pathogenesis in human cells. Maeda et al. (2007) used ATRA to treat cells from (1) cell line 8E5, which contains one HIV proviral genome per cell, and (2) the fresh peripheral blood of three HIV-infected patients. ATRA suppressed HIV replication by inhibiting reverse transcriptase in both the cell line and in human cells. The effect was reported as dose dependent; however, only two concentrations, 10^{-5}-M ATRA and 10^{-7}-M ATRA were used. Additionally, ATRA reduced the measured HIV proviral load in 8E5 cells and in the cells from patients, similar to the effect of azidothymidine (AZT) treatment (using 64-μM AZT). In another study, Jiang et al. (2012) determined the effect of ATRA treatment on ATP-binding cassette transporter A1 (ABCA1) expression in CD4$^+$ T cells. ABCA1 allows cholesterol to efflux from macrophages and neuronal and intestinal cells and appears to be regulated by ATRA. When cholesterol effluxes out of cells due to enhanced ABCA1 expression, HIV cannot enter cells. In activated, antibody-primed CD4$^+$ T cells, ATRA unregulated ABCA1 expression at the transcription level in a time- and dose-dependent manner. The increase in ABCA1 resulted in higher cholesterol efflux from cells and yielded a 40% higher response to ATRA than the control, dimethyl sulfoxide (DMSO) ($p < 0.05$). With the decrease in intracellular cholesterol, a 30% reduction in HIV entry into cells was observed in comparison to control. These results show the robust effect of ATRA *in vitro* and support the role of vitamin A in improving HIV progression.

In vitro and *in vivo* studies (e.g., He et al., 2007; Lu et al., 2008) have explored the effect of ATRA supplementation in relation to HIV disease outcomes, such as kidney disease. He et al. (2007) used *in vitro* models and confirmed the results with *in vivo* models, ultimately finding that ATRA inhibits the proliferation and restores differentiation markers in HIV-1-infected renal podocytes, which are cells found in Bowman's capsule in the kidneys that aid in filtration (He et al., 2007). The putative mechanism is that ATRA halts the cell cycle at the G_1–S transition, inducing intracellular cAMP production. Additionally, He et al. (2007) discovered that podocytes have many major retinoic acid receptors (RARs), two of which HIV suppresses, offering insight into why nephropathy is often associated with HIV-1 infection. RAR-α is generally suppressed during HIV-1 infection; however, in this study, it was found that RAR-α still plays a role in the effect of ATRA on the podocyte genotype.

Confirming these *in vitro* results, ATRA administration also reduced proteinuria, cell differentiation, and glomerosclerosis in Tg26 transgenic mice in comparison with non-treated mice. Lu et al. (2008) continued exploring the HIV-1 *nef* gene and the role of the Nef protein in podocyte dedifferentiation through the Src-dependent mitogen-activated protein kinase 1 and 2 (MAPK1/2) pathways. ATRA stimulates mitogen-activated protein kinase phosphatase-1 (MKP1) expression, a protein that has anti-inflammatory and anti-apoptotic effects. MKP1 may be depressed in renal disease. Lu et al. (2008) found that ATRA activates MKP1 in HIV-infected podocytes, which suppresses Nef-induced activation of the Src-MAPK1/2 pathways (expressed during HIV infection), ultimately returning podocytes to a more differentiated state. These findings (summarized in Table 1.1) offer potential new avenues for treating HIV-associated nephropathy, the most common cause of renal failure in HIV-1 patients.

TABLE 1.1

Laboratory and Animal Studies

Study	Exposure Groups	Experiment Type		Results
		Model	Main Outcomes	
Jiang et al. (2012)	(1) ATRA (2) DMSO (control)	*In vitro*; donated blood and Jurkat E6.1 cell line IG5	ABCA1 expression in CD4+ T cells	(1) → ABCA1 expression ↑ (time-/dose-dependent) in activated CD4+ T cells → cholesterol efflux ↑ → HIV entry ↓ into cells
Maeda et al. (2007)	(1) ATRA (2) Ethanol (3) AZT (4) Distilled water	*In vitro*; 8E5 cell line and lymphocytes of 3 human patients	HIV replication HIV proviral load HIV reverse transcriptase activity	(1) → suppressed HIV replication in both cell line and human cells; (1) → proviral load ↓; (1), (3) → reverse transcriptase activity ↓
Watson et al. (2010)	(1) ATRA (2) ATRA + MPR	*In vivo*; Balb/c mice infected with HIV	Antibody responses	(1) → no antibody production (2) → IgG titers ↑
Yu and Vajdy (2011)	(1) HIVenvgp120cn54 + NIDS (2) HIVenvgp120cn54 + PBS	*In vivo*; Balb/c mice	Serum antibody responses Vaginal antibody responses Responses against gp120 Antibody neutralization titers Cytokine responses	(1) → serum anti-gp120 and IgG1 responses ↑; booster vaccination → IgG ↑, IgG2a ↑, and IgA ↑; vaginal antibody titers ↑; serum IgG1 responses ↑; enhanced serum neutralization; enhanced splenic Th$_1$/Th$_2$ responses
Royal et al. (2007)	(1) TgVA– (2) TgVA+ (3) WtVA– (4) WtVA+ (dietary deficiency)	*In vivo*; HIV-1 Tg rat model	MOR expression T-cell pro-inflammatory cytokine expression HIV gene expression (*env*, *tat*, *nef*, *vif*)	(1), (2), (3) → IFN-γ ↑, TNF-α ↑ (1), (2) Tg groups → *env*, *tat*, *nef*, mRNA ↑ (1), (2), (3) → IFN-γ ↑, TNF-α ↑ (activated T cells) (3) → TNF-α ↓; (1) → MOR expression ↓
Sultana et al. (2010)	(1) TgVA– (2) TgVA+ (3) WtVA– (4) WtVA+ (dietary deficiency) Treatment: morphine (M) or placebo (P)	*In vivo*; HIV-1 Tg rat model	# of parvalbumin-and NeuN-expressing neurons → relationship with HIV-regulatory proteins	(1), (2), (3), (4) ↔ # NeuN (1) + (M), (4), (4) + (P): ↔ # # parvalbumin (1) + (M) → HIV proteins expression ↑

Reference	Groups	Model	Outcome measured	Results
Guo et al. (2012)	(1) TgVA− (2) TgVA+ (3) WtVA− (4) WtVA+ (dietary deficiency) Treatment: morphine (M) or placebo (P)	In vivo; HIV-1 Tg rat model	# of parvalbumin-expressing GABA interneurons in hippocampus	(1), (3) → # hippocampal neurons ↓
Lu et al. (2008)	(1) ATRA (2) DMSO	In vitro; murine podocytes infected with HIV-1	MKP1 expression Podocyte differentiation and proliferation	(1) → MKP1 ↑ → net-induced activation ↓ → podocytes → differentiation ↑
He et al. (2007)	In vitro HIV-infected/non-infected + (1) ATRA (2) 9-cis-RA (3) DMSO In vivo (1) ATRA (2) corn oil (control)	Murine podocytes infected with HIV-1 HIV-1 Tg26 rat model	Podocyte differentiation and proliferation HIV-associated nephropathy (HIVAN) pathogenesis	(1) → inhibited proliferation, restored differentiation markers, induced ↑ in intracellular cAMP through RAR-α (1) → ↓ proteinuria, ↓ cell proliferation, ↓ glomerosclerosis

Note: ATRA, all-*trans*-retinoic acid; AZT, azidothymidine; DMSO, dimethyl sulfoxide; M, morphine; MOR, μ-opioid receptor; MPR, *N*-[4-methoxyphenyl]retinamide; NIDS, nutritive immune-enhancing delivery system; P, placebo; VA+, vitamin A replete or administration; VA−, vitamin A deficient; ↔, no effect/no differences among groups; ↓, decreased/reduced; ↑, increased; →, resulted/caused/activated.

ANIMAL STUDIES

Many animal studies, using mice and rats, have been conducted to better understand the effects of nutrition on HIV-related outcomes. These studies can be divided into two categories: the effect on HIV-related outcomes by either undergoing a vitamin A-deficient diet or administering dietary vitamin A.

Several studies have manipulated the diets of HIV transgenic rats in comparison to wild-type rats to demonstrate how dietary depletion of vitamin A might affect the course of HIV disease. Many studies have utilized the Tg transgenic rat model and pathogen-free, age-matched control rats (Royal et al., 2007; Sultana et al., 2010; Guo et al., 2012). This model, which uses a non-pathogenic viral genome that mimics the symptoms of HIV, is particularly useful for research on opioid users, given that one out of 125 acquire HIV through intravenous drug use (Degenhardt et al., 2010). Royal et al. (2007) determined the effects of vitamin A deficiency on the μ-opioid receptor (MOR), T-cell pro-inflammatory cytokines, and HIV gene expression. Activation of the MOR may mediate the clinical effects of vitamin A deficiency in opioid users infected with HIV. Female Tg and wild-type rats were fed a normal maintenance diet, mated, and then continued on the diet for two weeks of gestation. The female rats were then fed a diet either deficient or replete in vitamin A, and their pups were fed the same diets as their mothers. T cells were stimulated with phytohemagglutinin (PHA), a plant protein that can be used as a mitogen to trigger T-cell division and activate HIV-1 in lymphocytes. Stimulation resulted in increased interferon-gamma (IFN-γ) expression, with larger increases among the wild-type, vitamin A-deficient (WtVA−), Tg vitamin A-replete (TgVA+), and Tg vitamin A-deficient (TgVA−) mice. The pro-inflammatory cytokine TNF-α increased in the aforementioned groups and was reduced in the WtVA+ mice. TgVA− had the lowest expression of MOR at baseline and, after PHA stimulation, had the highest expression of the MOR from CD4+ and CD8+ T cells in comparison to both the other PHA-stimulated samples and non-stimulated samples. The expression of HIV genes *env*, *tat*, *nef*, and *vif* in whole blood varied among the groups of mice and diets. When stimulated with PHA, the Tg rats showed increased expression of *env*, *tat*, and *nef* mRNA, with TgVA− *tat* and *vif* expression similar to rats on the vitamin A-replete diet; however, the TgVa− rats had higher *env* and *nef* expression than what was observed in the TgVA+ rat. Although generalizable only to rats with this transgene, these studies showed that vitamin A deficiency alters T-cell phenotypes and immune responses in the presence of HIV-like infection and may offer clues to the mechanisms by which vitamin A deficiency affects HIV pathogenesis in humans.

Further experiments performed on this rat model include studies on parvalbumin+ neurons to investigate the increased frequency of cognitive impairment found in HIV-infected opioid users. Parvalbumin is a calcium-binding protein, and neurons that express parvalbumin modulate electrical activity involved in cognitive function. Sultana et al. (2010) used similar methodology in raising rats as described above, feeding them diets either replete or deficient in vitamin A with the addition of morphine or a placebo. In contrast to the placebo-treated, wild-type rats and morphine-treated TgVA− rats, fewer parvalbumin+ cells were found in the morphine-treated WtVA+ rats, placebo-treated WtVA− rats, and placebo-treated TgVA+ rats. The *tat* gene, which may induce toxicity, showed increased expression in vitamin A-deficient rats treated with morphine. These experiments suggest that vitamin A deficiency, exposure to opioids such as morphine, and HIV infection alone or in concert may alter neuronal metabolic activity and manifest in changed levels of parvalbumin expression in this rat model.

A study by Guo et al. (2012) that focused on similar outcomes also used the aforementioned Tg rat model with or without vitamin A-deficient diet and morphine to determine the effect on gamma-aminobutyric acid (GABA)-expression interneurons in the hippocampus of Tg rats. GABAergic interneurons express parvalbumin and mediate hippocampus activity, which regulates memory. Similar to the study of Sultana et al. (2010), parvalbumin levels were assessed. Overall, TgVA− rats, with or without morphine administration, had higher parvalbumin expression than placebo-treated WtVA− rats. TgVA− rats treated with morphine had higher expression than wild-type rats and placebo-treated TgVA– rats. From these studies, it appears that vitamin A deficiency and morphine can increase parvalbumin expression and affect cognition in this HIV infection rat model; further study in humans is warranted.

Using vitamin A as a vaccine adjuvant, Yu and Vajdy (2011) created a nutritive immune-enhancing delivery system (NIDS) vaccine that also included an emulsion of polyphenol–flavonoid, catechin hydrate, and mustard oil. Inoculation with HIV gp120 protein with the NIDS, or with placebo (phosphate-buffered saline solution) was tested on mice. Two mucosal and two systemic vaccinations in three- to six-month-old female BALB/c mice yielded both local and systemic increases in antibodies, as well as cytokine responses, in mice receiving the NIDS. Serum anti-gp120 IgG1 responses were enhanced 198-fold more in mice receiving the NIDS ($p < 0.002$). Vaginal IgG1 and IgA titers also increased significantly—255-fold ($p < 0.025$) and 8-fold ($p < 0.039$), respectively—with the NIDS preparation in comparison to gp120 alone. Also, NIDS appeared to augment local and systemic antibody responses against gp120 and was effective (i.e., induced high antibody response) against homologous and heterologous strains of HIV1, including BaL, CM, SF162, IIIB, and CN54 subtype C. Finally, NIDS appeared to increase T-cell responses in terms of cytokine production, specifically IFN-γ, IL-5, and IL-10. Overall, the results showed that the nutritive-based adjuvant was remarkably effective in enhancing immune responses.

A study by Watson et al. (2010) also used BALB/c mice to determine whether ATRA could promote antibody responses when co-delivered with a model antigen in the same formulation. A peptide derived from the membrane proximal region (MPR) of HIV-1 gp41 was selected: N-MPR. The MPR is a key target for development of a vaccine that elicits neutralizing antibodies (Montero et al., 2008). Mice were immunized with liposomes containing lipid-anchored N-MPR and either ATRA or monophosphoryl lipid A (MPL), a TLR4 agonist and potent liposomal vaccine adjuvant. In this study, ATRA alone did not stimulate the production of antibodies when co-delivered with MPR; however, if ATRA was delivered with MPL, IgG antibody titers to MPR were enhanced fourfold in comparison to 13-*cis*-RA and MPL. The interaction between ATRA and MPL remains to be explored further; the results of this and the study by Yu and Vajdy (2011) point toward ATRA as an effective vaccine adjuvant. Table 1.1 summarizes the studies discussed in this section.

OBSERVATIONAL STUDIES

It is well established from cross-sectional analyses that HIV-infected patients have suboptimal vitamin A concentrations in comparison to healthy populations (Kassu et al., 2007; Papathakis et al., 2007; Fufa et al., 2009; Mehta et al., 2011; Mulu et al., 2011; Obuseh et al., 2011; Loignon et al., 2012; Machado et al., 2013; Monteiro et al., 2014). Increasingly, observational studies focus on vitamin A status as a predictor of a range of outcomes, including HIV-related morbidity measurements, gynecological infections among HIV-infected women, metabolic syndrome symptoms among HIV-infected adults receiving ART, and mortality among HIV-infected children. Additionally, research in susceptibility to HIV at the genetic level has pinpointed polymorphisms that increase the risk of HIV infection, and one such study (Kuhn et al., 2006) that takes nutritional status into account is described in this section. Table 1.2 provides a summary of these studies.

In Addis Ababa, Ethiopia, 153 HIV-positive adults were enrolled into a cross-sectional study to determine correlations between micronutrients and HIV status (Fufa et al., 2009). The authors found a high prevalence of low vitamin A and zinc status in the initial stages of HIV (as measured by CD4+ T-cell count) and increased wasting and malnutrition as the disease progresses. Although this study found no significant association between vitamin A and CD4+ T-cell count ($r = 0.032$, $p > 0.722$), it was the first to characterize micronutrient and HIV status among HIV-infected adults living in Addis Ababa. Another study in Tanzania found no association between low serum retinol and the risk of seroconversion; more details are available in a previous review (Villamor et al., 2006; Mehta and Fawzi, 2007).

TABLE 1.2
Observational Studies

Study	Exposure	Study Design; Population	Main Outcomes	Results
Fufa et al. (2009)	Serum retinol	Cross-sectional; adults	CD4+ count	↔
Villamor et al. (2006)	Serum retinol	Case-control; adults	CRP concentration	↔
			Risk of seroconversion	↔
Tohill et al. (2007)	Serum vitamins A, B$_{12}$, C, and E; carotenoids; folate; RBC folate; several minerals	Cross-sectional substudy from HERS; women	Gynecological conditions	↑ α-Carotene → odds ↓ of trichomoniasis ↑ Vitamin A, β-carotene → risk ↓ of bacterial vaginosis
Chatterjee et al. (2010)	Vitamin A + vitamin B$_{12}$ plasma concentrations	Nested prospective cohort; children	Mortality Morbidity Birthweight	Highest vitamin A quartile → mortality ↓ ↔ ↔
Kuhn et al. (2006)	(1) Vitamin A + β-carotene + large vitamin A dose at delivery (2) Placebo	Retrospective; HIV+ mothers' neonates	MBL2-variant MTCT	(1) MBL2-variant → MTCT (2) MBL2-variant → MTCT ↑

Note: CRP, C-reactive protein; HERS, Heart and Estrogen/Progestin Replacement Study; MBL2, mannose binding lectin 2; MTCT, mother-to-child transmission; RBC, red blood cell; ↔, no effect/no differences among groups; ↓, decreased/reduced; ↑, increased; →, resulted/caused/activated.

Women infected with HIV are at higher risk for gynecological infections, and one study has shown that nutrition may play a role in the prevalence of such morbidities. In the United States, a cross-sectional sub-study was performed on data from 329 HIV-infected and 184 HIV-uninfected participants in the HIV Epidemiology Research Study (HERS) (Tohill et al., 2007). Blood was collected from the participants, ages 20 to 57 years, and assessed for 13 micronutrients, including vitamin A and carotenoids. Gynecological measurements were made on the core study cohort and included diagnoses of trichomoniasis, bacterial vaginosis, *Candida* colonization, human papilloma-virus (HPV) infection, and abnormal cervical cytology. By using population concentration quartiles to estimate four discrete nutrient concentrations, the authors produced an indirect standardization to population nutrient concentrations (instead of only assessing population nutrient deficiency). Increasing levels of α-carotene were associated with lower prevalence of trichomoniasis (95% CI for all analyses; adjusted odds ratio [AOR] of 0.88, 0.63, and 0.12 for Q2, Q3, and Q4, respectively). Additionally, higher concentrations of vitamin A, β-carotene, and vitamins C and E were associated with a lower risk of bacterial vaginosis (vitamin A odds ratios [ORs] of 0.60, 0.45, and 0.87 for Q2, Q3, and Q4, respectively; β-carotene ORs of 0.72, 1.46, and 0.40 for Q2, Q3, and Q4, respectively). Though the study had a large sample size, the authors acknowledge its limitations, including lack of acute phase reactants, inability to account for the cohort's high prevalence of infection and inflam-mation, and lack of causality due to the study design. Nonetheless, this study highlights the need for a future randomized controlled trial using vitamin A and/or carotenoid supplementation and measuring gynecological outcomes in HIV-infected women.

In Tanzania, a prospective cohort study nested within a large randomized controlled trial (Tanzania Vitamin and HIV Infection Trial) (Fawzi et al. 1999) assessed plasma concentrations of vitamin A and child mortality, child morbidity, infant birthweight, respiratory infections, diarrheal infections, and HIV infections in children born to HIV-infected mothers (Chatterjee et al., 2010). From 12 to 27 weeks gestation until the end of pregnancy, women took micronutrient supplements containing (1) vitamin A and β-carotene; (2) multiple micronutrients; (3) vitamin A, β-carotene, and multiple micronutrients; or (4) a placebo. Using Cox proportional hazards models, all children (both HIV-infected and uninfected) in the highest quartile of vitamin A status had a 49% lower risk of mortality (HR, 0.51; 95% CI, 1.29–0.90) up to 24 months of age. However, no associations were detected between the children's plasma vitamin A concentration and MTCT, symptoms of respira-tory disease, or diarrhea. The observational nature of this study may explain the lack of association between vitamin A status and MTCT. An alternative explanation is that a child's vitamin A status may not have any bearing on MTCT; rather, it is the action of vitamin A in the mother that increases MTCT, as seen in previous studies. This study supports vitamin A supplementation in HIV-infected mothers as being key to reducing deaths in their children.

A retrospective study explored mannose-binding lectin 2 (MBL-2) gene polymorphisms in South African infants born to HIV-positive mothers undergoing vitamin A/β-carotene supplementation (Kuhn et al., 2006). MBL-2 binds carbohydrate ligands, including those on the HIV envelope, opso-nizing the virus (Coutsoudis et al., 1999). Initially, the authors explored MBL-2 because previ-ous studies showed an increased frequency of MBL-2 alleles among adults with HIV and because MBL-2 has been associated with an increased risk of vertical transmission in Brazilian children (Boniotto et al., 2003). MBL-2 is part of the innate immune response, and polymorphisms in this gene result in lower concentrations of functional MBL-2 in serum (i.e., dampened acute phase response) and unexplained immunodeficiency (Turner, 1996). During data analysis, the authors observed that there were differences among the arms of the trial, and thus assessed gene–environ-ment interactions between the vitamin A and β-carotene supplementation and MBL-2 variants in relation to MTCT. The results were striking: After adjusting for maternal CD4+ T-cell count, low birthweight, and nonexclusive breastfeeding, there was a significant association between MBL-2 variants and susceptibility to HIV transmission among the placebo group only (OR, 2.97; 95% CI, 1.12–7.83). The vitamin A/β-carotene supplementation was significantly associated with a reduction in HIV transmission among infants with variant MBL-2 alleles (OR, 0.37; 95% CI, 0.15–0.91) in contrast to no reduction in non-variant MBL-2 alleles (OR, 1.25; 95% CI, 0.56–2.78). The authors also determined that pre-intervention maternal serum retinol and CD4+ T-cell counts modified associations between intervention group MBL-2 variants and HIV transmission, in that placebo group MBL-2 variants were associated with increased transmission if the mothers' serum retinol level was in the lowest third of the population (<22.4 ng/mL). Similarly, if the mothers' baseline CD4+ T-cell counts were within the lowest third (<335 counts), MBL-2 variants showed lower rates of transmission. From this study, it appears that serum retinol level impacts the risk of contracting HIV at the genetic level, specifically, the mannose-binding-lectin gene and associated polymorphisms.

RANDOMIZED CONTROLLED TRIALS

Adults

Some evidence from a clinical trial conducted in Canada points toward the possible benefits of using carotenoids to improve survival and mortality in advanced AIDS patients (Austin et al., 2006). In this randomized, double-blind, placebo-controlled, multi-center trial, 331 adults with advanced AIDS were treated with daily oral multivitamins containing vitamin A and other trace elements (the exact formulation was not described) while continuing other anti-HIV therapies. About half of the subjects ($n = 165$) also received mixed carotenoids (12,560 µmol/L β-carotene), equivalent to 630 µmol/L retinol four times per day. All were followed for a mean of 13 months (standard deviation, six months). The authors found no associations between increased β-carotene levels and new or recurrent AIDS-defining illness (hazard ratio [HR], 1.21; 95% CI, 0.65–2.25). After adjusting for carotenoid treatment in covariate analysis, the authors saw a trend toward decreased risk of death in those with higher baseline serum carotene concentrations (HR, 0.25; 95% CI, 0.10–0.63) and higher baseline CD4+ T-lymphocyte counts (HR, 0.60; 95% CI, 0.46–0.78). Viral load had no effect on death (HR, 1.76; 95% CI, 0.87–3.54). The authors concluded that β-carotene supplementation has a positive effect in AIDS patients, even though the β-carotene content of the supplement was uneven throughout the trial due to vitamin degradation.

Several recent trials have explored the impact of micronutrient-fortified food consumption on various HIV-related outcomes (Ndekha et al., 2009; Hummelen et al., 2011; Evans et al., 2013; Grobler et al., 2013; Motswagole et al., 2013; Ivers et al., 2014). In one trial, sorghum was mixed with a vitamin and mineral premix (Motswagole et al., 2013). The mixture contained 87 µmol vitamin A, 0.35 mg vitamin B_1, 0.50 mg vitamin B_2, 4.50 mg vitamin B_3, 0.50 mg vitamin B_6, 0.05 mg folate, and 2.80 mg elemental iron. Control (non-fortified) and fortified sorghum was provided to 67 HIV-positive adults for two months in a double-blind, randomized, placebo-controlled trial in Kanye, Botswana, to assess effects on immune function. The authors found no significant differences in serum retinol level, CD4+ cell count, or HIV viral load before and after intervention. The authors attributed the lack of effect to the possibility of low micronutrient content in the food, despite fortification. Although no effect was seen, the authors stressed the need for future HIV interventions using fortified foods (with, potentially, higher micronutrient levels), as well as maintaining macronutrient intake and proper weight in HIV patients as a vital part of disease management.

Pregnant or Lactating Women and Their Infants

Although previous studies have found that supplementing ART-naïve, HIV-infected, pregnant, or lactating women with vitamin A/β-carotene increases the risk of transmission through breastfeeding, the mechanism is not well understood. Several trials have explored the role of vitamin supplementation and MTCT, including HIV shedding in breast milk and subclinical mastitis, using data collected from the trial conducted by Fawzi et al. (1999) in Tanzania. One study aimed to evaluate the effect of vitamin A/β-carotene supplementation compared to multivitamins (B complex, C, and E) on HIV shedding in breast milk during the first two years postpartum to shed light on the mechanistic actions involved; 1319 breast milk samples from 594 women were analyzed for viral and proviral load (Villamor et al., 2010). Women assigned to the vitamin A/β-carotene arm had a significantly higher proportion of samples with detectable viral load at or after six months postpartum (51.3% vs. 44.8%, respectively; $p = 0.02$). The multivitamin arm and placebo arm did not differ significantly in viral load ($p = 0.69$), and neither vitamin A/β-carotene nor multivitamins impacted the proviral load ($p = 0.29$ and $p = 0.86$, respectively). After adjustment for β-carotene concentration, breast milk retinol concentration was not associated with viral load; however, β-carotene concentration was related to increased viral load in breast milk when quartile 1 (low β-carotene concentration) was compared to quartile 2 or higher ($p = 0.02$). Because the proviral load was not affected by vitamin A/β-carotene supplementation, the authors postulated that mechanisms other than maternal macro-phageal CCR5 upregulation are at work or that mastitis increases MTCT. A later study (Arsenault et al., 2010) characterized subclinical mastitis prevalence in this population, with moderate subclinical mastitis defined as ratio of sodium to potassium (Na:K) breast milk concentration between 0.6 and 1 or, in severe cases, as greater than 1. Both treatment arms—vitamin A/β-carotene and multivita-min supplements—had an increased risk of severe subclinical mastitis (45% and 75%, respectively) compared to placebo. This unexpected effect of multivitamins was apparent among women with higher baseline CD4+ cell counts but not in women with more advanced HIV. One explanation for this surprising outcome is that the vitamin intervention enhanced women's immunological and inflammatory response. Mastitis is caused by infection with *Staphylococcus aureus* or *Escherichia coli*, which increases the production of IFN-γ and IL-8, cytokines that enhance neutrophil oxidative burst capacity. Increased intake of vitamins in the presence of these pathogens might increase neu-trophil activity, leading to excessive oxidation and tissue damage in terms of opened tight junctions in the mammary epithelium. It is clear from these studies that, although nutrient supplementation generally positively impacts HIV-related morbidity, vitamin A/β-carotene and multivitamin adjunct therapy is not recommended for pregnant or lactating mothers, as the risk for HIV transmission to breastfeeding children is heightened, as described by the WHO Guidelines (2011d,e,f).

Although vitamin A/β-carotene and multivitamin supplementation increases the risk of MTCT, vitamin A/β-carotene and/or multivitamin supplementation in HIV-infected Tanzanian pregnant women had several positive impacts on health outcomes in their children. In one study, sex dif-ferences were apparent among the 959 mother–infant pairs analyzed (Kawai et al., 2010). Among girls, the multivitamin intervention lessened the risk of fetal death (risk ratio [RR], 0.68; 95% CI, 0.47–0.97) and low birthweight (RR, 0.39; 95% CI, 0.22–0.67). Compared to girls, low birthweight among boys was reduced by only 19% (RR, 0.81; 95% CI, 0.44–1.49). Small-for-gestational-age among both sexes was reduced non-differentially by sex (p for interaction = 0.66). Maternal mul-tivitamin supplementation also reduced their children's risks of diarrhea overall by 17%. However, vitamin A/β-carotene did not have any effects on fetal death, low birthweight, or gestational age, although this arm did see a reduction in the diarrhea risk among boys. This study conflicts with previous findings that showed a reduction in mortality only in boys. Overall, girls appeared to reap more benefits of maternal multivitamin supplementation than boys, which could be explained by a number of factors, including thymus size, susceptibility to malnutrition, low birthweight risk, and varying immune function among the sexes. Another study sought to uncover the effect of mater-nal multivitamin supplementation on HIV-1 vertical transmission and progression and found that, although multivitamin supplementation increased both psychomotor and mental development in children, vitamin A did not have any effects (McGrath et al., 2006); further details may be found in Mehta and Fawzi's review (2007).

Several studies analyzed data on pregnant or postpartum women with and without HIV from trials conducted in Zimbabwe (Zimbabwe Vitamin A for Mothers and Babies [ZVITAMBO] trial study group) and in Tanzania (Fawzi et al., 2007). The ZVITAMBO trial enrolled a total 14,110 mother–neonate pairs, wherein both mother and infant, mother only, infant only, or neither mother nor infant received vitamin A supplementation in a randomized, placebo-controlled trial with a 2 × 2 factorial design (Humphrey et al., 2006). A single dose of 41,880 µmol/L vitamin A or placebo given within 96 hours postpartum had no significant impact on HIV incidence in HIV-negative mothers, but those with low baseline serum retinol levels were 10.4 (95% CI, 3.00–36.28) times more likely to sexually acquire HIV during the postpartum year. More details can be found in a previous review (Mehta and Fawzi, 2007). In another study based on this cohort, no effect on HIV-positive or HIV-negative maternal mortality or morbidity was seen, and in HIV-positive women serum retinol increased only among those with a CD4$^+$ cell count less than 200×10^6 cells/L (Zvandasara et al., 2006). Both studies attribute the lack of effect to the fact that just 9% of the HIV-negative women were vitamin-A deficient at baseline. The ZVITAMBO trial results give further evidence that HIV alters metabolism, causing vitamin A deficiency that may not be necessarily corrected by supplementation.

The aforementioned randomized controlled trial in Tanzania, which enrolled 1078 HIV-positive pregnant women, has led to a number of studies. Smith Fawzi et al. (2007) assessed whether multivitamin supplementation in this cohort had any impact on health-related quality of life (QOL) and the risk of major depressive disorder (MDD), for depression has been shown to be prevalent among HIV-infected patients in observational studies (Cook et al., 2004; Ickovics et al., 2001). A psychosocial assessment was performed throughout the follow-up period, starting with two months after enrollment, two months after delivery, every six months until 2001, and every 12 months thereafter. Using the Hopkins Symptom Checklist-25 (HSCL-25) to assess MDD and the Medical Outcomes Study Short Form-36 to assess health-related QOL, the authors found that multivitamin supplementation reduced the incidence of elevated depressive symptoms (RR, 0.78; 95% CI, 0.66–0.99) and reduced the incidence of poor health-related QOL. However, no associations between vitamin A supplementation and depressive symptoms or QOL were found. Although vitamin A did not impact depressive symptoms in this study, no harmful effects were noted. Multivitamins appear to have more than just positive physical effects in HIV patients—they seem to improve mental and emotional health, thereby improving quality of life.

Children

In KwaZulu-Natal, South Africa, three studies were performed on both HIV-infected and uninfected infants that were enrolled in a large, randomized clinical trial and assessed for longitudinal growth, anemia, and diarrhea, as predicted by vitamin A, zinc, and multiple micronutrients (Luabeya et al., 2007; Chhagan et al., 2009, 2010). In this trial, four- to six-month-old infants were treated with vitamin A only, with vitamin A and zinc, or with vitamin A, zinc, and multiple micronutrients, including B-complex vitamins; vitamins C, D, E, and K; and minerals. Unfortunately, the lower-than-expected enrollment of HIV-positive children limited the possible analyses. Luabeya et al. (2007) found no difference in respiratory or diarrheal disease morbidity among the three cohorts. However, Chhagan et al. (2010) found that vitamin A, zinc, and multiple micronutrients had worse longitudinal growth than in the other two intervention arms ($p = 0.042$ for treatment by time interaction). Because these studies had only 25 HIV-infected children, individual subject plots were made to find influential subjects that may have contributed to the growth outcomes; censorship due to death or loss to follow-up was associated with poor growth. Chhagan et al. (2009) found that in contrast to vitamin A and zinc, with or without multiple micronutrients, vitamin A alone failed to improve growth in HIV-uninfected children with recurring diarrhea. However, these are *post hoc* analyses and must be interpreted with caution. Table 1.3 provides a summary of these studies.

Interaction with ART

In addition to other micronutrients, vitamin A is thought to complement ART in treating and reducing HIV symptoms and morbidities, as well as in slowing down HIV progression. Previous observational studies have shown differences in vitamin A status and immunity associated with ART. Drain et al. (2007) reviewed research regarding micronutrients and highly active antiretroviral therapy (HAART) prior to 2007. One six-month intervention showed that certain micronutrients, including daily doses of 150 µg of vitamin A (along with vitamins C and E), resulted in improvement in immunity among the HIV-positive adults receiving HAART (Jaruga et al., 2002). Another observational study found decreased serum retinol but increased retinol-binding protein (RBP) in HIV-positive adults receiving HAART (Toma et al., 2001); however, another cross-sectional study showed no differences in mean plasma vitamin A concentration between those adults receiving HAART and those not receiving the therapy (Rousseau et al., 2000). Below, we review recent studies examining interactions between vitamin A and ART/HAART.

A cross-sectional study in Addis Ababa was conducted among HIV/AIDS patients to determine the association between micronutrient levels, including serum retinol, and the response to HAART (measured by CD4+ T-cell count) (Eshetu et al., 2014). The study included 171 patients who had taken HAART for at least six months. Retinol deficiency was found to be the second highest nutrient deficiency at 14% prevalence (after zinc, at 46.8% prevalence), and statistically significantly lower CD4+ T-cell counts were found among patients with deficient retinol. When analyzed by quartiles, higher serum retinol in the fourth quartile was associated with lower T-cell counts in comparison to the third quartile. The authors noted that Jones et al. (2006) also found high $\log_{10}$ viral load levels in this same quartile. The effect may be due to retinol's function in increasing lymphoid cell differentiation and, hence, increasing CCR5 receptors, which allow HIV to attach to lymphocytes. Although causation cannot be determined in this study, caution is advised in supplementing patients on HAART with vitamin A.

Across-sectional study in São Paulo, Brazil, was conducted among adults undergoing three different HAART regimens (Kaio et al., 2013). Participants were divided into groups based on their treatment regimens: (1) a combination of nucleoside analog reverse transcriptase inhibitors (NRTIs) and non-NRTIs; (2) a combination of NRTIs, protease inhibitors, and ritonavir; and (3) a combination of NRTIs and other classes. The authors found that serum vitamin A and β-carotene concentrations did not differ by regimen after controlling for gender, age, educational level, smoking, physical activity, body mass index, time of infection with HIV, presence of comorbidities, CD4+ T-cell count, total cholesterol and fractions, and triglyceride levels.

In Uganda, 847 children ages 1 to 5 years were stratified by ART use ($n = 85$ using ART; $n = 762$ no ART), and each arm was randomized to a daily regimen of either twice the recommended dietary allowance (RDA) of 14 vitamins and minerals (including vitamin A at 800 μg per dose) or the standard RDA recommendation of six vitamins (400 μg vitamin A per dose) (Ndeezi et al., 2010). After the six-month intervention, all children received the standard-of-care regimen of six vitamins. Mortality, CD4+ T-cell count, and growth at 12 months after intervention were assessed. No significant differences between the ART/no ART groups receiving extra vitamins and those receiving the standard-of-care amounts of six multivitamins were found. Although the results were null, few adverse effects were reported, showing that vitamins did not cause harm, even if they did not have a statistically significant benefit. A beneficial effect may be observed should the limitations of the current study—the lack of a placebo group, perhaps giving vitamins at too low a dosage, and a shorter period of intervention—be resolved in future trials.

A trial conducted in Canada sought to determine whether β-carotene supplementation affects the action of the protease inhibitor antiretroviral drug nelfinavir and its active metabolite, M8, in HIV-1-infected individuals (Sheehan et al., 2012). Results from previous studies suggest that β-carotene may inhibit or induce cytochrome P450 enzymes and transporters. Nelfinavir pharmacokinetic analysis was performed at baseline and after 28 days of β-carotene supplementation; although serum carotene levels increased, no significant differences in nelfinavir and M8 concentrations were observed before or after β-carotene supplementation at the 90% confidence level. Though the result was null, it can be concluded that β-carotene supplementation was not detrimental to the action of the antiretroviral drug and may promote adherence to the antiretroviral regimen.

Once in the bloodstream, vitamin A is bound to RBP for transport in the circulation. RBP level may be a potential biomarker for the early detection of metabolic abnormalities associated with HAART treatment in HIV patients. A study conducted in Seoul sought to determine associations between RBP4, a recently identified adipokine thought to be linked to insulin resistance, obesity,

TABLE 1.3
Randomized Controlled Trials

Study	Exposure	Population	Main Outcomes	Results
Smith Fawzi et al. (2007)	(1) VA + βC (2) MMN (3) MMN + VA + βC (4) Placebo	Pregnant women	Quality of life Depression of symptoms	(1) ↔ (1) ↔
Zvandasara et al. (2006)	(1) VA (2) Placebo	Postpartum women	Mortality Morbidity	(1) → Mortality (1) → Malaria ↓, vaginal infection ↓, pelvic inflammatory disease ↓, cracked or bleeding nipples sick visits ↓
Arsenault et al. (2010)	(1) VA + βC (2) MMN (3) VA + MMN + βC (4) Placebo	Breastfeeding women	Subclinical mastitis severity	(3) → Risk of incidence ↑
Villamor et al. (2010)	(1) VA + βC (2) VB + VC + VE (3) VB + VC + VA + βC (4) Placebo	Breastfeeding women	HIV viral load in breast milk HIV proviral load in breast milk	(1) → Detectable viral load ↑ (1) ↔
Humphrey et al. (2006)	(1) Maternal VA/infant VA (2) Maternal VA/infant placebo (3) Maternal placebo/infant VA (4) Maternal placebo/infant placebo	HIV+ mothers' neonates	HIV incidence HIV risk Seroconversion	↔ Per 1 mmol/L serum retinol, 87% decline in risk Serum retinol < 0.7 mmol/L → seroconversion likelihood ↑

Reference	Intervention groups	Population	Outcomes
McGrath et al. (2006)	(1) VA + βC (2) MMN (3) MMN + VA + βC (4) Placebo	Children born to HIV+ mothers	Mental development ↔ Psychomotor development ↔
Kawai et al. (2010)	(1) VA + βC (2) VB + VC + VE (3) VB + VC + VA + βC (4) Placebo	Children	All-cause child mortality ↔ HIV infection ↔ Birth outcomes (stillbirths, low birth weight, preterm, small for gestational age) ↔ Morbidity (diarrhea and respiratory infection) ↔
Chhagan et al. (2009)	(1) VA (2) VA + zinc (3) MMN + VA + zinc	Children	Incidence of diarrhea (1) → Persistent and severe diarrhea ↓
Chhagan et al. (2010)	(1) VA (2) VA + zinc (3) MMN + VA + zinc	Children	Length-for-age z-score ↔ Weight-for-age z-score ↔
Luabeya et al. (2007)	(1) VA (2) VA + zinc (3) MMN + VA + zinc	Children	Diarrhea morbidity ↔ Respiratory disease morbidity ↔
Motswagole et al. (2013)	(1) MMN-fortified sorghum meal porridge (2) Non-fortified sorghum meal porridge	Adults	Serum retinol ↔ HIV load ↔ CD4+ cell count ↔
Austin et al. (2006)	(1) MMN + βC (2) MMN	Adults	Mortality (2) MMN → risk of death ↑

Note: βC, β-carotene; MMN, multiple micronutrients; VA, vitamin A; VB, vitamin B; VC, vitamin C; VE, vitamin E; ↔, no effect/no differences among groups; ↓, decreased/reduced; ↑, increased; →, resulted/caused/activated.

and type 2 diabetes (Kotnik et al., 2011), and metabolic disease outcomes in HIV-infected patients receiving HAART (Han et al., 2009). HAART has been shown to contribute to the development of metabolic disease symptoms, including insulin resistance, dyslipidemia, and lipodystrophy, and thus there is an increased prevalence of metabolic syndrome and cardiovascular disease in this population. This study enrolled 113 patients who had received HAART for at least six months; patients receiving certain other medications, anti-obesity drugs, or having chronic disease were excluded. A fasting blood sample was taken and analyzed for RBP4 levels. Waist circumference ($p = 0.011$), waist-to-hip-ratio ($p = 0.004$), body mass index ($p = 0.014$), and total body fat mass ($p = 0.024$) were significantly increased with increasing RBP4 quartiles. Subjects with higher RBP4 had significantly higher triglycerides ($p = 0.011$). However, the authors did not state whether subjects were taking dietary supplements such as vitamin A, and serum retinol was not established. Thus, advising patients receiving HAART to take vitamin A supplementation must be elucidated further in future studies. Table 1.4 provides a summary of these studies.

PROGRAMS WITH VITAMIN A-SPECIFIC PLANS FOR COMBATING HIV/AIDS AND RECOMMENDATIONS

Programs that have specific recommendations regarding vitamin A supplementation are highlighted here. Many countries simply follow the guidelines of the World Health Organization (WHO), such as Papua New Guinea (PNG NDoH, 2011). Some countries, including Kenya and India, indicate specific recommendations, as described below (NASCOP, 2006; NACO, 2012, 2013).

The Government of Kenya provides HIV/AIDS treatment guidelines with specific nutrition recommendations. The *Kenyan National Guidelines on Nutrition and HIV/AIDS* (NASCOP, 2006) recommends that both HIV-infected and HIV-negative pregnant women and new mothers receive the same micronutrient interventions; specific to vitamin A, this includes the consumption of vitamin A- and pro-vitamin A-rich foods and a single dose of vitamin A (200,000 IU) within eight weeks postpartum. Infants who require replacement formula (instead of breast milk) should consume milk with micronutrients added at the level of the RDA, including vitamin A. Both HIV-exposed and HIV-infected children should receive vitamin A, along with deworming and routine vaccinations. These guidelines were last updated in 2006, however, and may require revision in accordance with the WHO's latest guidelines (see below).

The National AIDS Control Organisation (NACO) of India has also published specific recommendations for vitamin A supplementation for both children (NACO, 2013) and adults (NACO, 2012). According to NACO, all children 6 to 60 months of age, both HIV-infected and uninfected, are to receive vitamin A supplements (100,000 IU every six months until 12 months of age; 200,000 IU every six months from 12 months to 5 years of age). Recommendations for adults, including pregnant women, are to take vitamin A at levels based on the RDA (adults, 600 µg/day retinol; pregnant women in India, 800 µg/day retinol).

SUMMARY OF WORLD HEALTH ORGANIZATION GUIDELINES AND RECOMMENDATIONS

The World Health Organization is a global health leader operating within the United Nations (UN) and provides norms, standards, health and disease statistics, and support to countries for monitoring trends in health. The WHO offers guidelines for overall HIV prevention, diagnosis, treatment, and care (WHO, 2014b) and also has specific recommendations for vitamin A supplementation among specific populations who are HIV positive (WHO, 2011a–f). These guidelines are compiled from several documents that were published in 2011 and can be accessed online (http://www.who.int/elena/titles/full_recommendations/vitamina_supp/en/). The WHO vitamin A supplementation and HIV recommendations are based on systematic reviews from the Cochrane Collaboration (Imdad et al., 2010; Irlam et al., 2010, 2013).

TABLE 1.4
Vitamin A and ART/HAART

Study	Exposure	Study Design; Population	Main Outcomes	Results
Eshetu et al. (2014)	Serum retinol, iron, zinc	Cross-sectional; adults on HAART	CD4+ T-cell counts	Retinol deficiency → CD4+ ↓
Kaio et al. (2013)	Serum retinol, β-carotene	Cross-sectional; adults on HAART	—	↔ ↔ ↔
Ndeezi et al. (2010)	(1) 2× RDA vitamins A, B_1, B_2, B_6, B_{12}, C, D, E, and niacin; folate; zinc; copper; iodine + selenium (2) 1× RDA vitamins A, C, D, B_1, B_2, and niacin	Randomized control trial; children	Mortality Anthropometry CD4+ count	1) CD4+ and CD4+:CD8+ ↑
Sheehan et al. (2012)	β-carotene	Randomized control trial; adults	Steady-state plasma pharmacokinetics of nelfinavir and its metabolite M8	CD4+ and CD4+:CD8+ ↑
Han et al. (2009)	Serum RBP4	Cross-sectional; adults on HAART	Body measurements; insulin resistance; lipid profiles; obesity; lipodystrophy	(+): Waist circumference, waist:hip ratio, BMI, total body fat mass, total cholesterol, log triglycerides, insulin resistance, intraabdominal fat distance (−): Insulin sensitivity

Note: ↔, No effect/no differences among groups; ↓, decreased/reduced; ↑, increased; →, resulted/caused/activated.

Recommendations

- Vitamin A supplementation is not recommended for newborns and infants up to 5 months of age (WHO, 2011a,b). In locales where night blindness prevalence is ≥1% among children 12 to 24 months of age or where vitamin A deficiency (serum retinol < 0.70 µmol) is ≥ 20% among children 6 to 59 months of age, WHO *recommends* that infants 6 to 11 months of age, including those who are HIV positive, receive one dose of vitamin A (100,000 IU or 300 mg RE) in an oral liquid, oil-based preparation of retinyl palmitate or retinyl acetate (WHO, 2011c).
- For children 12 to 59 months of age, including HIV-positive individuals, WHO *recommends* 200,000 IU (60 mg RE) of vitamin A every four to six months (WHO, 2011c).
- For pregnant women, it is *not recommended* that they receive routine vitamin A supplementation to prevent maternal and infant morbidity and mortality, as vitamin A is a known teratogen. However, in settings where night blindness ≥ 5% in pregnant women or in children 24 to 59 months of age, vitamin A supplementation *is recommended* during pregnancy to prevent night blindness (WHO, 2011d).
- WHO does *not recommend* that HIV-positive pregnant women receive vitamin A supplementation for reducing the risk of mother-to-child transmission (MTCT) of HIV (WHO, 2011e). Several studies have shown an *increased* risk for MTCT when vitamin A is administered, as discussed in this chapter and in Mehta and Fawzi's review (2007).
- Vitamin A supplementation is *not recommended* for postpartum women for the prevention of maternal and infant morbidity and mortality (WHO, 2011f). Again, studies have shown that vitamin A supplementation increases the risk of HIV transmission from mothers to their babies via horizontal transmission (i.e., through breastfeeding).

WHO guidelines for vitamin A supplementation among HIV-positive adults require further research, and WHO does not have specific recommendations for vitamin A supplementation among non-pregnant, HIV-positive adults. Because low levels of serum vitamin A have been associated with increased disease progression and risk of mortality, providing vitamin A supplements may delay disease progression. However, inconsistent results show no clear indication of benefits resulting from vitamin A supplementation among HIV-positive adults (last updated July 2015, accessible at http://www.who.int/elena/titles/vitamina_hiv_adults/en/).

SUMMARY OF PRESIDENT'S EMERGENCY PLAN FOR AIDS RELIEF RECOMMENDATIONS

The President's Emergency Plan for AIDS Relief (PEPFAR) is the largest U.S. bilateral health assistance program and government initiative. It is part of the U.S. President's Global Health Initiative created during President George W. Bush's term (2001–2009), beginning with a commitment of $15 million toward fighting HIV/AIDS. The initiative is entering its second phase, focusing on transitioning from an emergency response to promoting sustainable country-level programs. PEPFAR's published guidelines, specific to vitamin A, include the following (Sadr et al., 2011):

- Vitamin A (and zinc) supplementation is recommended for HIV-infected children, according to national guidelines (PEPFAR, 2006).
- Components of an integrated care package for newborns, infants, and children up to 5 years of age should include vitamin A and other micronutrient supplementation (PEPFAR, 2011).

These recommendations, too, will require expansion to more populations, with revisions and updating as more research comes to light.

CONCLUSIONS

Despite the efforts of researchers, organizations, and agencies around the world, HIV/AIDS continues to affect millions of people, including children. Vitamin A administration influences the course of disease in adults, children, and pregnant women, as well as in mouse models in laboratory settings. Additional research has demonstrated several possible mechanisms to explain why vitamin A appears to increase the risk of mother-to-child transmission, such as exacerbated mastitis in mothers leading to infected children; these susceptible populations should avoid vitamin A supplementation. What remains to be determined is the proper dosages of micronutrients necessary for at-risk populations and how the supplementation should be delivered—by pill, through fortified foods, or by other methods. Genetic polymorphisms of MBL-2 appear to modulate the association between vitamin A status and HIV risk, thus highlighting the need for further research into genetic differences in the link between nutrition and HIV. Research regarding how vitamin supplementation can impact the prognosis of diseases that increase the risk of HIV co-infection, such as tuberculosis, is also a priority. Additionally, vitamins B, C, D, and E must be better characterized in the context of HIV; Fawzi's Trial of Vitamins and HAART in HIV Disease Progression (Clinicaltrials.gov identifier: NCT00383669) is one study examining the effects of multivitamins on HIV disease progression. The complexity of vitamin A's role in HIV pathogenesis, with its both helpful and harmful effects, warrants more study to determine the most effective and efficient use of this micronutrient. Further research and international collaborations are crucial in the continuing fight against HIV/AIDS.

REFERENCES

Arsenault, J.E., S. Aboud, K. P. Manji, W. W. Fawzi, and E. Villamor. (2010). Vitamin supplementation increases risk of subclinical mastitis in HIV-infected women. *Journal of Nutrition* 140(13): 1788–92.

Austin, J., N. Singhal, R. Voigt et al.; CTN 09/CRIT Cartenoids Study Group. (2006). A community randomized controlled clinical trial of mixed carotenoids and micronutrient supplementation of patients with acquired immunodeficiency syndrome. *European Journal of Clinical Nutrition* 60(11): 1266–76.

Baeten, J. M., R. S. McClelland, J. Overbaugh et al. (2002). Vitamin A supplementation and human immunodeficiency virus type 1 shedding in women: results of a randomized clinical trial. *Journal of Infectious Diseases* 185(8): 1187–91.

Baeten, J. M., R. S. McClelland, M. H. Wener et al. (2007). Relationship between markers of HIV-1 disease progression and serum beta-carotene concentrations in Kenyan women. *International Journal of STD & AIDS* 18(3): 202–6.

Boniotto, M., L. Braida, D. Pirulli, L. Arraes, A. Amoroso, and S. Crovella. (2003). MBL2 polymorphisms are involved in HIV-1 infection in Brazilian perinatally infected children. *AIDS* 17(5): 779–80.

Buccigrossi, V., G. Laudiero, E. Nicastro, E. Miele, F. Esposito, and A. Guarino. (2011). The HIV-1 transactivator factor (Tat) induces enterocyte apoptosis through a redox-mediated mechanism. *PloS One* 6(12): e29436.

Chatterjee, A., R. J. Bosch, D. J. Hunter, K. Manji, G. I. Msamanga, and W. W. Fawzi. (2010). Vitamin A and vitamin B-12 concentrations in relation to mortality and morbidity among children born to HIV-infected women. *Journal of Tropical Pediatrics* 56(1): 27–35.

Chhagan, M. K., J. Van den Broeck, K.-K. A. Luabeya, N. Mpontshane, K. L. Tucker, and M. L. Bennish. (2009). Effect of micronutrient supplementation on diarrhoeal disease among stunted children in rural South Africa. *European Journal of Clinical Nutrition* 63(7): 850–7.

Chhagan, M. K., J. Van den Broeck, K.-K. A. Luabeya, N. Mpontshane, A. Tomkins, and M. L. Bennish. (2010). Effect on longitudinal growth and anemia of zinc or multiple micronutrients added to vitamin A: a randomized controlled trial in children aged 6–24 months. *BMC Public Health* 10: 145.

Cook, J. A., D. Grey, J. Burke et al. (2004). Depressive symptoms and AIDS-related mortality among a multisite cohort of HIV-positive women. *American Journal of Public Health* 94(7): 1133–40.

Coutsoudis, A., K. Pillay, E. Spooner, L. Kuhn, and H. M. Coovadia. (1999). Randomized trial testing the effect of vitamin A supplementation on pregnancy outcomes and early mother-to-child HIV-1 transmission in Durban, South Africa. South African Vitamin A Study Group. *AIDS* 13(12): 1517–24.

Degenhardt, L., B. Mathers, P. Vickerman, T. Rhodes, C. Latkin, and M. Hickman. (2010). Prevention of HIV infection for people who inject drugs: why individual, structural, and combination approaches are needed. *The Lancet* 376(9737): 285–301.

Drain, P. K., R. Kupka, F. Mugusi, and W. W. Fawzi. (2007). Micronutrients in HIV-positive persons receiving highly active antiretroviral therapy. *American Journal of Clinical Nutrition* 85(2): 333–45.

Epple, H.-J., K. Allers, H. Tröger et al. (2010). Acute HIV infection induces mucosal infiltration with CD4+ and CD8+ T cells, epithelial apoptosis, and a mucosal barrier defect. *Gastroenterology* 139(4): 1289–300.

Eshetu, A., A. Tsegaye, and B. Petros. (2014). Selected micronutrient levels and response to highly active antiretroviral therapy (HAART) among HIV/AIDS patients attending a teaching hospital in Addis Ababa, Ethiopia. *Biological Trace Element Research* 162(1–3): 106–12.

Evans, D., L. McNamara, M. Maskew et al. (2013). Impact of nutritional supplementation on immune response, body mass index and bioelectrical impedance in HIV-positive patients starting antiretroviral therapy. *Nutrition Journal* 12(1): 111.

Fawzi, W. W., G. I. Msamanga, D. Spiegelman, E. J. Urassa, and D. J. Hunter. (1999). Rationale and design of the Tanzania Vitamin and HIV Infection Trial. *Controlled Clinical Trials* 20(1): 75–90.

Fawzi, W. W., G. I. Msamanga, D. Hunter, B. Renjifo, G. Antelman, H. Bang, K. Manji, S. Kapiga, D. Mwakagile, M. Essex, and D. Spiegelman. (2002). Randomized trial of vitamin supplements in relation to transmission of HIV-1 through breastfeeding and early child mortality. *AIDS* 16(14): 1935–44.

Fawzi, W. W., G. I. Msamanga, R. Kupka et al. (2007). Multivitamin supplementation improves hematologic status in HIV-infected women and their children in Tanzania. *American Journal of Clinical Nutrition* 85(5): 1335–43.

Fufa, H., M. Umeta, S. Taffesse, N. Mokhtar, and H. Aguenaou. (2009). Nutritional and immunological status and their associations among HIV-infected adults in Addis Ababa, Ethiopia. *Food and Nutrition Bulletin* 30(3): 227–32.

Grobler, L., N. Siegfried, M. E. Visser, S. S. N. Mahlungulu, and J. Volmink. (2013). Nutritional interventions for reducing morbidity and mortality in people with HIV. *Cochrane Database of Systematic Reviews* 2: CD004536.

Guo, M., J. Bryant, S. Sultana, O. Jones, and W. Royal III. (2012). Effects of vitamin A deficiency and opioids on hippocampal neuronal numbers and parvalbumin expression in the HIVA-1 transgenic rat. *Current HIV Research* 10(5): 463–68.

Han, S. H., B. S. Chin, H. S. Lee et al. (2009). Serum retinol-binding protein 4 correlates with obesity, insulin resistance, and dyslipidemia in HIV-infected subjects receiving highly active antiretroviral therapy. *Metabolism: Clinical and Experimental* 58(11): 1523–9.

He, J. C., T.-C. Lu, M. Fleet et al. (2007). Retinoic acid inhibits HIV-1-induced podocyte proliferation through the cAMP pathway. *Journal of the American Society of Nephrology* 18(1): 93–102.

Hummelen, R., J. Hemsworth, J. Changalucha et al. (2011). Effect of micronutrient and probiotic fortified yogurt on immune-function of anti-retroviral therapy naive HIV patients. *Nutrients* 3(10): 897–909.

Humphrey, J. H., J. W. Hargrove, L. C. Malaba et al.; ZVITAMBO Study Group. (2006). HIV incidence among post-partum women in Zimbabwe: risk factors and the effect of vitamin A supplementation. *AIDS* 20(10): 1437–46.

Ickovics, J. R., M. E. Hamburger, D. Vlahov et al.; HIV Epidemiology Research Study Group. (2001). Mortality, CD4 cell count decline, and depressive symptoms among HIV-seropositive women. *JAMA* 285(11): 1466–74.

Imdad, A., K. Herzer, E. Mayo-Wilson, M. Y. Yakoob, and Z. A. Bhutta. (2010). Vitamin A supplementation for preventing morbidity and mortality in children from 6 months to 5 years of age. *Cochrane Database of Systematic Reviews*, 12: CD008524.

Irlam, J. H., M. M. Visser, N. N. Rollins, and N. Siegfried. (2010). Micronutrient supplementation in children and adults with HIV infection. *Cochrane Database of Systematic Reviews* 12: CD003650.

Irlam, J. H., N. Siegfried, M. E. Visser, and N. C. Rollins. (2013). Micronutrient supplementation for children with HIV infection. *Cochrane Database of Systematic Reviews* 10: CD010666.

Ivers, L. C., J. E. Teng, J. G. Jerome, M. Bonds, K. A. Freedberg, and M. F. Franke. (2014). A randomized trial of ready-to-use supplementary food versus corn–soy blend plus as food rations for HIV-infected adults on antiretroviral therapy in rural Haiti. *Clinical Infectious Diseases* 58(8): 1176–84.

Jaruga, P., B. Jaruga, D. Gackowski et al. (2002). Supplementation with antioxidant vitamins prevents oxidative modification of DNA in lymphoctyes of HIV-infected patients. *Free Radical Biology and Medicine* 32(5): 414–20.

Jiang, H., Y. Badralmaa, J. Yang, R. Lempicki, A. Hazen, and V. Natarajan. (2012). Retinoic acid and liver X receptor agonist synergistically inhibit HIV infection in CD4+ T cells by up-regulating ABCA1-mediated cholesterol efflux. *Lipids in Health and Disease* 11: 69.

Jones, C. Y., A. M. Tang, J. E. Forrester et al. (2006). Micronutrient levels and HIV disease status in HIV-infected patients on highly active antiretroviral therapy in the Nutrition for Healthy Living cohort. *Journal of Acquired Immune Deficiency Syndromes* 43(4): 475–82.

Kaio, D. J., P. H. Rondó, J. M. Souza, A. V. Firmino, L. A. Luzia, and A. A. Segurado. (2013). Vitamin A and beta-carotene concentrations in adults with HIV/AIDS on highly active antiretroviral therapy. *Journal of Nutritional Science and Vitaminology* 59(6): 496–502.

Kantarci, S., I. N. Koulinska, S. Aboud, W. W. Fawzi, and E. Villamor. (2007). Subclinical mastitis, cell-associated HIV-1 shedding in breast milk, and breast-feeding transmission of HIV-1. *Journal of Acquired Immune Deficiency Syndromes* 46(5): 651–4.

Kassu, A., B. Andualem, N. Van Nhien et al. (2007). Vitamin A deficiency in patients with diarrhea and HIV infection in Ethiopia. *Asia Pacific Journal of Clinical Nutrition* 16(Suppl. 1): 323–8.

Katona, P. and J. Katona-Apte. (2008). The interaction between nutrition and infection. *Clinical Infectious Diseases* 46(10): 1582–8.

Kawai, K., G. Msamanga, K. Manji et al. (2010). Sex differences in the effects of maternal vitamin supplements on mortality and morbidity among children born to HIV-infected women in Tanzania. *British Journal of Nutrition* 103(12): 1784–91.

Kotnik, P., P. Fischer-Posovszky, and M. Wabitsch. (2011). RBP4: a controversial adipokine. *European Journal of Endocrinology* 165(5): 703–11.

Kuhn, L., A. Coutsoudis, D. Trabattoni et al. (2006). Synergy between mannose-binding lectin gene polymorphisms and supplementation with vitamin A influences susceptibility to HIV infection in infants born to HIV-positive mothers. *American Journal of Clinical Nutrition* 84(3): 610–5.

Loignon, M., H. Brodeur, S. Deschênes, D. Phaneuf, P. V. Bhat, and E. Toma. (2012). Combination antiretroviral therapy and chronic HIV infection affect serum retinoid concentrations: longitudinal and cross-sectional assessments. *AIDS Research and Therapy* 9(1): 3.

Long, K. Z., J. L. Rosado, J. I., Santos et al. (2010). Associations between mucosal innate and adaptive immune responses and resolution of diarrheal pathogen infections. *Infection and Immunity* 78(3): 1221–8.

Lu, T.-C., Z. Wang, X. Feng et al. (2008). Retinoic acid utilizes CREB and USF1 in a transcriptional feed-forward loop in order to stimulate MKP1 expression in human immunodeficiency virus-infected podocytes. *Molecular and Cellular Biology* 28(18): 5785–94.

Luabeya, K.-K. A., N. Mpontshane, M. Mackay et al. (2007). Zinc or multiple micronutrient supplementation to reduce diarrhea and respiratory disease in South African children: a randomized controlled trial. *PloS One* 2(6): e541.

Machado, R. H. V., S. Bonafe, A. Castelo, and R. V. Patin. (2013). Vitamin profile of pregnant women living with HIV/AIDS. *e-SPEN Journal* 8(3): e108–12.

Maeda, Y., T. Yamaguchi, Y. H. Ata et al. (2007). All-*trans* retinoic acid attacks reverse transcriptase resulting in inhibition of HIV-1 replication. *Hematology* 12(3): 263–6.

McGrath, N., D. Bellinger, J. Robins, G. I. Msamanga, E. Tronick, and W. W. Fawzi. (2006). Effect of maternal multivitamin supplementation on the mental and psychomotor development of children who are born to HIV-1-infected mothers in Tanzania. *Pediatrics* 117(2): e216–25.

Mda, S., J. M. van Raaij, U. E. Macintyre, F. P. de Villiers, and F. J. Kok. (2010). Improved appetite after multi-micronutrient supplementation for six months in HIV-infected South African children. *Appetite* 54(1): 150–5.

Mehta, S. and W. Fawzi. (2007). Effects of vitamins, including vitamin A, on HIV/AIDS patients. *Vitamins and Hormones* 75: 355–83.

Mehta, S., D. Spiegelman, S. Aboud, E. L. Giovannucci, and G. I. Msamanga. (2011). Lipid-soluble vitamins A, D, and E in HIV-infected pregnant women in Tanzania. *European Journal of Clinical Nutrition* 64(8): 808–17.

Monteiro, J. P., M. L. Santos Cruz, M. M. Mussi-Pinhata et al. (2014). Vitamin A, vitamin E, iron and zinc status in a cohort of HIV-infected mothers and their uninfected infants. *Revista Da Sociedade Brasileira de Medicina Tropical* 47(6): 692–700.

Montero, M., N. E. van Houten, X. Wang, and J. K. Scott. (2008). The membrane-proximal external region of the human immunodeficiency virus type 1 envelope: dominant site of antibody neutralization and target for vaccine design. *Microbiology and Molecular Biology Reviews* 72(1): 54–84.

Mora, J. R., M. Iwata, and U. H. von Andrian. (2008). Vitamin effects on the immune system: vitamins A and D take centre stage. *Nature Reviews. Immunology* 8(9): 685–98.

Motswagole, B. S., T. C. Mongwaketse, M. Mokotedi et al. (2013). The efficacy of micronutrient-fortified sorghum meal in improving the immune status of HIV-positive adults. *Annals of Nutrition and Metabolism* 62(4): 323–30.

Mulu, A., A. Kassu, K. Huruy et al. (2011). Vitamin A deficiency during pregnancy of HIV infected and non-infected women in tropical settings of Northwest Ethiopia. *BMC Public Health* 11: 569.

NACO. (2012). *National Guidelines for Providing Nutritional Care and Support for Adults Living with HIV and AIDS*. New Delhi: National AIDS Control Organisation, Ministry of Health and Family Welfare, Government of India, pp. 1–65

NACO. (2013). Nutrition guidelines for HIV-exposed and infected children (0–14 years of age). In: *Children's Guideline Book*. New Delhi: National AIDS Control Organisation, Ministry of Health and Family Welfare, Government of India, pp. pp. 2–48.

NASCOP. (2006). *Kenyan National Guidelines on Nutrition and HIV/AIDS*. Nairobi: National AIDS and STI Control Programme (http://www.ilo.org/wcmsp5/groups/public/---ed_protect/---protrav/---ilo_aids/documents/legaldocument/wcms_127535.pdf).

Ndeezi, G., T. Tylleskär, C. M. Ndugwa, and J. K. Tumwine. (2010). Effect of multiple micronutrient supplementation on survival of HIV-infected children in Uganda: a randomized, controlled trial. *Journal of the International AIDS Society* 13: 18.

Ndekha, M. J., J. J. G. van Oosterhout, E. E. Zijlstra, M. Manary, H. Saloojee, and M. J. Manary. (2009). Supplementary feeding with either ready-to-use fortified spread or corn–soy blend in wasted adults starting antiretroviral therapy in Malawi: randomised, investigator blinded, controlled trial. *BMJ* 338: b1867.

Neves, F. F., H. Vannucchi, A. A. Jordão, Jr., and J. F. Figueiredo. (2006). Recommended dose for repair of serum vitamin A levels in patients with HIV infection/AIDS may be insufficient because of high urinary losses. *Nutrition* 22(5): 483–9.

Nunnari, G., C. Coco, M. R. Pinzone et al. (2012). The role of micronutrients in the diet of HIV-1-infected individuals. *Frontiers in Bioscience (Elite Edition)* E4: 2442–56.

Obuseh, F. A., P. E. Jolly, A. Kulczycki et al. (2011). Aflatoxin levels, plasma vitamins A and E concentrations, and their association with HIV and hepatitis B virus infections in Ghanaians: a cross-sectional study. *Journal of the International AIDS Society* 14: 53.

Papathakis, P. C., N. C. Rollins, C. J. Chantry, M. L. Bennish, and K. H. Brown. (2007). Micronutrient status during lactation in HIV-infected and HIV-uninfected South African women during the first 6 mo after delivery. *American Journal of Clinical Nutrition* 85(1): 182–92.

PEPFAR. (2006). *Guidance for United States Government In-Country Staff and Implementing Partners for a Preventive Care Package for Children Aged 0–14 Years Old Born to HIV-Infected Mothers*. Washington, DC: The President's Emergency Plan for AIDS Relief (https://2009-2017.pepfar.gov/documents/organization/77005.pdf).

PEPFAR. (2011). *PEPFAR Guidance on Integrating Prevention of Mother to Child Transmission of HIV, Maternal, Neonatal, and Child Health and Pediatric HIV Services*. Washington, DC: The President's Emergency Plan for AIDS Relief (https://2009-2017.pepfar.gov/documents/organization/158963.pdf).

PNG NDoH. (2009). *Guidelines for HIV Care and Treatment in Papua New Guinea*. Port Moresby: Papua New Guinea National Department of Health (http://www.who.int/hiv/pub/guidelines/papua_art.pdf).

Purnomo, J., S. Jeganathan, K. Begley, and L. Houtzager. (2012). Depression and dietary intake in a cohort of HIV-positive clients in Sydney. *International Journal of STD & AIDS* 23(12): 882–6.

Reilly, L., N. Nausch, N. Midzi, T. Mduluza, and F. Mutapi. (2012). Association between micronutrients (vitamin A, D, iron) and schistosome-specific cytokine responses in Zimbabweans exposed to *Schistosoma haematobium*. *Journal of Parasitology Research* 2012: 128628.

Rousseau, M. C., C. Molines, J. Moreau, and J. Delmont. (2000). Influence of highly active antiretroviral therapy on micronutrient profiles in HIV-infected patients. *Annals of Nutrition and Metabolism* 44(5–6): 212–6.

Royal, III, W., H. Wang, O. Jones, H. Tran, and J. L. Bryant. (2007). A vitamin A deficient diet enhances pro-inflammatory cytokine, Mu opioid receptor, and HIV-1 expression in the HIV-1 transgenic rat. *Journal of Neuroimmunology* 185(1–2): 29–36.

Sadr, W. E., M. Cohen, K. DeCock et al. (2011). *PEPFAR Scientific Advisory Board Recommendations for the Office of the US Global AIDS Coordinator: Implications of HPTN 052 for PEPFAR's Treatment Programs*. Washington, DC: The President's Emergency Plan for AIDS Relief, pp. 1–34.

Scrimshaw, N. S., C. E. Taylor, and J. E. Gordon. (1968). *Interactions of Nutrition and Infection*, WHO Monograph Series No. 57. Geneva: World Health Organization.

Semba, R. D. (1994). Vitamin A, immunity, and infection. *Clinical Infectious Diseases* 19(3): 489–99.

Sheehan, N. L., R. P. G. van Heeswijk, B. C. Foster et al. (2012). The effect of β-carotene supplementation on the pharmacokinetics of nelfinavir and its active metabolite M8 in HIV-1-infected patients. *Molecules* 17(1): 688–702.

Smith Fawzi, M. C., S. F. Kaaya, J. Mbwambo et al. (2007). Multivitamin supplementation in HIV-positive pregnant women: impact on depression and quality of life in a resource-poor setting. *HIV Medicine* 8(4): 203–12.

Solomons, N.W. (2012). Vitamin A. In: *Present Knowledge in Nutrition*, 10th ed., edited by J. W. Erdman, I. A. MacDonald, and S. H. Zielsel, pp. 149–184. Ames, IA: Wiley-Blackwell.

Srinivas, A., and B. F. Dias. (2008). Antioxidants in HIV positive children. *Indian Journal of Pediatrics* 75(4): 347–50.

Sultana, S., H. Li, A. Puche, O. Jones, J. L. Bryant, and W. Royal. (2010). Quantitation of parvalbumin+ neurons and human immunodeficiency virus type 1 (HIV-1) regulatory gene expression in the HIV-1 transgenic rat: effects of vitamin A deficiency and morphine. *Journal of Neurovirology* 16(1): 33–40.

Tohill, B. C., C. M. Heilig, R. S. Klein et al. (2007). Nutritional biomarkers associated with gynecological conditions among US women with or at risk of HIV infection. *American Journal of Clinical Nutrition* 85(5): 1327–34.

Toma, E., D. Devost, N. Chow Lan, and P. V. Bhat. (2001). HIV-protease inhibitors alter retinoic acid synthesis. *AIDS* 15(15): 1979–84.

Turner, M. W. (1996). Mannose-binding lectin: the pluripotent molecule of the innate immune system. *Immunology Today* 17(11): 532–40.

UNAIDS. (2013). *Global Report: UNAIDS Report on the Global AIDS Epidemic 2013*. Geneva: Joint United Nations Programme on HIV/AIDS. (http://www.unaids.org/sites/default/files/media_asset/UNAIDS_Global_Report_2013_en_1.pdf).

Villamor, E. and W. W. Fawzi. (2005). Effects of vitamin A supplementation on immune responses and correlation with clinical outcomes effects of vitamin A supplementation on immune responses and correlation with clinical outcomes. *Clinical Microbiology Reviews* 18(3): 446–64.

Villamor, E., R. Mbise, D. Spiegelman et al. (2002). Vitamin A supplements ameliorate the adverse effect of HIV-1, malaria, and diarrheal infections on child growth. *Pediatrics* 109(1): e6.

Villamor, E., S. Kapiga, and W. Fawzi. (2006). Vitamin A serostatus and heterosexual transmission of HIV: case-control study in Tanzania and review of the evidence. *International Journal of Vitamin and Nutrition Research* 76(2): 81–5.

Villamor, E., I. N. Koulinska, S. Aboud et al. (2010). Effect of vitamin supplements on HIV shedding in breast milk. *American Journal of Clinical Nutrition* 92(4): 881–6.

Watson, D. S., Z. Huang, and F. C. Szoka, Jr. (2010). All-*trans* retinoic acid potentiates the antibody response in mice to a lipopeptide antigen adjuvanted with liposomal lipid A. *Immunology and Cell Biology* 87(8), 630–3.

Webb, A. L., S. Aboud, J. Furtado et al. (2011). Effect of vitamin supplementation on breast milk concentrations of retinol, carotenoids, and tocopherols in HIV-infected Tanzanian women. *European Journal of Clinical Nutrition* 63(3): 332–9.

WHO. (2003). *Nutrient Requirements for People Living with HIV/AIDS*. Geneva: World Health Organization.

WHO. (2009). *Global Prevalence of Vitamin A Deficiency in Populations at Risk 1995–2005*. Geneva: World Health Organization.

WHO. (2011a). *Guideline: Neonatal Vitamin A Supplementation*. Geneva: World Health Organization (http://www.who.int/nutrition/publications/micronutrients/guidelines/vas_neonatal/en/).

WHO. (2011b). *Guideline: Vitamin A Supplementation for Infants 1–5 Months of Age*. Geneva: World Health Organization (http://www.who.int/nutrition/publications/micronutrients/guidelines/vas_infants_1-5/en/).

WHO. (2011c). *Guideline: Vitamin A Supplementation for Infants and Children 6–59 Months of Age*. Geneva: World Health Organization (http://www.who.int/nutrition/publications/micronutrients/guidelines/vas_6to59_months/en/).

WHO. (2011d). *Guideline: Vitamin A Supplementation in Pregnant Women*. Geneva: World Health Organization (http://www.who.int/nutrition/publications/micronutrients/guidelines/vas_pregnant/en/).

WHO. (2011e). *Guideline: Vitamin A Supplementation During Pregnancy for Reducing the Risk of Mother-to-Child Transmission of HIV*. Geneva: World Health Organization (http://www.who.int/nutrition/publications/micronutrients/guidelines/vas_mtct_hiv/en/).

WHO. (2011f). *Guideline: Vitamin A Supplementation in Postpartum Women*. Geneva: World Health Organization (http://www.who.int/nutrition/publications/micronutrients/guidelines/vas_postpartum/en/).

WHO. (2014a). *Nutrition: Micronutrient Deficiencies*. Geneva: World Health Organization (http://www.who.int/nutrition/topics/vad/en/).

WHO. (2014b). *Consolidated Guidelines for HIV Prevention, Diagnosis, Treatment and Care for Key Populations*. Geneva: World Health Organization (http://apps.who.int/iris/bitstream/10665/128048/1/9789241507431_eng.pdf?ua=1&ua=1).

WHO. (2014c). *Global Health Observatory (GHO) Data: HIV/AIDS*. Geneva: World Health Organization (http://www.who.int/gho/hiv/en/).

WHO and CDC. (2007). *Nutrition: Assessing the Iron Status of Populations*, 2nd ed. Report of a Joint World Health Organization/Centers for Disease Control and Prevention Technical Consultation on the Assessment of Iron Status at the Population Level, Geneva, April 6–8, 2004.

Yu, M. and M. Vajdy. (2011). A novel retinoic acid, catechin hydrate and mustard oil-based emulsion for enhanced cytokine and antibody responses against multiple strains of HIV-1 following mucosal and systemic vaccinations. *Vaccine* 29(13): 2429–36.

Zvandasara, P., J. W. Hargrove, R. Ntozini et al.; ZVITAMBO Study Group. (2006). Mortality and morbidity among postpartum HIV-positive and HIV-negative women in Zimbabwe: risk factors, causes, and impact of single-dose postpartum vitamin A supplementation. *Journal of Acquired Immune Deficiency Syndromes* 43(1): 107–16.

2 B-Vitamins and HIV/AIDS

Alexander J. Layden and Julia L. Finkelstein

CONTENTS

INTRODUCTION

B-Vitamins

B-vitamins are a class of water-soluble micronutrients that are required for cell metabolism. These include thiamin (vitamin B_1), riboflavin (vitamin B_2), niacin (vitamin B_3), pantothenic acid (vitamin B_5), pyridoxine (vitamin B_6), biotin (vitamin B_7), folate (vitamin B_9), and vitamin B_{12}. B-vitamins serve as cofactors in the metabolism of amino acids, fatty acids, and sugars, as well as the synthesis and methylation of DNA (McCormick et al., 1999; Powers, 2003; Kamanna and Kashyap, 2008; Stover, 2009; Allen, 2012; Combs, Jr., 2012). In particular, folate, vitamin B_6, and vitamin B_{12} are required in one-carbon metabolism, including *de novo* purine biosynthesis and production of *S*-adenosyl methionine, the universal methyl donor required in over 100 methylation processes (Stover, 2009; Finkelstein et al., 2015). Requirements for B-vitamins are increased during periods of rapid growth and development, including during pregnancy and early childhood (Stover, 2009; Finkelstein et al., 2015).

B-vitamins and Immune Function

B-vitamins are required for innate and adaptive immunity and the maintenance of processes underlying immune function. For example, folate, vitamin B_6, and vitamin B_{12} are important for lymphocyte maturation and proliferation, T-cell cytotoxicity, and protection against oxidative stress (Dhur et al., 1991; Gay and Meydani, 2001). In observational studies among patients with megaloblastic anemia, intramuscular vitamin B_{12} injections restored CD8 T-cell counts, total leukocyte counts, and natural killer cell activity (Tamura et al., 1999; Erkurt et al., 2008), and folic acid supplementation improved cell-mediated immunity (Gross et al., 1975). Another study found that increased dietary intake of vitamin B_6 was associated with elevated lymphocyte proliferation (Kwak et al., 2002). During elevated interferon-gamma (IFN-γ) activity, riboflavin and vitamin B_6 may be depleted, given the role of these nutrients as cofactors for tryptophan catabolism, a metabolic process that is increased during IFN-γ-mediated immune activity (Christensen et al., 2012; Theofylaktopoulou et al., 2014). Few studies have been conducted to investigate the associations of other B-vitamins and immune function.

B-vitamins and HIV/AIDS: Evidence from Observational Studies

B-vitamin deficiencies are common in HIV-infected individuals and have been associated with increased risk of HIV disease progression and adverse health outcomes in observational studies. HIV disease may itself contribute to the etiology of certain B-vitamin deficiencies through a number of potential mechanisms, such as gut epithelial damage (Brenchley and Douek, 2007), infection of marrow stromal cells (Koka et al., 1999), impaired hematopoietic progenitor cell growth (Moses et al., 1996), and bone marrow pathologies, autoimmune hemolysis, and intestinal blood loss (Coyle, 1997; Kreuzer and Rockstroh, 1997; Sullivan et al., 1998). For example, riboflavin, folate, and vitamin B_{12} are absorbed across the villi of enterocytes through carrier-mediated transport (Sundaram, 2000; Milman, 2012; Finkelstein et al., 2015); damage to the intestinal lining and changes in lumen pH caused by the acute phase of HIV infection and chronic inflammation reduce the efficacy of gut absorption, which may result in these deficiencies.

Conversely, B-vitamins, such as vitamin B_6, folate, and vitamin B_{12}, could influence HIV disease progression via restoration of lymphocyte counts and promotion of lymphocyte maturation. Vitamin B_6, folate, and vitamin B_{12} are critical methyl donors or coenzymes in one-carbon metabolism, a process necessary for DNA *de novo* synthesis (McCormick and Chen, 1999; Powers, 2003; Stover, 2009; Finkelstein et al., 2015); inadequate concentrations of these nutrients could hamper proper DNA synthesis for CD4$^+$ lymphocytes, a primary host target of HIV. HIV promotes apoptosis of host cells through over-activation of the pro-apoptotic proteins p53 and capsase 3 (Lương and Nguyễn, 2013). Animal studies report that thiamin treatment may reduce the activity of p53 and capsase 3, suggesting a protective role of thiamin against HIV-induced cell apoptosis (Lương and Nguyễn, 2013). To date, however, there is limited evidence of the role of niacin, biotin, and panto-thenic acid in HIV infection or disease progression. Several observational human studies have been conducted to examine the associations between B-vitamins and HIV/AIDS, although the potential mechanisms have not been elucidated.

Vitamin B_6, Vitamin B_{12}, and Folate

Inadequate status or intake of vitamin B_6, vitamin B_{12}, and folate have been associated with increased HIV disease progression in several studies, including the Multicenter AIDS Cohort Study (MACS), the first and largest study to date of the natural history of AIDS (Tang et al., 1993, 1996, 1997). Among men having sex with men (MSM), lower serum vitamin B_{12} (<120 pmol/L vs. ≥120 pmol/L) was associated with increased risk of HIV disease progression to AIDS by 9 years follow-up (RR, 1.89; 95% CI, 1.15–3.10; $p < 0.05$); neither impaired serum vitamin B_6 (<88 nmol/L) nor folate (<3.4 nmol/L) status was associated with AIDS progression (Tang et al., 1997). In the same MACS cohort, men with higher dietary intake of vitamin B_6 (i.e., ≥2 times the RDA level) had a reduced risk of AIDS-related mortality (relative hazard [RH], 0.60; 95% CI, 0.39–0.93; $p < 0.05$) compared to men with lower intake (i.e., <2 times the RDA level) (Tang et al., 1996). In a cohort of antiretroviral therapy (ART)-naïve, HIV-infected homosexual men, individuals who became vita-min B_{12}-deficient (plasma vitamin B_{12} < 200 pg/mL) during the 18-month follow-up period had a significant decrease in CD4 T-cell counts ($p = 0.038$) (Baum et al., 1995).

HIV may also impair B-vitamin absorption or metabolism. Case-control studies from Rwanda and Brazil found that HIV-infected individuals had lower serum vitamin B_{12} and plasma folate concentrations compared to healthy HIV-uninfected controls (Masaisa et al., 2011; Deminice et al., 2013). A cross-sectional study of patients with AIDS found that 87% ($n = 13/15$) had impaired vitamin B_{12} absorption (i.e., <7% absorption by the Shillings test) (Goodgame et al., 1995). Another study found that 35.8% of patients with AIDS (including CD4 T-cell counts < 200 cells/mL) had impaired vitamin B_{12} absorption (i.e., <30 mg/dL of D-xylose) (Knox et al., 2000).

Evidence regarding the associations between B-vitamins and HIV/AIDS among individuals receiving antiretroviral therapy has been limited and conflicting. A study in Spain found that HIV-infected adults who received highly active antiretroviral therapy (HAART) for at least three months had a significantly lower prevalence of vitamin B_{12} insufficiency (serum vitamin B_{12} ≤ 200 pmol/L; 8.7% vs. 27%; $p < 0.0001$) and folate insufficiency (erythrocyte folate ≤ 580 nmol/L; 10.3% vs. 22%; $p < 0.0001$) compared to HAART-naïve, HIV-infected adults (Remacha et al., 2003). However, another study among asymptomatic HIV-infected adults reported that longer HAART duration was correlated with lower plasma vitamin B_{12} ($r = -0.62$; $p < 0.05$) and folate ($r = -0.39$; $p < 0.05$) concentrations (Deminice et al., 2013). Among HIV-infected adults from the Nutrition for Healthy Living (NFHL) cohort, patients who took a protease inhibitor (PI) from baseline to follow-up (mean = six months) had smaller changes in serum vitamin B_{12} (+0.12 pg/mL) concentrations for each μg/day increase in the dietary intake of vitamin B_{12} compared to non-PI users (+1.06 pg/mL; $p < 0.05$) (Woods et al., 2003). However, patients taking PIs had overall higher median serum vitamin B_{12} concentrations at baseline compared to non-PI users (median [interquartile range, IQR]: 491 pg/mL [82–667] vs. 462 pg/mL [369–617]; $p = 0.0077$) (Woods et al., 2003).

Other B-vitamins

Limited data are available regarding the role of other B-vitamins in the context of HIV/AIDS, including thiamin, riboflavin, niacin, pantothenic acid, or biotin. In a study among homosexual men in Florida, HIV-infected individuals had significantly lower mean riboflavin concentrations, as defined by erythrocyte glutathione reductase activity (activity coefficient, 1.19 ± 0.14 vs. 1.37 ± 0.20; $p < 0.0001$) compared to HIV-uninfected controls (Beach et al., 1992). Several observational studies have examined the associations of dietary intake of B-vitamins and HIV-related outcomes, with conflicting results. As part of the MACS of men who have sex with men (MSM), individuals who had higher dietary intake of thiamin (>4.9 vs. <2.4 mg/day; relative hazard [RH], 0.60; 95% CI, 0.36–0.98; $p < 0.05$) and niacin (>61.0 vs. ≤ 61.0 mg/day; RH, 0.52; 95% CI, 0.31–0.86; $p < 0.05$) at baseline had a lower rate of HIV disease progression to AIDS during follow-up (median = 6.8 years) (Tang et al., 1993). Similarly, men who consumed at least five times the recommended dietary allowance (RDA) levels of thiamin (RH, 0.61; 95% CI, 0.38–0.98; $p < 0.05$) or riboflavin (RH, 0.60; 95% CI, 0.37–0.97; $p < 0.05$) had significantly lower risk of AIDS-related mortality (RH, 0.61; 95% CI, 0.38–0.98; $p < 0.05$) compared to men with lower intake (i.e., <5 times the RDA level) (Tang et al., 1996). Other observational studies have reported no significant differences in the dietary intake of thiamin or riboflavin in HIV-infected women compared to HIV-uninfected women (Addo et al., 2011) and no significant associations between dietary intake of thiamin, riboflavin, or niacin and HIV disease progression to AIDS at 6 years follow-up (Abrams et al., 1993). In a study among children and young adults (1 to 25 years old), HIV-infected individuals had mean suboptimal intake of folate and pantothenic acid compared to the RDA cutoffs (both $p < 0.0001$) (Ziegler et al., 2014).

OBJECTIVES

Findings from observational studies to date suggest that B-vitamin deficiencies are common in HIV-infected populations and are associated with increased risk of adverse health outcomes. Several randomized clinical trials have been conducted to examine the effects of B-vitamins (as the B-complex or single nutrients) on HIV-related health outcomes. The objective of this review is to examine the evidence that links B-vitamins and HIV/AIDS, with an emphasis on randomized trials. We examine the efficacy and safety of B-vitamin supplementation (i.e., B-complex or single vitamin) on health outcomes in HIV-infected individuals, including mortality, HIV disease progression, anemia and B-vitamin status, adverse pregnancy outcomes, and child growth, morbidity, and development. We then discuss research gaps and implications of findings for clinical care and public health practice, with an emphasis on resource-limited settings.

METHODS: SEARCH STRATEGY AND SELECTION PROCESS

A structured literature search was conducted using MEDLINE® electronic databases. Relevant Medical Subject Heading (MeSH®) terms were used to identify published studies through February 14, 2015. The MeSH terms used are included in Figure 2.1, in which the search strategy is summarized. Initial inclusion criteria for this review were the availability of an abstract and inclusion of data on B-vitamin intake, status, or supplementation and HIV/AIDS. The following B-vitamins were included in this review: vitamin B_1 (thiamin), vitamin B_2 (riboflavin), vitamin B_3 (niacin), vitamin B_5 (pantothenic acid), vitamin B_6 (pyridoxine), vitamin B_7 (biotin), vitamin B_9 (folate), and vitamin B_{12} (cobalamin).

B-Vitamin Biomarkers

Biomarkers for the following B-vitamins were included in this review:

- Vitamin B_1—Whole blood thiamin and thiamin pyrophosphate
- Vitamin B_2—Erythrocyte, plasma, and whole blood riboflavin
- Vitamin B_3—Whole blood, serum, and plasma niacin and niacinamide
- Vitamin B_5—Whole blood, serum, and plasma pantothenic acid and pantothenate
- Vitamin B_6—Whole blood, serum, and plasma pyridoxine 5′-phosphate (PNP), pyridoxine, pyridoxal 5′-phosphate (PLP), pyridoxal, pyridoxamine 5′-phosphate (PMP), and pyridoxamine

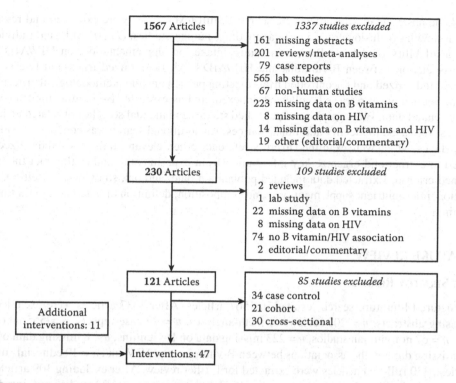

FIGURE 2.1 Diagrammatic representation of the search strategy used to identify and select studies for inclusion in the review.

- Vitamin B$_7$—Whole blood, serum, and plasma biotin
- Vitamin B$_9$ (folate)—Serum, plasma, and erythrocyte folate
- Vitamin B$_{12}$—Serum and plasma total vitamin B$_{12}$, methylmalonic acid (MMA), total homocysteine (tHcy), and holotranscobalamin (holoTC).

HIV-Related Outcomes

HIV-related outcomes included all-cause and AIDS-related mortality, World Health Organization (WHO) HIV stage disease progression, opportunistic infections, CD4 and CD8 T-cell counts, HIV RNA viral load, and HIV viral shedding. Perinatal outcomes evaluated included the following:

- *Maternal outcomes*—Weight gain during pregnancy, anemia and B-vitamin status, preeclampsia, and depression during pregnancy
- *Pregnancy outcomes*—Miscarriage (<28 weeks gestation), stillbirth (≥28 weeks gestation), fetal loss (miscarriage or stillbirth), gestational age at delivery, preterm birth (<37 weeks gestation), birthweight, low birthweight (<2500 g), small-for-gestational age (SGA; birthweight < 10th percentile for gestational age), mother-to-child transmission of HIV, breast milk micronutrient composition, and mastitis
- *Infant outcomes*—HIV infection; co-infections and clinical symptoms (i.e., measles, respiratory infections, diarrhea, malaria); anthropometry and growth (i.e., weight, length, head circumference, and mid-upper arm circumference), including weight for age (WAZ), weight for length (WLZ), and length for age (LAZ) WHO z-scores (underweight, WAZ < –2; wasting, WLZ < –2; stunting, LAZ < –2); cognitive and psychomotor development; and anemia and B-vitamin status.

Available abstracts of all studies were searched, full-text articles were extracted and reviewed, and the following inclusion criteria were applied: (1) human studies; (2) HIV-infected individuals; and (3) availability of data on B-vitamin status, intake, or supplementation, on HIV/AIDS, and on the association between B-vitamins and HIV/AIDS. All randomized trials and interventions and quasi-randomized and uncontrolled trials meeting participant and methodological criteria were included. Sources were retrieved, collected, indexed, and assessed for B-vitamin supplementation and HIV-related data. Bibliographies of published studies and manual searches of related articles in references were used to identify additional sources. An additional search was conducted to identify review articles, which were examined to cross-reference other relevant studies. A standardized table was used to extract and organize key information from experimental studies that met the above-mentioned criteria. Extracted data included publication date, authors, study design, setting, target population, micronutrient supplement type and composition, definition of outcomes, main findings, and limitations.

LITERATURE REVIEW

SEARCH STRATEGY RESULTS

The structured literature search resulted in 1567 articles. After 1337 articles were excluded ($n = 161$ missing abstracts, $n = 201$ reviews or meta-analyses, $n = 79$ case-reports, $n = 565$ laboratory studies, $n = 67$ non-human studies, $n = 223$ missing data on B-vitamins, $n = 8$ missing data on HIV, $n = 14$ missing data on the associations between B-vitamins and HIV, and $n = 19$ editorials or commentaries), 230 full-text articles were extracted for further review. After excluding 109 articles that did not meet inclusion criteria ($n = 2$ review, $n = 1$ laboratory study, $n = 22$ studies missing data on B-vitamins, $n = 8$ missing data on HIV, $n = 74$ missing data on the associations between B-vitamins and HIV, $n = 2$ editorial or commentary, and $n = 5$ full-text not available) and an additional 85 observational studies ($n = 30$ cross-sectional, $n = 34$ case-control, and $n = 21$ cohort studies), a total of 36 randomized trials or other types of intervention studies were included in this review. An additional 11 research articles were identified from references of included studies, for a total of 47 articles. The structured literature search was summarized in Figure 2.1, and micronutrient supplementation trial study design (Table 2.1) and findings are summarized in detail in Tables 2.2 and 2.3.

RANDOMIZED TRIALS OF MULTIPLE MICRONUTRIENT SUPPLEMENTATION

A total of 38 articles reported the effects of multiple-micronutrient supplementation (including B-vitamins) on health outcomes in HIV-infected individuals. Twenty of these articles came from the same study, the Trial of Vitamins (TOV) (Principal Investigator: Fawzi). The micronutrient interventions evaluated in these randomized trials were daily oral supplements containing B-vitamins (i.e., thiamin, riboflavin, niacin, vitamin B_6, folic acid, and vitamin B_{12}) in combination with other vitamins and minerals. The dose of specific micronutrients varied by trial. HIV-related outcomes included mortality, HIV disease progression, anemia and B-vitamin status, and co-morbidities; pregnancy outcomes; and pediatric micronutrient status, morbidity, growth, and development. Findings from these micronutrient supplementation trials are summarized in detail in Table 2.2.

HIV-RELATED OUTCOMES

Micronutrient supplementation with B-vitamins in combination with other vitamins and minerals has been associated with improved HIV-related outcomes in several randomized trials. B-vitamin supplementation decreased the risks of HIV disease progression and AIDS-related death (Jiamton et al., 2003; Fawzi et al., 2004b) and increased CD4 T-cell counts (Fawzi et al., 1998; Baum et al.,

2013) in randomized trials in both pregnant and non-pregnant HIV-infected women. Daily supplementation with B-vitamins also reduced the risk of HIV-related opportunistic infections, weight loss, and anemia in trials in HIV-infected pregnant women (Villamor et al., 2005b; Fawzi et al., 2007; Villamor et al., 2008; Olofin et al., 2014).

HIV Disease Progression and AIDS-Related Mortality

Several randomized trials have been conducted to examine the effects of micronutrient supplementation on HIV disease progression using the WHO HIV disease stage classifications (1 to 4) and AIDS-related mortality. The Trial of Vitamins (TOV), a randomized trial among HIV-infected, ART-naïve pregnant women (12 to 27 weeks gestation) in Tanzania, was conducted to determine the effects of maternal multivitamin supplementation on HIV disease progression, mother-to-child transmission (MTCT) of HIV, and adverse pregnancy outcomes among HIV-infected pregnant women and their children. In this randomized, double-blind, placebo-controlled trial, 1078 HIV-infected pregnant women were enrolled at 12 to 27 weeks gestation and randomized to receive one of four regimens daily: (1) vitamin A alone, (2) multivitamins (B-complex, C, and E) alone, (3) vitamin A and multivitamins, (4) or placebo, using a 2×2 factorial design. The multivitamin supplement included B-complex, C, and E vitamins in doses 6 to 10 times the RDA levels (multivitamins: 20 mg vitamin B_1, 20 mg vitamin B_2, 100 mg niacin, 25 mg vitamin B_6, 0.8 mg folic acid, 50 µg vitamin B_{12}, 500 mg vitamin C, and 30 mg vitamin E). The vitamin A intervention consisted of 5000 IU of vitamin A and 30 mg of β-carotene daily, with an additional 200,000 IU of vitamin A administered to women at delivery. Micronutrient supplementation with B-complex, C, and E vitamins did not significantly reduce the risk of HIV disease progression to AIDS or AIDS-related death (WHO stage 4; RR, 0.80; 95% CI, 0.64–1.01; $p = 0.06$) compared to receiving no multivitamins (Fawzi et al., 2004b). In the same trial, multivitamin supplementation reduced the risk of AIDS-related conditions, including oral ulcers ($p < 0.001$), angular cheilitis ($p < 0.001$), difficult or painful swallowing ($p < 0.001$), dysentery ($p = 0.03$), and fatigue ($p = 0.007$) during follow-up (median = 60 months) compared to no supplementation (Fawzi et al., 2004b).

Another randomized trial, Trial of Vitamins and HAART in HIV Disease Progression (TOV3) (Principal Investigator: Fawzi), was conducted to examine the effects of daily multivitamins at 6 to 10 times the RDA level (using the same B-complex, C, and E vitamin doses as TOV) compared to the single RDA level (i.e., 1.2 mg vitamin B_1, 1.2 mg vitamin B_2, 15 mg niacin, 1.3 mg vitamin B_6, 2.4 µg vitamin B_{12}, 0.4 mg folic acid, 80 mg vitamin C, and 15 mg vitamin E) on HIV progression and immune reconstitution among HIV-infected adult men and women initiating HAART in Tanzania (Isanaka et al., 2012). In contrast to the aforementioned TOV, multivitamin supplementation with B-complex, C, and E vitamins at multiple RDA levels did not significantly reduce the risk of HIV disease progression or AIDS-associated mortality, compared to multivitamins provided at the single RDA level ($p > 0.10$) (Isanaka et al., 2012).

Similarly, a randomized trial in Thailand (Principal Investigator: Jaffar) was conducted to assess the effects of daily micronutrient supplementation on the risks of hospital admission and mortality among HIV-infected adult men and women (Jiamton et al., 2003). HIV-infected adults were randomized to a daily multivitamin supplement (multivitamin: 24 mg vitamin B_1, 15 mg vitamin B_2, 40 mg pantothenic acid, 40 mg vitamin B_6, 30 µg vitamin B_{12}, 100 µg folacin, 3000 µg vitamin A, 6 mg β-carotene, 20 µg vitamin D_3, 80 mg vitamin E, 180 µg vitamin K, 400 mg vitamin C, 10 mg iron, 200 mg magnesium, 8 mg manganese, 30 mg zinc, 300 µg iodine, 3 mg copper, 400 µg selenium, 150 µg chromium, and 66 mg cysteine) or a placebo for 100 days. Multivitamin supplementation did not significantly reduce the risk of all-cause mortality ($p = 0.10$) compared to placebo (Jiamton et al., 2003). When participants were stratified by baseline CD4 T-cell counts ($<200 \times 10^6$ cells/L), multivitamin supplementation significantly reduced the risk of death (hazard ratio [HR], 0.37; 95% CI, 0.13–1.06; $p = 0.0052$) among individuals with lower CD4 T-cell counts compared to placebo (Jiamton et al., 2003).

TABLE 2.1
Summary of Multivitamin Trials

Principal Investigator	References	Trial Start	Treatment Comparisons
Falguera	Falguera et al. (1995)	September 1991	(ZDV+ folic acid + vitamin B_{12}) vs. ZDV alone Group 1: 250 mg ZDV 2× daily, 1000 µg of intramuscular vitamin B_{12}/month, and 15 mg of folic acid daily Group 2: 250 mg of ZVD 2× daily
Fawzi	Fawzi et al. (1998, 2000, 2002, 2003, 2004a,b, 2007), Villamor et al. (2002, 2005a,b, 2007, 2010), Baylin et al. (2005), Merchant et al. (2005), McGrath et al. (2006), Smith Fawzi et al. (2007), Webb et al. (2009), Arsenault et al. (2010), Kawai et al. (2010a), Olofin et al. (2014)	April 1995	2 × 2 factorial design Group 1: Vitamin A (30 mg β-carotene and 5000 IU preformed vitamin A) Group 2: Multivitamin (20 mg of vitamin B_1, 20 mg vitamin B_2, 25 mg vitamin B_6, 100 mg niacin, 50 µg vitamin B_{12}, 500 mg vitamin C, 30 mg vitamin E, 0.8 mg folic acid) Group 3: Vitamin A and multivitamin Group 4: Placebo
Friis	Friis et al. (2004)	1996	Multivitamin vs. placebo Multivitamin: 3000 µg RE vitamin A, 3.5 mg β-carotene, 1.5 mg thiamine, 1.6 mg riboflavin, 2.2 mg vitamin B_6, 4.0 µg vitamin B_{12}, 17 mg niacin, 80 mg vitamin C, 10 µg vitamin D, 10 µg vitamin E, 15 mg zinc, 1.2 µg copper, 65 µg selenium
McClelland	McClelland et al. (2004)	September 1998	Multivitamin vs. placebo Multivitamin: 20 mg vitamin B_1, 20 mg vitamin B_2, 25 mg vitamin B_6, 100 mg niacin, 50 µg vitamin B_{12}, 500 mg vitamin C, 30 mg vitamin E, 0.8 mg folic acid, 200 µg selenium
Jaffar	Jiamton et al. (2003)	March 2000	Multivitamin vs. placebo Multivitamin: 3000 µg vitamin A, 6 mg β-carotene, 20 µg vitamin D_3, 80 mg vitamin E, 180 µg vitamin K, 400 mg vitamin C, 24 mg vitamin B_1, 15 mg vitamin B_2, 40 mg vitamin B_6, 30 µg vitamin B_{12}, 100 µg folacin, 40 mg pantothenic acid, 10 mg iron, 200 mg magnesium, 8 mg manganese, 30 mg zinc, 300 µg iodine, 3 mg copper, 400 µg selenium, 150 µg chromium, 66 mg cysteine
Fawzi	Kawai et al. (2010b)	November 2002	Single-RDA multivitamin vs. multiple-RDA multivitamin Single-RDA: 1.4 mg thiamin, 1.4 mg riboflavin, 18 mg niacin, 1.9 mg of B_6, 2.6 µg B_{12}, 70 mg vitamin C, 10 mg vitamin E, 0.4 g of folic acid Multiple-RDA: 20 mg thiamin, 20 mg riboflavin, 100 mg niacin, 25 mg vitamin B_6, 50 µg vitamin B_{12}, 500 mg vitamin C, 30 mg vitamin E, 0.8 g folic acid

Fawzi	Villamor et al. (2008), Kawai et al. (2014)	March 2000	Multivitamin vs. placebo Multivitamin: 5000 IU retinol, 20 mg vitamin B_1, 20 mg vitamin B_2, 100 mg niacin, 25 mg vitamin B_6, 50 µg vitamin B_{12}, 500 mg vitamin C, 200 mg vitamin E, 0.8 mg folic acid, 100 µg selenium
Bennish	Luabeya et al. (2007)	August 2005	Group 1: 1250 IU vitamin A Group 2: 1250 IU vitamin A and 10 mg Zn Group 3: 1250 IU vitamin A, 10 mg Zn, and a multivitamin (0.5 mg vitamin B_1, 0.5 mg vitamin B_2, 0.5 mg vitamin B_6, 0.9 µg vitamin B_{12}, 35 mg vitamin C, 5 µg vitamin D, 6 mg vitamin E, 10 µg vitamin K, 0.6 mg copper, 150 µg folate, 50 µg iodine, 10 mg iron, 6 mg niacin)
Fawzi	Duggan et al. (2012), Kupka et al. (2013), Liu et al. (2013), Sudfeld et al. (2013), Manji et al. (2014)	June 2004	Multivitamin vs. placebo Multivitamin: 60 mg vitamin C, 8 mg vitamin E, 0.5 mg thiamine, 0.6 mg riboflavin, 4 mg niacin, 0.6 mg vitamin B_6, 130 µg folic acid, 1 mg vitamin B_{12} (children received double the treatment dosage after 6 months of age)
Baum	Baum et al. (2013)	December 2004	2 × 2 factorial design Group 1: Multivitamin (20 mg thiamin, 20 mg, riboflavin, 100 mg niacin, 25 mg vitamin B_6, 50 µg vitamin B_{12}, 800 µg folic acid, 500 mg vitamin C, 30 mg vitamin E) Group 2: 200 µg selenium Group 3: Multivitamin + selenium Group 4: Placebo
Mda	Mda et al. (2010)	November 2005	Multi-micronutrient vs. placebo Multi-micronutrient: 300 µg retinol, 0.6 mg thiamin, 0.6 mg riboflavin, 8 mg niacin, 0.6 mg pyridoxine, 1 µg vitamin B_{12}, 70 µg folic acid, 25 mg ascorbic acid, 5 µg vitamin D, 7 mg vitamin E, 700 µg copper, 8 mg iron, 30 µg selenium, 8 mg zinc
Ndeezi	Ndeezi et al. (2010, 2011)	June 2005	2-RDA multivitamin supplement vs. standard-of-care supplement 2-RDA multivitamin supplement: 800 µg vitamin A, 1.2 mg vitamin B_1, 1.2 mg vitamin B_2, 1.6 mg niacin, 1.2 mg vitamin B_6, 2.4 µg vitamin B_{12}, 50 mg vitamin C, 400 IU vitamin D, 14 mg vitamin E, 400 µg folate, 60 µg selenium, 10 mg zinc, 800 µg copper, 180 µg iodine Standard-of-care (1-RDA multivitamin): 400 µg vitamin A, 0.6 mg vitamin B_1, 0.6 mg vitamin B_2, 0.8 mg niacin, 25 mg vitamin C, 200 IU vitamin D
Fawzi	Isanaka et al. (2012)	November 2006	Multiple-RDA multivitamin vs. single-RDA multivitamin Multiple-RDA multivitamin: 20 mg thiamin, 20 mg riboflavin, 25 mg vitamin B_6, 100 mg niacin, 50 µg vitamin B_{12}, 0.8 mg folic acid, 500 mg vitamin C, 30 mg vitamin E Single-RDA multivitamin: 1.2 mg thiamin, 1.2 mg riboflavin, 1.3 mg vitamin B_6, 15 mg niacin, 2.4 µg vitamin B_{12}, 0.4 mg folic acid, 80 mg vitamin C, 15 mg vitamin E

TABLE 2.2

Randomized Trials of Multiple Micronutrient Interventions

Study	Sample	Enrollment	Methods	Exposure	Outcome	Main Findings
Falguera et al. (1995)	60 HIV-infected adults (CD4 < 500 cells/mm^3) initiating zidovudine (ZVD) therapy	September 1991–April 1992	Patients were randomized to one of two treatment groups for 12 months: (1) ZVD (n = 31) or (2) ZVD, folinic acid, and vitamin B_{12} (n = 29). At baseline and every 3 months follow-up, demographic and clinical data were recorded and blood was measured for CD4/CD8 counts, B_2-microglobulin, Hb, Hct, MCV, WBC, serum and RBC folate, and vitamin B_{12}	(ZVD + folinic acid + vitamin B_{12}) vs. ZVD alone. Group 1: 250 mg ZVD 2× daily, 15 mg of folinic acid daily, and 1000 μg of intramuscular vitamin B_{12}/month Group 2: 250 mg of ZVD 2× daily	Myelotoxicity : Hb < 8 g/dL or neutrophils < 1000 cells/mm^3 Vitamin B12 concentrations: low, <177 pmol/L; borderline, 177–200 pmol/L Serum folate concentrations: low, 8.2 nmol/L; borderline, 8.2–10 nmol/L RBC folate: low, <272 nmol/L; borderline, 272–300 nmol/L Differences in CD4 and CD8 counts CBC differences	Patients receiving (ZDV + folinic acid + vitamin B_{12}) compared to ZDV alone had significantly higher mean serum vitamin B_{12}, serum folate, and RBC folate concentrations at 3, 6, 9, and 12 months followup ($p < 0.05$ for all), and had no significant differences in Hb, Hct, MCV, leukocyte, or neutrophil count ($p > 0.05$). Vitamin B_{12} and folate concentrations were not associated with myelosuppression development ($p > 0.05$).
Fawzi et al. (1998)	1075 HIV-1-infected, ART-naïve pregnant women (12–27 weeks gestation)	April 1995–July 1997	Women were tested for HIV-1 serostatus and enrolled if positive. Women were randomized to 1 of 4 groups to receive a daily oral dose of: (1) vitamin A (n = 269); (2) multivitamin without vitamin A (n = 269); (3) vitamin A and multivitamin (n = 270); or (4) placebo (n = 267) from enrollment through pregnancy and lactation periods. All women received ferrous sulfate (400 μg) and folate (5 mg) daily and prophylactic chloroquine phosphate (500 mg) weekly.	2 × 2 factorial design Group 1: Vitamin A (30 mg β-carotene and 5000 IU preformed vitamin A) Group 2: Multivitamin (20 mg vitamin B_1, 20 mg vitamin B_2, 25 mg vitamin B_6, 100 mg niacin, 50 μg vitamin B_{12}, 500 mg vitamin C, 30 mg vitamin E, 0.8 mg folic acid)	*Maternal outcomes:* Mortality CD4, CD8, CD3, WBC counts, total lymphocytes, and CD4:CD8 ratio HIV-1 disease stage BMI Malaria status *Neonate outcomes:* Miscarriage < 28 weeks gestation Stillbirth ≥ 28 weeks gestation Preterm birth < 37 weeks gestation Severe preterm birth < 34 weeks gestation Low birthweight < 2500 g Very low birthweight < 2000 g	*Maternal outcomes:* Women receiving multivitamins compared to those not receiving multivitamins had • Greater increases in mean CD4 count from baseline to 6 weeks postpartum (+167 ± 210 cells vs. +112 ± 268 cells, $p < 0.001$) and 30 weeks postpartum (+99 ± 208 cells vs. +59 ± 167 cells, $p = 0.003$) • Greater increases in mean CD8 counts from baseline to 6 weeks postpartum (+385 ± 450 cells vs. +289 ± 404 cells, $p = 0.001$) but not at 30 weeks postpartum ($p = 0.06$)

At delivery, women receiving vitamin A received an additional 200,000 IU of vitamin A.

Interim medical issues were measured at baseline and monthly follow-up.

At baseline, STD status was determined and urine and stool samples were taken

Blood cell counts were measured at baseline and at 6 and 30 weeks postpartum.

At delivery, placental weight, neonate weight/length, and gestational age were recorded by a research midwife.

Group 3: Vitamin A and multivitamin

Group 4: Placebo

SGA birth weight < 10th percentile for gestational age

HIV vertical transmission (delivery or breastfeeding)

• Greater increases in mean CD3 counts from baseline to 6 weeks postpartum (+585 ± 648 cells vs. +411 ± 559 cells, $p < 0.001$) and 30 weeks postpartum (+345 ± 493 cells vs. +254 ± 475 cells, $p = 0.02$)

Birth outcomes:

Multivitamin supplementation:

• Decreased the risk of stillbirth (RR, 0.58; 95% CI, 0.33–1.02; $p = 0.05$)

• Decreased the risk of fetal death (RR, 0.61; 95% CI, 0.39–0.9; $p = 0.02$)

• Decreased the risk of LBW (RR, 0.56; 95% CI, 0.38–0.82; $p = 0.003$) and very LBW (RR, 0.42; 95% CI, 0.18–1.01; $p = 0.05$)

• Decreased the risk of severe preterm birth (RR, 0.61; 95% CI, 0.38–0.96; $p = 0.03$)

• Decreased the risk of combined LBW and preterm birth (RR, 0.55; 95% CI, 0.32–0.83; $p = 0.03$) and combined LBW and term birth (RR, 0.53; 95% CI, 0.29–0.99; $p = 0.04$)

• Decreased the risk of SGA (RR, 0.57; 95% CI, 0.29–0.82; $p = 0.002$)

• Was not associated with the risk of miscarriage ($p = 0.26$) or preterm birth ($p = 0.23$)

(continued)

TABLE 2.2 (continued)
Randomized Trials of Multiple Micronutrient Interventions

Study	Sample	Enrollment	Methods	Exposure	Outcome	Main Findings
Fawzi et al. (2000)	1074 HIV-1-infected, ART-naïve, pregnant women (12–27 weeks gestation)	April 1995–July 1997	See methods above. All infants received 100,000 IU of vitamin A at 6 months of age and 200,000 IU every 6 months after. Whole blood was collected from infants at birth, 6 weeks postpartum, and at 3-month intervals thereafter; blood was tested for HIV-1 status.	Exposure is described above.	*Infant outcomes:* Fetal loss: all miscarriages and still births HIV infection at birth and 6 weeks HIV infection at 6 weeks among infants uninfected at birth HIV infection or death before birth HIV infection or death from birth to 49 days among infants uninfected at birth	Maternal multivitamin supplementation: • Decreased the risk of fetal loss (RR, 0.59; 95% CI, 0.39–0.91; $p = 0.02$) • Was not associated with the risk of HIV infection at birth ($p = 0.08$) or at 6 weeks ($p = 0.39$) or at 6 weeks among children uninfected at birth ($p = 0.88$) • Was not associated with the risk of HIV infection or death at birth ($p = 0.89$) or HIV infection or death at 6 weeks among HIV-infected infants at birth ($p = 0.73$) LBW (<2500 g) altered the efficacy of multivitamin use on HIV infection at 6 weeks ($p = 0.02$). Among HIV-uninfected children, mothers receiving multivitamins compared to mothers not receiving multivitamins gave birth to heavier babies ($+94$ g, $p = 0.02$).
Fawzi et al. (2002)	898 HIV-1-infected, ART-naïve mothers and respective children	April 1995–July 1997	See methods above. At monthly visits postpartum, mothers were asked if child was being breastfed and, if not, when breastfeeding ended.	Exposure is described above.	*Infant outcomes:* HIV-transmission through breastfeeding; HIV infection after 6 weeks of age among children known not be HIV-infected at 6 weeks of age Child mortality by 24 months of age	Mothers receiving multivitamin supplementation compared to mothers not receiving multivitamin supplementation: • Did not have significantly lower risk of HIV-1 transmission (RR, 1.04; 95% CI, 0.82–1.32; $p = 0.72$) • Had children with a lower risk of mortality at 24 months of age (RR, 0.82; 95% CI, 0.66–1.02; $p = 0.08$)

| Villamor et al. (2002) | April 1995–July 1997 | 1069 HIV-1-infected, ART-naïve pregnant women (12–27 weeks gestation) | See methods above. Thin-smear blood films were analyzed for malaria parasites and stool samples were tested for parasitic worms in mothers. | Exposure is described above. | *Primary outcomes:* Continuous variables: overall and per-trimester weight gain; weekly rate of weight gain Categorical variables: risk of low total weight gain overall and per trimester (<25th percentile of total or specific trimester weight gain distribution); risk of low rate of weight gain (regression slope of person's weight gain per week or trimester < 25th percentile for population weight gain distribution); risk of weight loss

Secondary outcomes: Changes in mid-upper arm circumference

T-cell counts

HIV/AIDS stage (WHO definition) | • Did not have a significantly lower risk of HIV transmission through breastfeeding (RR, 0.85; 95% CI, 0.61–1.19; $p = 0.34$)
• Had a significantly lower risk of HIV transmission through breastfeeding (RR, 0.37; 95% CI, 0.16–0.85; $p = 0.02$) and child mortality at 24 months (RR, 0.30; 95% CI, 0.10–0.92; $p = 0.04$) among mothers with lymphocyte counts in the lowest quartile

Multivitamin supplementation:
• Significantly increased mean weight gain during 3rd trimester (+304 g; 95% CI, 17–590 g; $p = 0.04$) but did not affect weight gain throughout pregnancy or during 2nd trimester
• Reduced the risk of low total weight gain during 3rd trimester (RR, 0.70; 95% CI, 0.55–0.90; $p = 0.005$) but did not affect the risk throughout pregnancy or during 2nd trimester
• Reduced the risk of weight loss during 3rd trimester (RR, 0.69; 95% CI, 0.50–0.95; $p = 0.02$) but did not affect the risk throughout pregnancy or during 2nd trimester
• Reduced the risk of a low rate of weight gain (RR, 0.73; 95% CI, 0.58–0.93; $p = 0.01$) but did not affect the risk throughout pregnancy or during 2nd trimester |

(continued)

TABLE 2.2 (continued)
Randomized Trials of Multiple Micronutrient Interventions

Study	Sample	Enrollment	Methods	Exposure	Outcome	Main Findings
					Malaria, intestinal, and STD infection Hb, vitamin A, vitamin E, and selenium concentrations	The efficacy of multivitamin supplementation on weight gain was not altered by season of conception, WHO HIV stage, T-cell counts, malaria infection, or vitamin A, vitamin E, and Hb concentrations (p-interaction > 0.10).
Fawzi et al. (2003)	1075 HIV-1-infected, ART-naïve pregnant women (12–27 weeks gestation)	April 1995–July 1997	See methods above. At monthly clinic visits postpartum, mothers provided information on infant diarrheal or respiratory signs.	Exposure is described above.	*Infant outcomes:* HIV morbidity Episodes of diarrhea ≥ 3 watery stools/day Mucous/blood stool noted: acute, ≥1 days and <14 days; persistent, ≥14 days Respiratory complications: cough alone, cough and fever, cough with rapid respiratory rate, or cough and ≥1 additional symptoms (difficulty breathing, chest retractions, or refusal to eat, drink, or breastfeed) CD4 counts	Among infants, maternal multivitamin supplementation: • Decreased the risk of all-type diarrhea (RR, 0.83; 95% CI, 0.71–0.98; p = 0.03); acute diarrhea (RR, 0.83; 95% CI, 0.71–0.98; p = 0.03); and watery diarrhea with approaching significance (RR, 0.83; 95% CI, 0.68–1.02; p = 0.07) • Did not affect the risk of dysenteric diarrhea (p = 0.17) • Did not affect the risk of any respiratory complication (p > 0.20) Infant HIV status did not have an interactive effect with multivitamin supplementation for all diarrhea outcomes (p > 0.1) but did after multivitamin efficacy on the risk of cough (p = 0.054)

Study	Sample	Dates	Methods	Exposure	Outcomes	Results
Fawzi et al. (2004b)	1078 HIV-1-infected, ART-naïve pregnant women (12–27 weeks gestation)	April 1995–July 1997	See methods above. At monthly clinic visits during pregnancy and postpartum, a study nurse assessed HIV/AIDS stage, signs of diarrhea, HIV complications, and mortality; verbal autopsy was used for participants that traveled outside of study site.	Exposure is described above.	*Primary outcomes:* HIV progression I–IV (WHO guidelines) Time of progression to AIDS stage 4 and stage 3 or higher Mortality (death from AIDS related causes)	Among HIV-uninfected infants, maternal multivitamin supplementation: • Decreased risk of all-type diarrhea (RR, 0.80; 95% CI, 0.67–0.95; $p = 0.01$), acute diarrhea (RR, 0.81; 95% CI, 0.68–0.96; $p = 0.02$), and watery diarrhea (RR, 0.78; 95% CI, 0.63–0.97; $p = 0.03$) but not dysentery diarrhea ($p = 0.20$) Among children born prematurely (<37 weeks), maternal multivitamin supplementation: • Decreased risk of watery diarrhea (RR, 0.53; 95% CI, 0.33–0.84; $p = 0.007$, p-interaction $= 0.07$) Infants born to mothers taking a multivitamin compared to infants of mothers not taking a multivitamin had significantly higher mean overall CD4 counts during the first 2 years of life (+151 cells/µL; 95% CI, 64–273 cells/µL; $p = 0.0006$) and at 6 months (1711 ± 646 cells/µL vs. 1558 ± 576 cells/µL, $p = 0.0001$). Women taking only multivitamin supplement compared to placebo group: • Had decreased risk of progressing to AIDS or death by AIDS-related causes (RR, 0.71; 95% CI, 0.51–0.98; $p = 0.04$); progression to AIDS stage 4 (RR, 0.50; 95% CI, 0.58–0.90; $p = 0.003$); progression to AIDS stage 3 or higher (RR, 0.72; 95% CI, 0.58–0.90; $p = 0.003$); and all co-morbidities and clinical symptoms ($p \leq 0.02$ for all) except diarrhea ($p = 0.18$)

(continued)

TABLE 2.2 (continued)
Randomized Trials of Multiple Micronutrient Interventions

Study	Sample	Enrollment	Methods	Exposure	Outcome	Main Findings
			Blood was drawn at baseline and every 6 months follow-up and measured for CD4, CD8, and CD3 counts.		*Secondary outcomes:* CD4, CD8, and CD3 counts HIV-1 viral load Signs of disease: thrush, gingival erythema, angular cheilitis, oral ulcers, acute upper respiratory infection, mouth/throat ulcers, painful tongue/throat, diarrhea, dysentery, fatigue, and rash	• Had higher mean CD4 counts (+48 cells/mm³; 95% CI, 10–85 cells/ mm³; $p = 0.01$); higher mean CD3 counts (+88 cells/mm³; 95% CI, 14–161 cells/ mm³); and lower mean HIV-1 viral load (−0.18 log; 95% CI, −0.32 to −0.03; $p = 0.02$) for the overall study period Multivitamin supplementation (with or without vitamin A): • Significantly reduced signs of the following complications: oral ulcers (RR, 0.52; $p < 0.001$); angular cheilitis (RR, 0.44; $p < 0.001$); difficult or painful swallowing (RR, 0.47; $p < 0.001$); dysentery (RR, 0.75; $p = 0.03$); and fatigue (RR, 0.76; $p = 0.007$) • Significantly increased mean CD4 cell count (+50 cells/mm³, $p < 0.0001$) and lowered mean viral loads (−0.11 log, $p = 0.05$)
Fawzi et al. (2004a)	637 HIV-1-infected, ART-naïve pregnant women (12–27 weeks gestation)	April 1995–July 1997	See methods above. A cervicovaginal lavage (CVL) was obtained shortly before delivery (≥6 weeks after randomization) and measured for HIV-1 RNA and IL-1B levels	Exposure is described above.	Genital tract HIV shedding CVL IL-1B levels	Multivitamin supplementation: • Had no effect on HIV-1 viral shedding ($p > 0.50$) • Had no effect on mean CVL Il-1B concentrations ($p = 0.34$)

| Baylin et al. (2005) | 716 infants of HIV-1 infected, ART-naïve women | April 1995–July 1997 | See methods above. Stored blood from infants at 6 weeks and 6 months of age were analyzed for vitamin A, vitamin E, and vitamin B$_{12}$ | Exposure is described above. | *Infant outcomes:* Vitamin A status: deficiency < 0.70 and < 0.35 μmol/L Vitamin E status: deficiency < 11.6 μmol/L Vitamin B$_{12}$ status: deficiency < 150 pmol/L | Infants of mothers taking multivitamin supplements compared to infants of mothers not taking multivitamins: • At 5 weeks postpartum had lower mean vitamin A concentrations (0.45 ± 0.17 μmol/L vs. 0.50 ± 0.17, p = 0.0002), higher mean vitamin E (17.0 ± 7.7 μmol/L vs. 15.2 ± 6.5, p = 0.0008), and higher vitamin B$_{12}$ (423 ± 185 pmol/L vs. 247 ± 102 pmol/L, p < 0.0001) • At 6 months postpartum had higher vitamin E (15.7 ± 5.9 vs. 14.6 ± 6.1, p = 0.004) and higher vitamin B$_{12}$ (413 ± 165 pmol/L vs. 286 ± 138 pmol/L, p < 0.0001); vitamin A did not significantly differ (p = 0.27) • At 6 weeks postpartum had lower odds of vitamin B$_{12}$ deficiency (OR, 0.07; 95% CI, 0.02–0.22; p < 0.0001); multivitamins did not affect the odds of vitamin A deficiency or vitamin E deficiency (p ≥ 0.20) • At 6 months postpartum had greater odds of vitamin A deficiency (<0.35 μmol/L; OR, 1.44; 95% CI, 1.05–1.97; p = 0.02), lower odds of vitamin E deficiency (OR, 0.70; 95% CI, 0.50–0.97; p = 0.03), and lower odds of vitamin B$_{12}$ (OR, 0.13; 95% CI, 0.05–0.37; p < 0.0001); multivitamin supplementation did not significantly alter vitamin A, vitamin B$_{12}$, or vitamin E status from 6 weeks to 6 months postpartum |

(continued)

TABLE 2.2 (continued)
Randomized Trials of Multiple Micronutrient Interventions

Study	Sample	Enrollment	Methods	Exposure	Outcome	Main Findings
Villamor et al. (2005a)	886 infants of HIV-1-infected, ART-naïve women	April 1995–July 1997	See methods above. At monthly postnatal visits research nurses measured infant weight, length, mid-upper arm circumference (MUAC), and head circumference.	Exposure is described above. Supplementation continued to until the end of the trial (August 2003).	*Child growth from delivery to ≤24 months age:* Continuous variables: weight, length, MUAC, weight-for-age, weight-for length, length-for-age Categorical variables: wasting (<−2 z scores for weight for length), underweight (<−2 z scores weight for age), stunting (<−2 z scores length for age)	Mothers receiving multivitamins (without vitamin A) compared to the placebo group: • Had infants with significantly greater weight gain from birth to 24 months of age (+459 g; 95% CI, 35–882 g; p = 0.03), but there was no effect on length, head circumference, or MUAC • Had infants with greater weight-for-length scores (+0.38; 95% CI, 0.07–0.68; p = 0.01) and weight-for-age scores (+0.42; 95% CI, 0.07–0.77; p = 0.01), but there was no effect on length-for-age There was no effect on the risk of wasting, stunting, or an underweight infant at 24 months of age. Maternal vitamin A supplementation weakened the effect of multivitamins on infant weight gain (p-interaction = 0.0004), weight for age (p = 0.03), and weight for length (p = 0.02). Infant HIV infection increased the efficacy of maternal multivitamin status on infant weight gain (p-interaction < 0.001).

Study	Dates	Methods	Exposure/Outcomes	Results
				The combined multivitamin and vitamin A group compared to the placebo group had a significantly decreased risk of infant wasting from birth to 24 months of age (HR, 0.53; 95% CI, 0.32–0.88; $p = 0.01$) and risk of underweight infants at 24 months age (HR, 0.67; 95% CI, 0.46–0.97; $p = 0.03$), but there was no effect on stunting.
Villamor et al. (2005b)	April 1995–July 1997	See methods above. At monthly follow-up visits during pregnancy and postpartum (median follow-up: 68 months), nurses measured weight, MUAC, signs and symptoms of disease, and diarrhea status (≥3 watery stools/day).	Exposure is described above. *Primary outcomes:* MUAC, BMI. Wasting (BMI < 18 and MUAC < 22 cm). *Secondary outcomes:* Weight loss > 10% of weight at baseline. Weight loss periods (consecutive follow-up visits where weight was lost): long periods (> 4 months), short periods (≤ 4 months), severe periods (weight loss > 1 kg/month), moderate periods (weight loss ≤ 1 kg/month)	Multivitamin supplementation: • Decreased the risk of MUAC < 22 cm at first 2-year follow-up (HR, 0.71; 95% CI, 0.52–0.93; $p = 0.01$) and at first 4-year follow-up (HR, 0.79; 95% CI, 0.62–1.00; $p = 0.05$) but had no effect for the overall study period ($p = 0.10$) • Had no effect on the risk of BMI < 18 or weight loss > 10% at any time period • Reduced the risk of the first episode of MUAC < 22 cm by 41% at the first 2-year follow-up (95% CI, 13%–60%; $p = 0.008$), by 39% during the first 4-year follow-up (95% CI, 12%–57%; $p = 0.008$), and by 34% for the entire study period (95% CI, 6%–53%; $p = 0.02$)
Merchant et al. (2005)	955 HIV-1-infected, ART-naïve women / April 1995–July 1997	See methods above. Blood pressure was measured by a nurse at baseline and during monthly visits throughout the study.	Exposure is described above. Hypertension (systolic pressure ≥ 140 mmHg or diastolic pressure ≥ 90 mmHg)	Multivitamin supplementation decreased the risk of developing hypertension during pregnancy (RR, 0.62; 95% CI, 0.40–0.94, $p = 0.03$).

Villamor et al. (2005b): 1051 HIV-1-infected, ART-naïve women

(continued)

TABLE 2.2 (continued)
Randomized Trials of Multiple Micronutrient Interventions

Study	Sample	Enrollment	Methods	Exposure	Outcome	Main Findings
McGrath et al. (2006)	327 infants of HIV-1-infected, ART naïve mothers	April 1995–July 1997	See methods above. Infant mental and psychomotor development was assessed at 6, 12, and 18 months of age by the Bayley Scales of Infant and Toddler Development-II (BSID-II)	Exposure is described above.	*Infant outcomes:* Mental development and psychomotor development, both determined by index score on BSID-II	Infants of mothers taking multivitamins compared to infants of mothers not receiving multivitamins: • Did not significantly differ in mental development at 6 and 12 months of age • Had lower mean mental development indices at 18 months of age with approaching significance (78.4 vs. 82.0, $p = 0.09$) • Had higher mean psychomotor development indices at 6 months (95.9 vs. 92.8, $p = 0.03$) and at 12 months with approaching significance (95.4 vs. 90.6, $p = 0.07$); there was no difference at 18 months • Had overall higher psychomotor indices (+2.6; 95% CI, 0.1–5.1; $p = 0.04$) and raw motor scores (+0.8; 95% CI, 0.002–1.6; $p = 0.04$) • Had decreased risk of a psychomotor index < 70 (HR, 0.4; 95% CI, 0.2–0.7; $p = 0.004$), but there was no effect on mental indices

| Smith Fawzi et al. (2007) | 1013 HIV-1-infected, ART-naïve pregnant women | April 1995–July 1997 | See methods above. Depressive symptoms were measured by the Hopkins Symptoms Checklist 25, mental disorders were measured by DSM-IV criteria, and a Medical Outcomes Study Short Form-36 was used to assess health-related quality of life were measured 2 months after enrollment, 2 months postpartum, every 6 months until 2001, and every 12 months after 2001 | Exposure is described above. | *Maternal outcomes:* Depressive symptoms: feeling sad, feeling trapped, difficulty falling asleep, difficulty staying asleep, excessive worrying, heart racing, feelings of hopelessness, dizziness, weakness, or excessive crying; each symptom was scored 1 to 4, with 4 being the worst Quality of life: physical, role-physical, bodily pain, general health, vitality, social functioning, role-emotional, and mental health | Women receiving multivitamins compared to women who did not receive multivitamins:
• Had significantly higher indicators of quality of life at 2 months after enrollment ($p < 0.05$)
• Were not significantly different in prevalence of major depressive symptoms at 2 months post-enrollment (40% vs. 44.8%, $p = 0.14$)
• Had decreased risk of elevated level of depressive symptoms (Hopkins Symptoms score > 1.06; RR, 0.78; 95% CI, 0.66–0.92; $p = 0.005$)
• Had decreased risk of low quality-of-life dimension scores (< 25th percentile): physical functioning (RR, 0.76; 95% CI, 0.63–0.90; $p = 0.002$), role-physical (RR, 0.70; 95% CI, 0.57–0.88; $p = 0.002$), bodily pain (RR, 0.81; 95% CI, 0.69–0.95; $p = 0.008$), general health (RR, 0.77; 95% CI, 0.66–0.90; $p = 0.0007$), vitality (RR, 0.72; 95% CI, 0.61–0.84; $p = 0.0001$), social functioning (RR, 0.72; 95% CI, 0.59–0.88; $p = 0.001$), and mental health (RR, 0.82; 95% CI, 0.70–0.96; $p = 0.01$) |

(continued)

TABLE 2.2 (continued)
Randomized Trials of Multiple Micronutrient Interventions

Study	Sample	Enrollment	Methods	Exposure	Outcome	Main Findings
Fawzi et al. (2007)	906 HIV-1-infected, ART-naïve mothers and respective infants (*n* = 836)	April 1995–July 1997	See methods above.	Exposure is described above.	*Infant and maternal outcomes:* Hb concentrations: anemia (Hb < 11.0 g/dL), severe anemia (Hb < 8.5 g/dL) Presence of hypochromatic microcytic cells: severe anemia (hypochromasia ≥ 2+ and microcytic cells), moderate anemia (hypochromasia ≥ 1+ and microcytic cells), mild anemia (hypochromasia ≥ 1) Macrocytosis (presence of macrocytic cells)	Women receiving multivitamins compared to women who did not receive multivitamins: • Had significantly higher mean Hb concentrations at ≤70 days postpartum (*p* = 0.0002), at the first 2-years follow-up (*p* = 0.001), at the first 4-years follow-up (*p* = 0.01), and for the entire period with approaching significance (*p* = 0.07) • Had a lower risk of moderate hypochromic microcytosis with approaching significance (RR, 0.75; 95% CI, 0.60–1.16; *p* = 0.08); multivitamins did not affect the risk of anemia, severe anemia, mild and severe hypochromic microcytosis, or macrocytosis (*p* > 0.10) Infants of mothers receiving multivitamins compared to infants of mothers not receiving multivitamins: • Had significantly higher mean Hb concentrations at the first 2-years follow-up (*p* = 0.0009), at the first 4-years follow-up (*p* = 0.0001), and for the entire trial period (*p* = 0.0002); there were no significant differences at birth or 6 months postpartum (p > 0.10)

Study	Sample	Dates	Methods	Exposure/Outcomes	Results
Villamor et al. (2007)	829 children of HIV-1-infected, ART-naïve mothers	April 1995–July 1997	See methods above. Blood films were collected from children every 3 months or at interim clinic visits and tested for presence of malaria parasites.	*Infant outcomes:* Malaria infection (parasite density/ 200 leukocytes and 800 leukocytes) High parasitemia(≥5000/μL)	• Had a lower risk of severe hypochromic microcytosis (RR, 0.51; 95% CI, 0.31–0.84; $p = 0.004$); multivitamins did not affect the risk of infant anemia, severe anemia, mild and moderate hypochromic microcytosis, or macrocytosis Mothers taking multivitamin supplementation compared to mothers not taking multivitamin supplementation: • Did not significantly decrease risk of malaria parasitemia (RR, 0.95; 95% CI, 0.78–1.16; $p = 0.06$), high parasitemia (RR, 0.70; 95% CI, 0.48–1.02), or death from malaria (RR, 0.73; 95% CI, 0.33–1.60) at 2 years of age Mothers taking a multivitamin supplement compared to mothers taking a placebo: • Had a lower risk of children with clinical malaria by 2 years of age (RR, 0.29; 95% CI, 0.09–0.89; $p = 0.02$)
Webb et al. (2009)	626 HIV-1-infected, ART-naïve lactating mothers	April 1995–July 1997	See methods above. At delivery and every 3 months follow-up, breast milk was collected and measured for micronutrients.	Exposure is described above. Breast milk concentrations of retinol, carotenoids, tocopherols	Multivitamin supplementation: • Was not associated with changes in carotenoids or delta-tocopherol at any time point • Was not associated with changes in retinol at 3, 6, or 12 months postpartum Women taken multivitamins compared to women not taking multivitamins: • Had greater mean α-tocopherol at 3 months postpartum ($p < 0.05$)

(continued)

TABLE 2.2 (continued)
Randomized Trials of Multiple Micronutrient Interventions

Study	Sample	Enrollment	Methods	Exposure	Outcome	Main Findings
						• Had lower mean γ-tocopherol at delivery, 3 months, 6 months, and 12 months postpartum ($p < 0.05$) • Had lower mean retinol at delivery ($p < 0.05$)
Kawai et al. (2010b)	959 HIV-1-infected, ART-naive mothers and respective children	April 1995–July 1997	See methods above. Mortality and morbidity of children were assessed at monthly visits.	Exposure is described above.	*Primary outcomes:* All-cause child mortality HIV infection *Secondary outcomes:* Child morbidity (diarrhea or respiratory infection, as previously described) *Birth outcomes:* Stillbirth (death ≥ 28 weeks gestation) Birthweight LBW (< 2500 g) Preterm birth (< 37 weeks gestation) SGA (birthweight < 10th percentile for age) Infant vitamin B_{12} status	Infant sex did not significantly interact with the effect of maternal multivitamin supplementation on stillbirth, preterm birth, or small-for-gestational age ($p > 0.50$). Maternal multivitamin supplementation increased infant female birthweight more than for male infants with approaching significance (p-interaction = 0.10); multivitamins decreased the risk of LBW more so in females than males (p-interaction = 0.08). At 2 years of age among live-birth girls, childhood mortality was significantly reduced by maternal multivitamin use (RR, 0.68; 95% CI, 0.47–0.97; $p = 0.03$); no significant effect was found in male children ($p = 0.38$; p-interaction = 0.04).

| Arsenault et al. (2010) | 674 HIV-1-infected, ART-naive women | April 1995–July 1997 | See methods above. | Subclinical mastitis determined by ratio of breast milk sodium to potassium (Na:K): any form (Na:K > 0.6), moderate (Na:K > 0.6 and ≤ 1), severe (Na:K > 1.0) | Exposure is described above. | Infant sex did not significantly interact with maternal multivitamin supplementation for:
• Risk of HIV-transmission (p-interaction = 0.73) and HIV-free survival (p-interaction = 0.68)
• Diarrhea morbidity (p-interaction = 0.37)
• Respiratory infection (p-interaction ≥ 0.15 for all types of respiratory infections)
• Infant vitamin B_{12} concentrations at 6 weeks or 6 months ($p > 0.1$)
Women receiving multivitamins only compared to the placebo group had:
• A greater risk of any subclinical mastitis (RR, 1.33; 95% CI, 1.09–1.61; $p = 0.005$)
• A greater risk of severe subclinical mastitis (RR, 1.75; 95% CI, 1.27–2.41; $p = 0.0006$)
The risk of moderate and severe subclinical mastitis did not change from delivery to 2 years postpartum (p-interaction = 0.90 and 0.53, respectively).
Among women with ≥350 CD4 cells/μL, the multivitamin-only group compared to the placebo group had an increased risk of any subclinical mastitis (RR, 1.49; 95% CI, 1.12–1.98; $p = 0.006$). |

(continued)

TABLE 2.2 (continued)
Randomized Trials of Multiple Micronutrient Interventions

Study	Sample	Enrollment	Methods	Exposure	Outcome	Main Findings
Villamor et al. (2010)	594- HIV-1-infected, ART-naïve mothers and respective infants	April 1995–July 1997	See methods above. HIV-1 viral RNA was extracted from cell-free aqueous milk.	Exposure is described above.	Breast milk HIV-1 shedding: cell free HIV-1 RNA viral load and HIV-1 RNA proviral load	Maternal multivitamin supplementation: • Was not associated with the risk of cell-free HIV-1 RNA viral shedding at <6 months postpartum ($p = 0.61$) or ≥6 months postpartum ($p = 0.41$) • Had no effect on the risk of proviral HIV-1 RNA load in breast milk throughout 2-years postpartum ($p = 0.86$)
Olofin et al. (2014)	1050 HIV-infected, ART-naïve pregnant women	April 1995–July 1997	See methods above. At baseline and every 12 months follow-up, blood films of women were tested for malaria.	Exposure is described above.	*Primary outcomes:* First new episode of malaria parasitemia as determined by blood films screened for *P. falciparum, P. malariae, P. vivax,* and *P. ovale* eggs. First presumptive diagnosis of clinical malaria by doctor or nurse, with symptoms of high-grade fevers associated with chills, rigors, and sweating and axillary temperatures ≥ 37.5°C	Micronutrient supplementation: • Decreased the risk of presumptive malaria (RR, 0.78; 95% CI, 0.67–0.92; $p = 0.003$) • Increased the risk of malaria parasitemia (RR, 1.24; 95% CI, 1.02–1.50; $p = 0.03$) • Had no effect on the risk of severe parasitemia (≥10,000 parasites; RR, 1.23; 95% CI, 0.66–2.29)
Friis et al. (2004)	1106 pregnant women (22–36 gestational weeks) and respective infants	1996–1997	Women were tested for HIV-1/2, and obstetric, medical, and demographic data were recorded at baseline. Women were randomized to receive a daily micronutrient ($n = 564$) or placebo ($n = 542$) from enrollment to delivery	Multivitamin (single RDA) vs. placebo	*Gestational age:* Preterm birth (<37 gestational weeks) *Birth size (weight, length, head circumference):* Low birthweight (<2500 g)	There were no significant differences for gestational length, birthweight, birth length, ponderal index, head circumference, preterm delivery, birth weight, or IUGR–LBW ($p > 0.05$). There were no significant interactions between multivitamin supplementation and HIV infection for any outcome ($p > 0.10$).

Reference	Dates	Population	Methods	Intervention	Outcomes	Results
			All women received iron and folic acid supplementation as part of standard care. At delivery, infants were weighed and their length and head circumference were measured by a research nurse; antenatal and birth records were used for deliveries not seen by research nurse.	Multivitamin: 3000 µg RE vitamin A, 3.5 mg β-carotene, 1.5 mg thiamine, 1.6 mg riboflavin, 2.2 mg vitamin B_6, 4.0 µg vitamin B_{12}, 17 mg niacin, 80 mg vitamin C, 10 µg vitamin D, 10 µg vitamin E, 15 mg zinc, 1.2 µg copper, 65 µg selenium	Intrauterine growth restriction (IUGR)–LBW (gestational age < 37 weeks and birthweight < 2500 g) Infant ponderal index	Among HIV-infected mothers, the intervention arm mothers gave birth to infants of mean greater birthweight than the placebo group infants with approaching significance (3017 g vs. 2916 g; $p = 0.056$).
McClelland et al. (2004)	September 1998–June 2000	400 HIV-1-infected, ART naïve women (18–45 yr)	Women were interviewed for demographic, sexual, obstetric, and medical history; blood was drawn for HIV-1 RNA concentrations, lymphocyte subsets, and micronutrient analysis; and vaginal/cervical specimens were collected. Women were randomly assigned to receive a daily micronutrient or placebo for 6 weeks At 6 weeks follow-up, a clinical history was taken, a physical examination was performed, and blood and genital tract specimens were acquired.	Multivitamin vs. placebo Multivitamin: 20 mg vitamin B_1, 20 mg vitamin B_2, 25 mg vitamin B_6, 100 mg niacin, 50 µg vitamin B_{12}, 500 mg vitamin C, 30 mg vitamin E, 0.8 mg folic acid, 200 µg selenium	*Primary outcome*: Cervical/vaginal viral shedding (presence of HIV-infected cells and HIV-1 RNA loads) *Secondary outcomes*: Plasma HIV-1 viral load CD4 count (low count < 200 cells/µL)	Vaginal shedding: Micronutrient supplementation increased the odds of the presence of HIV-1-infected cells (AOR, 2.5; 95% CI, 1.4–4.4; $p = 0.001$) and a 0.37-$\log_{10}$ copies/swab higher amount of HIV-1 RNA ($B = 0.37$; 95% CI, 0.11–0.62; $p = 0.004$). Cervical shedding: Micronutrient supplementation had no significant effects on percent of HIV-1-infected cells ($p = 0.20$) or HIV-1 RNA viral loads ($p = 0.20$). At 6 weeks follow-up, the micronutrient arm compared to the placebo arm had significantly higher CD4 counts (+23 cells/µL; 95% CI, 3–43 cells/µL; $p = 0.03$) and higher CD8 counts (+74 cells/µL; 95% CI, 23–126 cells/µL; $p = 0.005$); there were no significant differences in viral load ($p = 0.8$).

(continued)

TABLE 2.2 (continued)
Randomized Trials of Multiple Micronutrient Interventions

Study	Sample	Enrollment	Methods	Exposure	Outcome	Main Findings
Jiamton et al. (2003)	481 HIV-1-infected, ART-naïve adults (≥18 years) with CD4 counts of 50E6–550E6 cells/L	March 2000–January 2001	HIV status was confirmed and participants were randomly assigned to a daily micronutrient ($n = 242$) or placebo ($n = 239$) for 100 days. At baseline, a physical exam was administered by a physician; blood was drawn and plasma was assessed for vitamin E and selenium. Every 4 weeks follow-up, a nurse collected general health status data from participants by phone. Every 12 weeks follow-up, a physical exam was given; data on ART and prophylaxis medication usage and treatment compliance were recorded. CD4 count was tested at 24 and 48 weeks postpartum; HIV-1 viral load was tested at 48 weeks postpartum. General health status was recorded every 4 weeks; AIDS-defining illnesses were confirmed by the hospital and deaths were reported by next of kin.	Multivitamin vs. placebo Multivitamin: 3000 µg vitamin A, 6 mg β-carotene, 20 µg vitamin D_3, 80 mg vitamin E, 180 µg vitamin K, 400 mg vitamin C, 24 mg vitamin B_1, 15 mg vitamin B_2, 40 mg vitamin B_6, 30 µg vitamin B_{12}, 100 µg folacin, 40 mg pantothenic acid, 10 mg iron, 200 mg magnesium, 8 mg manganese, 30 mg zinc, 300 µg iodine, 3 mg copper, 400 µg selenium, 150 µg chromium, 66 mg cysteine	Mortality HIV plasma viral load AIDS progression CD4 count	Micronutrient supplementation: • Decreased the risk of mortality (HR, 0.53; 95% CI, 0.22–1.23; $p = 0.1$) • Decreased the risk of mortality among adults with a CD4 count < 200 E6 cells/L (HR, 0.37; 95% CI, 0.13–1.06; $p = 0.0052$) and among adults with a CD4 count < 100 E6 cells/L (HR, 0.26; 95% CI, 0.07–0.97; $p = 0.03$) • Did not effect the risk of first admission to hospital ($p = 0.4$) Participants taking multivitamins compared to the placebo group: • Did not significantly differ in CD4 count from baseline to final follow-up ($p > 0.3$) • Did not significantly differ in mean plasma viral load at 48 weeks follow-up ($p = 0.4$)

Reference	Population	Dates	Methods	Outcomes	Results
Kawai et al. (2010a)	1129 HIV-1-infected pregnant women (12–27 weeks gestation)	November 2002–June 2004	After their HIV-1-positive serostatus was confirmed, women were randomized to receive a daily dose of either a single RDA ($n = 565$) or multiple RDA ($n = 564$) multivitamin from enrollment to 6 weeks postpartum. All subjects received standard prenatal care: daily 60 mg of elemental Fe and 0.25 mg folic acid, and malaria prophylaxis at 20 and 30 weeks gestation. At the start of labor, 200 mg of nevirapine was given to the mother. At delivery, 2 mg per kg of infant weight of nevirapine was given to the infant. At baseline and every month following, physical examinations of the women were performed for anthropometric measurements, general health, and treatment compliance. Sociodemographic data and obstetric history were obtained at baseline. Infant anthropometry and gestational age were measured by a midwife. Single-RDA multivitamin vs. multiple-RDA multivitamin Single RDA: 1.4 mg thiamin, 1.4 mg riboflavin, 18 mg niacin, 1.9 mg of vitamin B_6, 2.6 µg of vitamin B_{12}, 70 mg of vitamin C, 10 mg of vitamin E, 0.4 g of folic acid Multiple RDA: 20 mg thiamin, 20 mg riboflavin, 100 mg niacin, 25 mg of vitamin B_6, 50 µg of vitamin B_{12}, 500 mg of vitamin C, 30 mg of vitamin E, 0.8 g of folic acid	*Primary outcome:* Infant: LBW (< 2500 g), preterm birth < 37 weeks gestation *Secondary outcomes:* Maternal: Hb concentrations, anemia (Hb < 11 g/dL), T-cell counts, HIV-1 viral load Infant: very LBW (<2000 g), severe preterm birth (<34 weeks gestation), SGA birthweight <10th percentile of weight-for-gestational age, fetal death (miscarriage/stillbirth), infant death < 6 weeks life, birthweight/length, gestational age, head circumference, placental weight	Maternal multivitamin supplementation compared to single multivitamin supplementation: • Did not affect the risk of LBW ($p = 0.75$), preterm birth ($p = 0.73$), small-for-gestational age ($p = 0.18$), fetal death ($p = 0.99$), perinatal death ($p = 0.25$), early infant death ($p = 0.19$), or fetal or early infant death ($p = 0.63$) • Did not result in significant differences in birth weight, length, head circumference, and placental weight ($p > 0.1$ for all) • Did not result in significant differences in T-cell counts, viral load, or Hb concentrations ($p > 0.1$ for all)

(continued)

TABLE 2.2 (continued)
Randomized Trials of Multiple Micronutrient Interventions

Study	Sample	Enrollment	Methods	Exposure	Outcome	Main Findings
			Women (n = 312) co-enrolled in a selenium supplement trial had blood drawn ≤10 weeks after delivery and were assessed for CD4, CD8, and CD3 counts; viral load; and Hb status.			Multivitamin supplementation: • Reduced the risk of TB reoccurrence between 1 and 8 months post-treatment by 45% overall (RR, 0.55 [0.33–0.93]; p = 0.02) and by 63% in HIV-infected patients (RR, 0.37 [0.15–0.92]; p = 0.02) • Among HIV-infected patients did not have significant differences with the patients receiving a placebo in CD4, CD8, or CD3 or HIV viral load for the entire follow-up period (p ≥ 0.1 for all), though during the first 8 months the CD8 count was higher among patients receiving micronutrients with approaching significance (mean difference: 76 E6 cells/L; 95% CI, –12E6–163 E6 cells/L; p = 0.09) • Among HIV-1-infected patients there were no significant differences in BMI, albumin, or Hb concentrations for the entire period or during the first 8 months follow-up compared to the placebo group (p > 0.1 for all)
Villamor et al. (2008)	887 adults with pulmonary tuberculosis (471 HIV-infected and 416 HIV-uninfected)	April 2000–April 2005	TB status confirmed by sputum tests. Patients were stratified by HIV infection after blood tests. Patients were randomized to receive a daily micronutrient or a placebo from baseline to last follow-up (median 43 months); all patients received standard anti-TB treatment. At baseline, nurses recorded socioeconomic data, marital status, and age. At monthly follow-ups, anthropometric and body mass data were obtained. Sputum and blood samples were obtained at baseline; 1, 2, 5, 8, and 12 months; and every 6 months following for a AFB test, Hb status, T-cells, and viral load. Physical examinations were given every 3 months follow-up, and stage of HIV disease was determined.	Multivitamin vs. placebo Multivitamin: 5000 IU retinol, 20 mg vitamin B1, 20 mg vitamin B2, 100 mg niacin, 25 mg vitamin B6, 50 ug vitamin B12, 500 mg vitamin C, 200 mg vitamin E, 0.8 mg folic acid, 100 μg selenium	*Primary outcomes:* Culture negativity at 1-month follow-up Mortality at ≥24 months follow-up TB recurrence during follow-up *Secondary outcomes:* Viral load among HIV-infected patients CD4 counts Body weight Clinical diagnoses and signs: fever, nausea/vomiting, diarrhea, fatigue, skin rashes, oral thrush, painful swallowing, extrapulmonary TB, peripheral neuropathy, genital ulcers	

Kawai et al. (2014)	887 adults with pulmonary tuberculosis (471 HIV-infected and 416 HIV-uninfected)	April 2000–April 2005	See methods above. Blood was collected and tested for cell-mediated immune lymphocyte proliferation.	Exposure is described above.	Cell-mediated immune response: lymphocyte proliferation to TB antigens or T-cell mitogens	No effects of micronutrient supplements were found on lymphocyte proliferation in HIV-uninfected and HIV-infected TB patients ($p > 0.1$).
Luabeya et al. (2007)	373 children (4–6 months) stratified into 3 groups: 32 HIV-1-infected, 154 HIV-exposed uninfected, and 187 HIV-non-exposed uninfected	June 2003–October 2004	At enrollment, a physical examination and HIV blood testing were performed of mothers and children. Children were randomized to receive daily treatments from baseline to 24 months of age: (1) vitamin A, (2) vitamin A plus zinc, and (3) vitamin A, zinc, and multiple micronutrients. At weekly visits, a questionnaire was given to mothers on infant diarrhea and respiratory morbidity. Growth and morbidity were assessed at hospital visits at 7, 8, 9, 12, 15, 18, 21, and 24 months follow-up. When ART became available in clinics in 2005, all HIV-infected children were referred for treatment.	Group1: 1250 IU vitamin A Group 2: 1250 IU vitamin A and 10 mg Zn Group 3: 1250 IU vitamin A, 10 mg Zn, and a multivitamin (0.5 mg vitamin B_1, 0.5 mg vitamin B_2, 0.5 mg vitamin B_6, 0.9 µg vitamin B_{12}, 35 mg vitamin C, 5 µg vitamin D, 6 mg vitamin E, 10 µg vitamin K, 0.6 mg copper, 150 µg folate, 50 µg iodine, 10 mg iron, 6 mg niacin)	*Primary outcome:* Percentage of days with diarrhea (stool more frequent or looser than normal or with blood/water) *Secondary outcomes:* Severity of diarrhea, as measured by duration of episodes, maximum number of stools during an episode, episode lasting ≥14 days, diarrhea with blood, clinic visits for diarrhea Distribution of diarrheal morbidity Proportion of children who ever had diarrhea and number of episodes *Respiratory outcomes:* Percentage of weeks with upper respiratory symptoms Percentage of children who ever had pneumonia by maternal report and by fieldwork confirmation	Among HIV-infected children, there were no significant differences detected for any diarrheal disease or respiratory complication outcomes between treatment groups ($p > 0.10$). Among all three cohorts combined, there were no significant differences in median values for diarrheal diseases or respiratory outcomes ($p > 0.05$) between treatment groups.

(continued)

TABLE 2.2 (continued)
Randomized Trials of Multiple Micronutrient Interventions

Study	Sample	Enrollment	Methods	Exposure	Outcome	Main Findings
Duggan et al. (2012)	2387 children born to HIV-infected women	February 2004–June 2007	Infants of HIV-infected, pregnant women presenting to clinic for prenatal care (≤32 weeks gestation) were enrolled in the study. Children were randomized to daily multivitamin ($n = 1193$) or placebo ($n = 1194$) from 6 weeks of age to 24 months. All mothers received multivitamins, standard antenatal care, and malaria prophylaxis. Mothers and infants were followed monthly to receive standard care, and child morbidity, anthropometry, and clinical symptoms were recorded; mortality was determined by verbal autopsy. Physical examinations were given to children every 3 months.	Multivitamin vs. placebo Multivitamin: 60 mg vitamin C, 8 mg vitamin E, 0.5 mg thiamine, 0.6 mg riboflavin, 4 mg niacin, 0.6 mg vitamin B_6, 130 µg folic acid, 1 mg vitamin B_{12} (children received double the treatment dosage after 6 months of age)	*Primary outcome:* All-cause mortality *Secondary outcomes:* Hospitalization Clinical symptoms, including diarrhea (≥3 loose stools/day), rapid respiratory rate, cough, fever, vomiting, pus draining from ears, or combination of both, refusal to eat, drink, or breastfeed	Multivitamin supplementation: • Did not affect the risk of all-cause mortality ($p = 0.33$) • Did not affect the risk of hospitalization, diarrhea, respiratory-related symptoms, pus draining from ears, or refusal to eat, drink, or breastfeed ($p > 0.1$) • Decreased the risk of fever (RR, 0.92; 95% CI, 0.55–0.99; $p = 0.02$) and vomiting (RR, 0.78; 95% CI, 0.65–0.93; $p = 0.007$) Among HIV exposed children, multivitamin supplementation: • Decreased the risk of hospitalizations (RR, 0.48; 95% CI, 0.24–0.95; $p = 0.035$), fever (RR, 0.79; 95% CI, 0.67–0.93; $p = 0.005$), and combined cough and fever (RR, 0.79; 95% CI, 0.65–0.96; $p = 0.019$) Among infants with LBW, micronutrient supplementation: • Increased the risk of fever (RR, 1.28; 95% CI, 0.97–1.70; p-interaction = 0.013) and combined risk of fever and cough (RR,146; 95% CI, 1.04–2.05; p-interaction = 0.006) • Decreased the risk of diarrhea (RR, 0.65; 95% CI, 0.42–0.99; p-interaction = 0.016)

| Liu et al. (2013) | 2387 children born to HIV-infected women | February 2004–June 2007 | See methods above. Duration of exclusive breastfeeding (no other food) and infant feeding were measured every month. At baseline for mothers and children, and at every 6 months follow-up in children, blood was collected and measured for CBC, Hb, and T-cell subset counts. | Exposure is described above. | *Primary outcomes:* Infant mortality Infant morbidity *Secondary outcomes:* Mother-to-child transmission of HIV ($n = 1753$) Infant Hb concentrations Anemia development: Hb < 10.0 g/dL at baseline or 11.0 g/dL at follow-up; severe (Hb < 8.5 g/dL), macrocytic (MCV > 86 fL), microcytic (MCV < 70 fL), microcytic (MCV < 70 fL) | Infant multivitamin supplementation: • Had no effect on mother-to-child HIV transmission ($p = 0.39$) • Decreased the risk of infant anemia (RR, 0.88; 95% CI, 0.79–0.99; $p = 0.03$), severe anemia (RR, 0.79; 95% CI, 0.65–0.95; $p = 0.01$), and microcytic anemia (RR, 0.76; 95% CI, 0.61–0.93; $p = 0.009$); baseline infant HIV status or maternal CD4 count did not affect the efficacy of multivitamin supplementation The infant multivitamin supplementation compared to the placebo group: • Had significantly higher mean Hb concentrations at 12 months follow-up (9.77 vs. 9.64 g/dL, $p = 0.03$), 18 months follow-up (9.76 vs. 9.57 g/dL, $p = 0.004$), and 24 months follow-up (9.93 vs. 9.75 g/dL, $p = 0.02$) • Did not significantly differ in Hb concentrations at any time point among HIV-infected children (p-interaction = 0.07) |
| Kupka et al. (2013) | 2387 children born to HIV-infected women | February 2004–June 2007 | See methods above. | Exposure is described above. | *Primary outcomes:* Length for age (LAZ) Weight for age (WAZ) Weight for length (WLZ) *Secondary outcomes:* Stunting, LAZ < −2 Wasting, WLZ < −2 Underweight, WAZ < −2 | Infant multivitamin supplementation: • Had no effect on LAZ ($p = 0.15$), WLZ ($p = 0.87$), or WAZ ($p = 0.86$) at 104 weeks follow-up • Had no effect on stunting ($p = 0.30$), wasting ($p = 0.29$), or underweight ($p = 0.48$) at 104 weeks follow-up |

(continued)

TABLE 2.2 (continued)
Randomized Trials of Multiple Micronutrient Interventions

Study	Sample	Enrollment	Methods	Exposure	Outcome	Main Findings
Sudfeld et al. (2013)	225 HIV-exposed, uninfected children with measles vaccine	February 2004–June 2007	See methods above. Infants at 9 months age were administered the measles vaccine. Between 15 months and 18 months of age, plasma was collected from infants and tested for measles IgG concentrations and measles IgG avidity.	Exposure is described above.	*Infant measles vaccine response:* Measles IgG seropositivity (≥200 mIU/mL) Measles IgG concentrations Measles IgG avidity index	Infant multivitamin supplementation: • Did not significantly affect measles IgG seropositivity ($p = 0.842$), measles IgG concentrations ($p = 0.291$), or measles IgG avidity ($p = 0.526$) In an ancillary analysis, HIV-infected children had a lower risk of measles IgG seroconversion compared to HIV-uninfected children (RR, 0.57; 95% CI, 0.42–0.78; $p = 0.008$).
Manji et al. (2014)	192 HIV-exposed, uninfected children	February 2004–June 2007	See methods above. At 15 months of age, infant cognition, language, and motor scales were assessed by the Bayley Scales of Infant and Toddler Development (BSID-III) by trained nurses.	Exposure is described above.	Raw BSID-III scores for the following: cognition, language, and motor scales	Infant multivitamin supplementation: • Did not significantly affect cognition ($p = 0.42$), expressive language ($p = 0.70$), receptive language ($p = 0.56$), or gross motor ($p = 0.32$) BSID-III raw scores • Improved mean fine motor scores with approaching significance (mean difference = 0.38; 95% CI, –0.01–0.78; $p = 0.06$) • Did not significantly decrease the risk of a BSID-III raw score in the 25th percentile or lower for any category ($p > 0.10$ for all)
Baum et al. (2013)	878 HIV-infected, ART-naïve adults (≥18 years)	December 2004–July 2009	Participants were randomized to one of four daily treatment groups for 24 months: (1) multivitamin ($n = 219$), (2) selenium ($n = 220$), (3) multivitamin and selenium ($n = 220$), or (4) placebo ($n = 219$)	2 × 2 factorial design	*Primary outcome:* Disease progression to CD4 counts <200/µL (until May 2008) and <250/µL (until July 2009)	The multivitamin supplementation only group compared to the placebo group had • Significantly lowered risk of a CD4 count <250 cells/µL (HR, 0.54; 95% CI, 0.30–0.98; $p = 0.04$)

Author (year)	Population	Dates	Methods	Intervention	Outcomes	Results
			HIV viral load, CBC, renal/liver function, plasma micronutrient concentrations, and lipid profiles were taken at baseline and every 6 months. A physical examination, CD4 count, and medical history were taken at baseline and every 3 months follow-up by nurses. Questionnaires on morbidity were collected at monthly follow-up visits.	Group 1: Multivitamin: 20 mg thiamin, 20 mg riboflavin, 100 mg niacin, 25 mg vitamin B_6, 50 μg vitamin B_{12}, 800 μg folic acid, 500 mg vitamin C, 30 mg vitamin E. Group 2: 200 μg selenium. Group 3: Multivitamin + selenium. Group 4: Placebo	*Secondary outcomes:* Combined outcome of CD4 < 250 cells/μL, AIDS-defining condition, or AIDS-related death. Combined outcome of CD4 < 350 cells/μL, AIDS-defining condition, or AIDS-related death. HIV viral load	• Lowered risk of a CD4 count < 350 cells/μL with approaching significance (HR, 0.68; 95% CI, 0.44–1.06; $p = 0.09$). Neither HIV viral load nor a combined outcome was associated with multivitamin supplementation only ($p ≥ 0.10$).
Mda et al. (2010)	118 HIV-infected, ART-naïve children (4 months–2 years) hospitalized for diarrhea or respiratory infection	November 2005–May 2007	HIV status was confirmed, patient body weight and lengths were recorded, and patients were randomized to 1 of 2 daily treatment groups: (1) multi-micronutrient ($n = 54$), or (2) placebo ($n = 52$) from baseline to hospital discharge. Fasting blood samples were drawn 1–2 days from discharge and tested for zinc, retinol, iron, ferritin, CRP, Hb, CD4/CD8 counts, and severity of HIV.	Multi-micronutrient vs. placebo. Multi-micronutrient: 300 μg retinol, 0.6 mg thiamin, 0.6 mg riboflavin, 8 mg niacin, 0.6 mg pyridoxine, 1 μg vitamin B_{12}, 70 μg folic acid, 25 mg ascorbic acid, 5 μg vitamin D, 7 mg vitamin E, 700 μg copper, 8 mg iron, 30 μg selenium, 8 mg zinc	*Primary outcome:* Duration of hospitalization for diarrhea (≥3 loose stools in 24 hours) or pneumonia (temperature ≥ 38°C, cough, and age-specific elevated respiratory rate). *Secondary outcomes:* Serum zinc, retinol iron, ferritin, and Hb concentrations. CD4 lymphocyte percentages. Anthropometric measurements. Inflammation (CRP > 10 mg/L)	Children taking multivitamins compared to those taking the placebo: • Had shorter mean hospitalization duration (7.3 ± 3.9 days vs. 9.0 ± 4.9 days, $p < 0.05$) • Had no significant differences in mean hospitalization duration among patients admitted for diarrhea ($p > 0.05$) or for respiratory ($p > 0.05$) • Did not significantly differ in serum zinc, vitamin A, iron, ferritin, and CD4 concentrations ($p > 0.05$) • Did not significantly differ in inflammation ($p > 0.05$)

(continued)

TABLE 2.2 (continued)
Randomized Trials of Multiple Micronutrient Interventions

Study	Sample	Enrollment	Methods	Exposure	Outcome	Main Findings
Sudfeld et al. (2013)	225 HIV-exposed, uninfected children with measles vaccine	February 2004–June 2007	See methods above. Infants at 9 months age were administered the measles vaccine. Between 15 months and 18 months of age, plasma was collected from infants and tested for measles IgG concentrations and measles IgG avidity.	Exposure is described above.	*Infant measles vaccine response:* Measles IgG seropositivity ($\geq$200 mIU/mL) Measles IgG concentrations Measles IgG avidity index	Infant multivitamin supplementation: • Did not significantly affect measles IgG seropositivity ($p = 0.842$), measles IgG concentrations ($p = 0.291$), or measles IgG avidity ($p = 0.526$) In an ancillary analysis, HIV-infected children had a lower risk of measles IgG seroconversion compared to HIV-uninfected children (RR, 0.57; 95% CI, 0.42–0.78; $p = 0.008$).
Ndeezi et al. (2010)	875 HIV-infected children (12–59 months)	June 2005–June 2008	Upon confirmation of HIV status, children were randomized to receive treatment or standard care for 6 months followed by standard care for another 12 months. Children were stratified by ART (85 ART mature, 762 ART-naïve). At baseline, caretakers provided data on children's previous medical, nutritional, and symptom history; a physical examination was given, and anthropometry and HIV/AIDS stage (WHO criteria) were measured. At baseline, venous blood was drawn and analyzed for CBC, CD4 count, CRP, zinc, and other trace minerals.	2-RDA multivitamin supplement vs. standard-of-care supplement 2-RDA multivitamin supplement: 800 μg vitamin A, 1.2 mg vitamin B_1, 1.2 mg vitamin B_2, 1.6 mg niacin, 1.2 mg vitamin B_6, 2.4 μg vitamin B_{12}, 50 mg vitamin C, 400 IU vitamin D, 14 mg vitamin E, 400 μg folate, 60 μg selenium, 10 mg zinc, 800 μg copper, 180 μg iodine	*Infant mortality:* Verbal autopsy or clinical records Side effects of supplement Serious adverse event (conditions that resulted in hospitalization, required medical attention, or were life-threatening/fatal) *Anthropometric measurements:* Weight for age (WAZ) Height for age (HAZ) Weight for height (WHZ)	At 12 months follow-up, infants in the treatment group compared to the standard-of-care group: • Were not significantly different in incidence of mortality (5.9% vs. 6.7%; RR, 0.9; 95% CI, 0.5–1.5). No significant differences were found among ART-mature or ART-naïve subsets • Were not significantly different in mean survival time ($p = 0.64$) • Were not significantly different in mean CD4 count ($p = 0.53$) or WHZ ($p = 0.39$) • Had higher mean HAZ z-scores (-2.17 ± 1.60 vs. -2.42 ± 1.50, $p = 0.08$) and higher mean WAZ (-0.78 ± 1.30 vs. 0.97 ± 1.03, $p = 0.07$) with approaching significance

Ndeezi et al. (2011)

214 HIV-infected children (12–59 months)

June 2005–June 2008

See methods above. Blood samples were collected at baseline and 6 months follow-up, and serum was analyzed for folate and vitamin B₁₂.

Children were followed up monthly for the first 6 months at the clinic and at 9 and 12 months to assess record of illness, anthropometry, and physical examination.

Standard-of-care supplement (1-RDA multivitamin): 400 µg vitamin A, 0.6 mg vitamin B₁, 0.6 mg vitamin B₂, 0.8 mg niacin, 25 mg vitamin C, 200 IU vitamin D

Exposure is described above.

Serum vitamin B_{12} status: low (<221 pmol/L), marginal (148–221 pmol/L), very low (<148 pmol/L)

Serum folate status: low (<13.4 nmol/L), marginal (6.8–13.4 nmol/L), very low (<6.8 nmol/L)

2-RDA multivitamin supplementation compared to standard-of-care supplementation:

• Had greater increases in median vitamin B_{12} status from baseline to 6 months (+90.5 [−0.8–203.5] pmol/L vs. +10 [−73.8–83.8] pmol/L, $p < 0.001$)

• Had greater increases in median folate status from baseline to 6 months (+8.0 [−0.3–17.1] nmol/L vs. −0.6 [−3.5 to −5.8] nmol/L, $p < 0.001$); among ART-treated infants there were significant increases in vitamin B_{12} ($p = 0.002$) and folate ($p = 0.040$) in the 2-RDA multivitamin group

• Had significantly lower odds of low vitamin B_{12} (OR, 4.5; 95% CI, 2.0–10.0) and low folate (OR, 10.8; 95% CI, 4.1–28.9)

(continued)

TABLE 2.2 (continued)
Randomized Trials of Multiple Micronutrient Interventions

Study	Sample	Enrollment	Methods	Exposure	Outcome	Main Findings
Isanaka et al. (2012)	3418 HIV-infected adults (≥18 years) initiating HAART	November 2006–November 2008	HIV status was confirmed, and a clinical examination and questionnaire were conducted for sociodemographic and socioeconomic data. Patients were randomized to receive either a high dose or standard dose of a daily multivitamin supplement for 24 months. At baseline and monthly follow-up visits, a physical examination was given, medical history and anthropometry were taken, HIV status was determined, and illnesses from the previous month were recorded.	Multiple-RDA multivitamin vs. 1-RDA multivitamin Multiple-RDA multivitamin: 20 mg thiamin, 20 mg riboflavin, 25 mg vitamin B_6, 100 mg niacin, 50 µg vitamin B_{12}, 0.8 mg folic acid, 500 mg vitamin C, 30 mg vitamin E	*Primary outcome:* HIV disease progression, defined as new or recurring episode of pulmonary tuberculosis, pneumonia, chronic diarrhea, cryptococcal meningitis, cytomegalovirus retinitis, TB meningitis, mucocutaneous herpes simplex virus, leukoencephalopathy, encephalopathy, histoplasmosis, coccidiomycosis, esophageal candidiasis mycobacterial infection, extrapulmonary TB, lymphoma, or Kaposi sarcoma	Study was stopped in March 2009 due to increased levels of alanine transaminase in patients receiving the high-dose multivitamin (RR = 1.44; 95% CI, 1.11–1.87; $p = 0.006$). High-dose multivitamin compared to a low-dose multivitamin: • Did not effect the risk of HIV disease progression, death from any cause, or AIDS-related death ($p > 0.10$) • Did not significantly change CD4 count, HIV viral count, BMI, or Hb concentrations • Lowered the risk of clinical neuropathy (RR, 0.81; 95% CI, 0.70–0.94; $p = 0.004$); no other clinical outcome was associated with multivitamin supplementation dosage

At baseline and every 4 months follow-up, blood was drawn and tested for CD4 count, absolute T-cell counts, HIV viral load, ALT levels, and hepatitis B/C.

At baseline and every 12 months follow-up, a semi-food frequency questionnaire (FFQ) was used to determine dietary and alcohol intake.

Cause of death was determined from medical records and verbal autopsies.

1-RDA multivitamin: 1.2 mg thiamin, 1.2 mg riboflavin, 1.3 mg vitamin B_6, 15 mg niacin, 2.4 µg vitamin B_{12}, 0.4 mg folic acid, 80 mg vitamin C, 15 mg vitamin E

Secondary outcomes:
AIDS-related death, defined as death from one of the aforementioned episodes Changes in CD4 count, plasma viral load, BMI, or Hb concentrations

Note: ART, antiretroviral therapy; BMI, body mass index; BSID-II, Bayley Scales of Infant and Toddler Development; BSID-III, Bayley Scales of Infant and Toddler Development; CBC, complete blood count; CI, confidence interval; CVL, cervicovaginal lavage; FFQ, food frequency questionnaire; HAART, highly active antiretroviral therapy; HAZ, height for age z-score; Hb, hemoglobin; Hct, hematocrit; HR, hazard ratio; IUGR, intrauterine growth restriction; LAZ, length for age z-score; LBW, low birthweight; MCV, mean corpuscular volume; MUAC, mid-upper arm circumference; OR, odds ratio; RBC, red blood cell; RDA, recommended dietary allowance; RR, risk ratio; SGA, small for gestational age; TB, tuberculosis; WAZ, weight for age z-score; WBC, white blood cell; WHZ, z-score; WLZ, weight for length z-score; ZVD, zidovudine.

TABLE 2.3

Randomized Trials of Single Micronutrient Interventions

Study	Sample	Period	Methods	Exposure	Outcomes	Main Findings
Safrin et al. (1994)	92 AIDS patients with *Pneumocystis carinii* pneumonia (PCP)	October 1989–May 1992	PCP was confirmed by bronchoalveolar lavage or sputum sample, and patients received folinic acid ($n = 47$) or placebo ($n = 45$) in conjunction with trimethoprim–sulfamethoxazole (TMP–SMZ) for the duration of TMP–SMZ treatment. RBC folate and arterial blood gas levels were measured at baseline; CD4 counts were measured within 2 months of study. At 3, 5, 7, 10, 14, 17, and 21 days of TMP–SMZ treatment, clinical response, CBC, and serum LDH were measured. TMP and SMZ were measured on day 3 and 1-month follow-up.	Daily 1-folinic acid (7.5 mg) vs. placebo	*Primary outcome:* TMP–SMZ failure/ dose-limited toxicity, defined as treatment discontinuation/ substitution *Secondary outcomes:* Anemia: major (>25% Hct drop), minor (10–25% Hct drop) Neutropenia: major (<0.7 × 10^9 cells/L), minor (>50% drop in neutrophil field) Thrombocytopenia: major (<40 × 10^9 cells/L), minor (40–100 × 10^9 cells/L) Azotemia: major (creatinine > 265 μmol/L), minor: creatinine > 44.2 μmol/L) Hepatotoxicity: major (AST/ALT > 5× study entry), minor (AST/ALT 2–5× greater than entry) Rash: major (severe and intolerable), minor (tolerable) Nausea: major (severe and intolerable), minor (tolerable)	Folinic acid supplementation: • Increased the probability of therapy failure compared to those taking a placebo ($p = 0.005$) • Increased the probability of death compared to placebo patients taking a placebo ($p = 0.02$) Patients taking folinic acid compared to the placebo group: • Did not significantly differ in TMP–SMZ dose-limiting toxicity ($p = 0.4$) or time of discontinuation of TMP–SMZ ($p = 0.7$) • Did not significantly differ in frequencies of rash, elevated ALT/ AST, thrombocytopenia, or nausea • Had a lower frequency of neutropenia (23% vs. 47%, $p = 0.03$) • Did not significantly differ in anemia overall ($p = 0.4$)

| Brossard et al. (1994) | 30 HIV patients (CD4 < 200/mm³, stages 2 and 3) | January 1990–September 1990 | Patients were randomized to three treatment groups administered 3× per week for 180 days: (1) low-dose folic acid (n = 9), (2) high-dose folic acid (n = 12), (3) placebo group (n = 9); all patients received 50 mg of pyrimethaminie 3× a week, 600 mg/d zidovudine, and pentamidine isothionate aerosol 300 mg/month. Blood was drawn and tested for CBC and lymphocytes at baseline and at 30, 90, and 180 days follow-up. | Group 1: 5 mg folic acid 3× per week Group 2: 25 mg folic acid 3× per week Group 3: Placebo | Differences in Hb, neutrophils, and platelets from baseline to 90 and 180 days follow-up Anemia (Hb < 10 g/dL) | At baseline, there were no significant differences among the three groups in mean Hb, neutrophil, or platelet concentrations. At 90 days follow-up, there were no significant mean differences in Hb, neutrophil, or platelet concentrations. At 180 days follow-up, mean Hb concentrations were significantly different among the three groups ($p <$ 0.05). At 180 days follow-up, the placebo group had significantly lower Hb concentrations compared to baseline (difference: -1.66 ± 1.07 g/dL; $p <$ 0.05). |
| Grigoletti et al. (2013) | 30 HIV-infected adults (≥18 years) on stable HAART therapy ≥6 months | August 2009–September 2011 | Patients were randomized to receive a daily folic acid supplement (n = 15) or placebo (n = 15) for 4 weeks. Blood pressure, heart rate, forearm blood flow, and endothelium-independent vasodilation in the brachial artery were measured at baseline and at 4 weeks follow-up. Blood was drawn and measured for plasma homocysteine (Hcy), serum folate, serum vitamin B$_{12}$, glucose, creatine, and lipids at baseline and 4 weeks postpartum. | Folic acid supplement (5 mg) vs. placebo | *Primary outcome:* Brachial artery vascular responses during hyperemia *Secondary outcome:* Changes in biochemical and hemodynamic variables | Participants receiving folic acid supplementation: • Had significantly increased serum folate (p-interaction < 0.001) and decreased Hcy (p-interaction < 0.001) from baseline to 4 weeks • Improved reactive hyperemia (from 14.9 ± 0.7 to 21.2 ± 1.4 mL/min/100 mL; p-interaction < 0.001) • Did not affect endothelium-independent vasodilation (p-interaction = 0.834) Increased folic acid concentrations were correlated with improved reactive hyperemia response ($r =$ 0.707; $p <$ 0.001). |

(continued)

TABLE 2.3 (continued)
Randomized Trials of Single Micronutrient Interventions

Study	Sample	Period	Methods	Exposure	Outcomes	Main Findings
Gerber et al. (2004)	14 HIV-infected, HAART-stable adults (>18 years) with dyslipidemia	July 2001–May 2002	Treatment for dyslipidemia was discontinued for 4 weeks, all participants received ER-niacin for 14 weeks, and participants were observed for another 4 weeks. Lipid profile, uric acid level, metabolic panel, CD4 count, and HIV load were measured at 0, 4, 10, 14, 18, and 22 weeks follow-up. Oral glucose tolerance test (OGTT) was conducted at 0 and 14 weeks follow-up.	ER-niacin treatment for 14 weeks: weeks 4–6 (500 mg/d niacin), weeks 6–12 (1000 mg/d niacin), weeks 12–16 (1500 mg/d niacin), weeks 16–18 (2000 mg/d niacin)	Treatment of dyslipidemia: defined as fasting triglycerides ≥ 200 mg/dL or LDL ≥ 130 mg/dL Glucose tolerance: intolerance (2-hr OGTT > 140 mg/dL), insulin sensitivity, as determined by minimal model of glucose disposal Lipid profile	From week 4 to week 18, ER-niacin: • Significantly decreased median total cholesterol (−14 mg/dL; 95% CI, −9 to −25; $p = 0.005$), triglycerides (−34 mg/dL; 95% CI, −17 to −42; $p = 0.019$), and non-HDL cholesterol (−19 mg/dL; 95% CI, −10 to −31; $p = 0.004$); median values increased after discontinuation of ER-niacin from week 18 to week 22 ($p < 0.05$ for all) • Increased median HDL with approaching significance (+3 mg/dL; 95% CI, 0 to +13; $p = 0.091$); LDL cholesterol did not significantly change ($p > 0.1$) • Increased median HOMA-IR (1.54–3.36; $p = 0.05$), B-cell sensitivity to basal glucose (7.0×10^{-9} vs. 11.2×10^{-9}/min; $p = 0.01$), B-cell secretion rate (152–262 pmol/min; $p = 0.01$)
Souza et al. (2010)	10 HIV-infected, HAART-treated adults with triglycerides > 200 mg/dL	August 2001–November 2003	Participants with triglycerides >200 mg/dL after 4 weeks of Step-1/Step-2 diet regimens were assigned to ER-niacin for 24 weeks.	ER-niacin treatment for 24 weeks: weeks 4–8 (500 mg/d), weeks 8–12 (1000 mg/d), weeks 12–32 (1500 mg/d)	Safety of treatment: nature and rate of adverse events (clinical signs, symptoms, lab tests) Tolerability of treatment: dose modifications or dropout Liver function (AST/ALT concentrations)	ER-niacin treatment from baseline to end of treatment: • Decreased median triglycerides (516.2 vs. 293.5 mg/dL; $p < 0.05$); cholesterol, HDL, or LDL did not significantly change ($p > 0.05$)

Study	Population		Methods	Intervention	Outcomes	Results
			Blood was drawn and measured for a lipid panel, liver function panel, and glucose metabolism at baseline (week 4) and at 24 weeks follow-up (week 32); adverse events (signs, symptoms, lab tests) were recorded throughout the intervention.		Fasting glucose/insulin HOMO-IR	• Did not significantly change tests of liver function, glucose metabolism, HOMO-IR ($p > 0.05$), or CD4 count No participants developed grade 3 or higher adverse events; flushing was most common adverse event.
Dube et al. (2006)	33 HIV-infected, ART-treated adults ($\geq$18 years) with HDL-C $\geq$ 4.66 nmol/L and triglycerides $\geq$ 2.26 mmol/L	Unknown	ER-niacin was administered daily for 44 weeks. Blood was collected and measured for fasting glucose, uric acid, creatinine, ALT/ AST, lipid profiles at baseline, and at 4, 8, 12, 18, 24, 32, 40, and 48 weeks follow-up. OGTT was conducted at 4, 12, 24, and 48 weeks follow-up. Lipoprotein testing, lipoprotein(a), and CRP were measured at 4, 24, and 48 weeks.	ER-niacin treatment for 44 weeks: weeks 4–8 (500 mg/d niacin), weeks 8–14 (1000 mg/d niacin), weeks 14–20 (1500 mg/d niacin), weeks 20–48 (2000 mg/d niacin); if non-LDLs < 4.14 mmol/L, LDL-C < 3.37 mmol/L, and triglycerides < 5.65 mmol/L week 8 or after, participants did not increase niacin dosage	*Primary outcomes:* Changes in glucose metabolism Changes in hepatic transaminases, fructosamine, and uric acid Onset of diabetes mellitus Safety/tolerability of ER-niacin *Secondary outcome:* Efficacy of ER-niacin (changes in lipid parameters, changes in anthropometry)	After 44 weeks of ER-niacin treatment: • Median fasting glucose increased (5.47–5.59 mmol/L; $p = 0.041$) • Median fasting insulin increased (66–99 pmol/L; $p = 0.016$) and median HOMO-IR increased (2.4–3.5 µU/mL·mmol/L; $p = 0.009$) • Median total cholesterol decreased (−0.21 mmol/L; $p < 0.001$), HDL-C increased (+0.13 mmol/L; $p = 0.002$), apo-A1 increased (+0.08 g/L; $p = 0.001$), non-HDL-C decreased (−0.49 mmol/L; $p < 0.001$), apo-B-100 decreased (−0.13g/L; $p = 0.002$), triglycerides decreased (−1.73 mmol/L; $p < 0.001$), lipoproteins decreased (−2.0 mmol/L; $p = 0.01$), large HDL particles increased (+0.9 µmol/L; $p = 0.003$), and large VLDL particles decreased (−9.9 nmol/L; $p < 0.001$)

(continued)

TABLE 2.3 (continued)
Randomized Trials of Single Micronutrient Interventions

Study	Sample	Period	Methods	Exposure	Outcomes	Main Findings
						After 44 weeks of treatment, 22% of participants had reached the composite lipid goal, 25% had achieved non-HDL cholesterol < 1.14 mmol/L, 34% had achieved LDL cholesterol < 3.37 mmol/L, and 84% had obtained triglycerides < 5.65 mmol/L.
Balasubramanyam et al. (2011)	191 HIV-infected, ART-treated adults (21–65 years) with hypertriglyceridemia (>150 mg/dL)	January 2004–September 2009	Participants were randomized to 5 groups (n = 10/group) to receive diet, exercise routine, and drug treatment or usual care with placebo for 24 weeks. Three-day food logs were recorded and confirmed by a dietitian at baseline and at 8, 16, and 24 weeks follow-up. Fitness and body composition (body cell mass/fat) were measured at baseline and at 8, 16, and 24 weeks follow-up. Fasting triglycerides were measured at 2, 4, 8, 12, 16, and 24 weeks follow-up. OGTT, indirect calorimetry, fasting plasma adiponectin, FFA, high-sensitivity C-reactive protein, and TSH were measured at baseline and final visit.	Group 1: Usual care and 2 placebo pills Group 2: Low-saturated-fat diet and exercise (D/E) and 2 placebo pills Group 3: D/E and active fenofibrate (145 mg) and 1 placebo pill Group 4: D/E and niacin (50 mg) and 1 placebo pill Group 5: D/E + fenofibrate + niacin Participants were stratified by ART class.	*Primary outcomes:* Fasting cholesterol, HDL-C, and non-HDL-C *Secondary outcomes:* Insulin sensitivity Glycemia Adiponectin CRP Energy expenditure Body composition	Participants taking niacin compared to controls: • Had increased mean HDL-C (43.3 ± 1.5 vs. 39.7 ± 1.3 mg/dL; p = 0.03) and decreased mean total cholesterol (HDL-C ratio 4.3 ± 0.02 vs. 4.8 ± 0.2; p = 0.01) Participants in Group 4 compared to Group 2: • Had increased mean plasma glucose (95.4 ± 3.2 vs. 88.7 ± 3.0 mg/dL; p = 0.002); increased mean OGTT for glucose (18,113 ± 1110 vs. 17,207 ± 1022 mg/dL over 120 min; p = 0.02), increased mean plasma insulin (11.9 ± 3.0 vs. 6.7 ± 1.6 µU/mL; p = 0.03), increased mean HOMA-IR (2.76 ± 0.75 vs. 1.38 ±0 .36; p = 0.008), decreased mean insulin sensitivity index (2.88 ± 0.67 vs. 4.95 ± 1.10; p = 0.007), and increased mean adiponectin (11.01 vs. 6.04 ng/mL; p <0.0001)

| Chow et al. (2010) | 19 HIV-infected, HAART-treated adults (≤18 years) with HDL-C < 40 mg/dL and LDL-C < 130 mg/dL | November 2007–April 2010 | Blood counts and liver and kidney function were measured at 2, 4, 8, 12, and 24 weeks follow-up. Adults were randomized to receive ER-niacin ($n = 10$) or a placebo ($n = 9$) daily for 12 weeks. At baseline and 12 weeks follow-up, participants were tested for CD4 count, HIV-RNA viral load, flow-mediated-vasodilation (FMD), lipid profile, insulin sensitivity, and CRP. Endothelial function (brachial artery reactivity testing, brachial artery diameter, and forearm blood flow scans) were also measured at baseline and at 12 weeks follow-up. | ER-niacin vs. placebo ER-niacin: 500 mg/d titrated to a maximum 1500 mg/d niacin over 8 weeks and continued for 4 weeks at 1500 mg/d | Change in FMD | ER-niacin supplementation:
• Did not significantly affect FMD ($p = 0.67$) or brachial diameters ($p = 0.56$); FMD significantly increased after adjusting for baseline FMD and HDL-C ($p = 0.048$)
• Increased median HDL-C (+3.0 mg/dL; IQR, 0.75–5.0), while there was no increase in the placebo group (p-interaction = 0.04)
• Did not significantly effect nitroglycerin-mediated dilation |

(continued)

TABLE 2.3 (continued)
Randomized Trials of Single Micronutrient Interventions

Study	Sample	Period	Methods	Exposure	Outcomes	Main Findings
Lin et al. (2013)	17 HIV-infected, HAART-treated adults (≤18 years) with HDL-C < 40 mg/dL and LDL-C <130 mg/dL	November 2007–April 2010	See methods above.	Exposure is described above.	Changes in lipid profile	ER-niacin supplementation compared to the placebo group: • Had higher median HDL concentrations at 12 weeks follow-up (44.0 vs. 30.5 mg/dL; $p = 0.03$), but there was no significant differences at baseline ($p = 0.15$) • Had no significant differences in total cholesterol, LDL, or triglycerides at baseline or at 12 weeks follow-up ($p > 0.1$) • Had significantly greater median decreases in small LDL particles (−17.02% vs. +21.42%; $p = 0.03$) and greater increases in LDL size (+1.22% vs. −1.96%; $p = 0.04$)

Note: ALT, alanine transaminase; ART, antiretroviral therapy; AST, aspartate transaminase; CRP, C-reactive protein; D/E, diet and exercise; ER-niacin, extended-release niacin; FFA, free fatty acid; FMD, flow-mediated vasodilation; HAART, highly active antiretroviral therapy; HDL, high-density lipoprotein; HOMA-IR, homeostatic model assessment of insulin resistance; LDL, low-density lipoprotein; OGTT, oral glucose tolerance test; PCP, *Pneumocystis carinii*; TMP–SMZ, trimethoprim–sulfamethoxazole; TRBC, red blood cell; TSH, thyroid-stimulating hormone; VLDL, very low-density lipoprotein.

HIV Viral Load and Viral Shedding

Evidence regarding the effects of multivitamin supplementation on circulating HIV RNA viral load has been conflicting. In TOV, HIV-infected, ART-naïve pregnant women who received daily multivitamin supplementation at multiple RDA levels (containing 20 mg of vitamin B_1, 20 mg vitamin B_2, 25 mg vitamin B_6, 100 mg niacin, 50 µg vitamin B_{12}, and 0.8 mg folic acid) had significantly lower mean HIV-1 viral load (-0.11 log; $p = 0.05$) during follow-up (median = 71 months) compared to no multivitamin supplementation (Fawzi et al., 2004a). However, in other randomized trials in HIV-infected adults or patients co-infected with HIV and tuberculosis (TB), multivitamin supplementation had no significant effects on HIV RNA viral load ($p > 0.05$) (Jiamton et al., 2003; Villamor et al., 2008; Baum et al., 2013). For example, in TOV3, among HIV-infected adults initiating HAART in Tanzania, B-complex, C, and E vitamin supplementation at multiples of the RDA level did not significantly reduce plasma HIV-1 viral load concentrations compared to multivitamins at the single RDA level ($p = 0.66$) (Isanaka et al., 2012). Findings regarding the effects of B-vitamin supplementation on HIV vaginal viral shedding have been divergent (Fawzi et al., 2004a; McClelland et al., 2004; Villamor et al., 2010). In a randomized trial in Mombasa, Kenya (Principal Investigator: McClelland), the effects of micronutrient supplementation on the risk of vaginal infections were examined among HIV-1-infected, ART-naïve nonpregnant women (McClelland et al., 2004). Daily micronutrient supplementation (20 mg vitamin B_1, 20 mg vitamin B_2, 100 mg niacin, 25 mg vitamin B_6, 50 µg vitamin B_{12}, 0.8 mg folic acid, 500 mg vitamin C, 30 mg vitamin E, and 200 µg selenium) for six weeks resulted in twofold greater odds of vaginal shedding of HIV-1 infected cells (adjusted odds ratio [AOR], 2.50; 95% CI, 1.40–4.40; $p = 0.001$) at six weeks of follow-up compared to placebo, after adjusting for baseline number of vaginal and cervical HIV-1 infected cells, vaginal and cervical HIV-1 RNA copies ($\log_{10}$ copies/swab), and body mass index (McClelland et al., 2004). However, there were no significant changes in plasma HIV-1 viral load ($p = 0.80$) (McClelland et al., 2004).

Immunological Factors

Findings regarding the effects of multivitamin supplementation on immunological factors have been conflicting. In the TOV, HIV-infected, ART-naïve pregnant women who received daily multivitamin supplementation (B-complex, C, and E vitamins at multiple RDA levels) had significantly greater mean increases in CD4 T-cell counts from baseline (12 to 27 weeks gestation) to six weeks postpartum (mean [SD]; +167 [210] vs. +112 [268] cells; $p < 0.001$) and 30 weeks postpartum (+99 [208] vs. +59 [167] cells; $p = 0.003$); CD8 T-cell counts from baseline to six weeks postpartum (+385 [450] vs. +289 [404] cells; $p = 0.001$); and CD3 T-cell counts from baseline to six weeks postpartum (+585 [648] vs. +411 [559] cells; $p < 0.001$) and 30 weeks postpartum (+345 [493] vs. +254 [475] cells; $p = 0.02$) compared to women who did not receive multivitamin supplements (Fawzi et al., 1998).

In a randomized trial in Botswana (Principal Investigator: Baum), the effects of multivitamin or selenium supplementation on immune function and time of progression to AIDS or mortality were examined among ART-naïve, HIV-infected adults (Baum et al., 2013). Adults were randomized to receive daily supplements of (1) multivitamins alone, (2) selenium alone, (3) multivitamins and selenium, or (4) a placebo in a 2×2 factorial design and were followed for 24 months. Adults receiving a multivitamin supplement (20 mg thiamin, 20 mg, riboflavin, 100 mg niacin, 25 mg vitamin B_6, 50 µg vitamin B_{12}, 800 µg folic acid, 500 mg vitamin C, and 30 mg vitamin E) had a significantly decreased risk of having low CD4 T-cell counts (<250 cells/µL; HR, 0.54; 95% CI, 0.30–0.98; $p = 0.04$) during the 24 months of follow-up compared to the placebo group (Baum et al., 2013). However, in other randomized trials among ART-naïve, HIV-infected adults, with or without TB co-infection, there were no significant effects of multivitamin supplementation on mean CD4, CD8, or CD3 T-cell counts ($p > 0.05$) compared to the placebo group (Jiamton et al., 2003; Villamor et al., 2008). Further, in TOV3, the aforementioned trial among HIV-infected adults initiating HAART, multivitamins at multiples of the RDA level did not significantly change CD4 T-cell counts from baseline to 24 months of follow-up compared to multivitamins at the single RDA level (Isanaka et al., 2012).

Hematological Status

To date, only one randomized trial has evaluated the effects of B-vitamin supplementation on hematologic status in HIV-infected individuals. In the aforementioned TOV, HIV-infected pregnant women receiving multivitamin supplementation (B-complex, C, and E vitamins at multiple RDA levels) during pregnancy had significantly higher mean hemoglobin concentrations within the first 70 days postpartum ($p = 0.0002$), at two years of follow-up ($p = 0.001$), and at four years of follow-up ($p = 0.01$) compared to women who did not receive multivitamin supplements (Fawzi et al., 2007). However, there were no significant effects of multivitamins on the risk of anemia (Hb < 11.0 g/dL), microcytic anemia (hypochromasia ≥ 1 or presence of microcytic cells), or macrocytic anemia (presence of any macrocytic cells) compared to no multivitamins ($p > 0.05$).

Comorbidities

In the TOV study, maternal multivitamin supplementation (B-complex, C, and E vitamins at multiple RDA levels) during pregnancy was associated with significantly lower risk of clinically diagnosed malaria (RR, 0.78; 95% CI, 0.67–0.92; $p = 0.003$) but also with increased risk of malaria parasitemia being detected in blood films (RR, 1.24; 95% CI, 1.02–1.50; $p = 0.03$) compared to no multivitamin supplementation (Olofin et al., 2014). In a randomized trial among patients with pulmonary TB (with or without HIV co-infection) (Principal Investigator: Fawzi), investigators examined the effects of multivitamin supplementation on TB sputum conversion, relapse, reinfection, and survival (Villamor et al., 2008). Adults with pulmonary TB on anti-tuberculosis treatment were randomized to receive a daily micronutrient (20 mg vitamin B_1, 20 mg vitamin B_2, 100 mg niacin, 25 mg vitamin B_6, 0.8 mg folic acid, 50 μg vitamin B_{12}, 5000 IU retinol, 500 mg vitamin C, 200 mg vitamin E, and 100 μg selenium) or a placebo throughout follow-up (median = 43 months), stratified by HIV co-infection. Among participants with HIV/TB co-infection at baseline, daily multivitamin supplementation reduced the risk of tuberculosis reoccurrence at the end of follow-up (RR, 0.37; 95% CI, 0.15–0.92; $p = 0.02$) compared to the placebo group (Villamor et al., 2008). An additional analysis from the same trial found no effects of multivitamin supplementation on lymphocyte proliferation to T-cell antigens ($p > 0.10$) in HIV/TB co-infected individuals compared to the placebo (Kawai et al., 2014).

PERINATAL OUTCOMES

Several randomized trials have been conducted among HIV-infected pregnant women to examine the effects of daily B-vitamin supplementation on maternal, pregnancy, and infant outcomes. Multivitamin supplementation including B-vitamins may decrease the risk of maternal preeclampsia (Merchant et al., 2005), increase maternal weight gain during pregnancy (Villamor et al., 2008), and reduce the risk of adverse pregnancy outcomes, including miscarriage, fetal loss, preterm birth, low birthweight, and small-for-gestational age (Fawzi et al., 1998). Prenatal multivitamin supplementation may also increase breast milk (Webb et al., 2009) and infant serum or plasma (Baylin et al., 2005) micronutrient concentrations.

Maternal Outcomes

Several papers published from the TOV study focused on the effects of multivitamin supplementation (B-complex, C, and E vitamins at multiple RDA levels) during pregnancy on the risks of adverse perinatal outcomes in HIV-infected, ART-naïve women in Tanzania. Daily multivitamin supplementation significantly reduced the risk of low maternal weight gain (<25th percentile) (RR, 0.73; 95% CI, 0.58–0.93; $p = 0.01$) and weight loss (RR, 0.69; 95% CI, 0.50–0.95; $p = 0.02$) during the third trimester compared to receiving no multivitamins; however, findings were not significant over the entire course of pregnancy (Villamor et al., 2002). In a subset of participants ($n = 955$) who were normotensive and had blood samples available at baseline from the same trial, women receiving a multivitamin had a lower risk of hypertension (systolic pressure $\geq$ 140 mmHg or diastolic pressure $\geq$ 90 mmHg) during pregnancy (RR, 0.62; 95% CI, 0.40–0.94; p = 0.03) compared to receiving no multivitamins (Merchant et al., 2005). Similarly, in the TOV study, HIV-infected pregnant women receiving multivitamins had a lower risk of depressive symptoms (Hopkins Symptom Checklist score > 1.06; RR, 0.78; 95% CI, 0.66–0.92; p = 0.005) and decreased the risk of scoring in the lowest quartile for various psychosocial dimensions of health-related quality of life, including physical functioning (RR, 0.76; 95% CI, 0.63–0.90; p = 0.002), role-physical (RR, 0.70; 95% CI, 0.57–0.88; p = 0.002), bodily pain (RR, 0.81; 95% CI, 0.69–0.95; p = 0.008), general health (RR, 0.77; 95% CI, 0.66–0.90; p = 0.0007), vitality (RR, 0.72; 95% CI, 0.61–0.84; p = 0.0001), social functioning (RR, 0.72; 95% CI, 0.59–0.88; p = 0.001), and mental health (RR, 0.82; 95% CI, 0.70–0.96; p = 0.01) domains compared to women who did not receive multivitamins (Smith Fawzi et al., 2007).

Pregnancy Outcomes

The effects of daily multivitamin supplementation containing B-vitamins on the risks of adverse pregnancy outcomes have been evaluated in several trials, including mother-to-child transmission of HIV, miscarriage, stillbirth, fetal loss, gestational age at delivery, preterm birth, birthweight, low birthweight, and small-for-gestational age. The safety and efficacy of micronutrient supplementation on perinatal outcomes in HIV-infected pregnant women are discussed in detail in Chapter 6 of this volume.

In the TOV study, daily prenatal multivitamin supplementation significantly decreased the risks of low birthweight (<2500 g; RR, 0.56; 95% CI, 0.38–0.82; p = 0.003), very low birthweight (<2000 g; RR, 0.42; 95% CI, 0.18–1.01; p = 0.05), and small-for-gestational age (RR, 0.57; 95% CI, 0.29–0.82; p = 0.002) (Fawzi et al., 1998); severe preterm birth (<34 weeks gestation; RR, 0.61; 95% CI, 0.38–0.96; p = 0.03); and fetal loss (RR, 0.59; 95% CI, 0.39–0.91; p = 0.02) compared to receiving no multivitamins (Fawzi et al., 1998, 2000). There were no significant effects of multivitamins on the risks of other adverse pregnancy outcomes, including stillbirth (RR, 0.58; 95% CI, 0.33–1.02; p = 0.05), miscarriage (RR, 0.66; 95% CI, 0.32–1.36; p = 0.26), or preterm birth (RR, 0.86; 95% CI, 0.68–1.10; p = 0.23) compared to no multivitamins (Fawzi et al., 1998, 2000).

A second randomized trial of multivitamin supplementation (TOV2) (Principal Investigator: Fawzi), was conducted among ART-naïve pregnant women (12 to 27 weeks gestation) in Tanzania to determine the effects of multivitamin supplementation with B-complex, C, and E vitamins at multiples of the RDA level (20 mg thiamin, 20 mg riboflavin, 100 mg niacin, 25 mg vitamin B_6, 0.8 g folic acid, 50 µg vitamin B_{12}, 500 mg vitamin C, 30 mg vitamin E) on the risk of adverse pregnancy outcomes compared to receiving multivitamins at the single RDA level (1.4 mg thiamin, 1.4 mg riboflavin, 18 mg niacin, 1.9 mg vitamin B_6, 0.4 g folic acid, 2.6 µg vitamin B_{12}, 70 mg vitamin C, and 10 mg vitamin E). There were no significant effects of the higher dose multivitamins on the risks of low birthweight (RR, 1.07; 95% CI, 0.70–1.62; p = 0.75), fetal death (RR, 1.00; 95% CI, 0.63–1.58; p = 0.99), preterm birth (RR, 1.04; 95% CI, 0.81–1.35; p = 0.73), SGA (RR, 1.30; 95% CI, 0.89–1.90; p = 0.18), or perinatal death (RR, 0.75; 95% CI, 0.47–1.21; p = 0.25) compared to multivitamin supplements at the single RDA level (Kawai et al., 2010a).

Lactation Period

The effects of daily multivitamin supplementation from pregnancy through two years postpartum on micronutrient concentrations of breast milk and the risk of mastitis were examined in several analyses in the TOV study. Daily multivitamin supplementation with B-complex, C, and E vitamins increased the risk of subclinical mastitis (sodium-to-potassium ratio [Na:K] > 0.6; RR, 1.33; 95% CI, 1.09–1.61; p = 0.005) and severe subclinical mastitis (Na:K > 1.0; RR, 1.75; 95% CI, 1.27–2.41; p = 0.0006) during lactation (from <2 weeks to >12 months postpartum) compared to no multivitamin supplementation (Arsenault et al., 2010).

CHILD OUTCOMES

Randomized trials of B-vitamin supplementation have been conducted among HIV-infected pregnant women and children to examine the effects on mother-to-child HIV transmission, co-infections and clinical symptoms (i.e., measles, respiratory infections, and diarrhea), anthropometry and growth (i.e., weight, length, head circumference, and mid-upper arm circumference), including weight for age (WAZ), weight for length (WLZ), and length for age (LAZ) WHO z-scores (underweight, WAZ < –2; wasting, WLZ < –2; stunting, LAZ < –2); cognitive and psychomotor development; and micronutrient status in children.

HIV Transmission and Mortality

The effects of maternal B-vitamin supplementation on the risk of MTCT of HIV was examined in three analyses conducted within the TOV study. There were no significant effects of maternal multivitamin supplementation on the risk of HIV transmission at birth (RR, 1.54; 95% CI, 0.94–2.51; $p = 0.08$), six weeks postpartum (RR, 1.17; 95% CI, 0.81–1.71; $p = 0.39$), or two years postpartum ($p > 0.05$) compared to no multivitamin supplementation (Fawzi et al., 2000; Kawai et al., 2010b). In overall analyses, maternal multivitamin supplementation did not significantly reduce the risk of MTCT of HIV through breastfeeding (RR, 0.85; 95% CI, 0.61–1.19; $p = 0.34$) (Fawzi et al., 2002). However, in analyses among a subgroup of women with lower immunological status (lymphocyte counts < 1340 cells/mm^3, lowest quartile), multivitamin supplementation significantly reduced the risk of MTCT of HIV (RR, 0.37; 95% CI, 0.16–0.85; $p = 0.02$) compared to no multivitamin supplementation (Fawzi et al., 2002). Similarly, among anemic women (Hb < 8.5 g/dL), multivitamin supplementation reduced the risk of MTCT of HIV (RR, 0.48; 95% CI, 0.24–0.93; $p = 0.03$) compared to no multivitamin supplementation (Fawzi et al., 2002). Maternal multivitamin supplementation was also associated with decreased risk of childhood mortality among female children at two years of age (RR, 0.68; 95% CI, 0.47–0.97; $p = 0.03$; p-interaction = 0.04) (Fawzi et al., 2000; Kawai et al., 2010b).

A randomized trial was conducted among children born to HIV-infected mothers (11%; $n = 264$) (Principal Investigator: Fawzi, Child1) to determine the effects of multivitamin supplementation on child morbidity and mortality (Duggan et al., 2012). Children were randomized to receive daily B-vitamin supplementation (0.5 mg thiamine, 0.6 mg riboflavin, 4 mg niacin, 0.6 mg vitamin B$_6$, 130 µg folic acid, and 1 mg vitamin B$_{12}$, with dose doubled at 6 months of age) or a placebo from 6 weeks to 24 months of age. Daily pediatric B-vitamin supplementation was not associated with lower risk of all-cause mortality in children (RR, 1.13; 95% CI, 0.88–1.14; $p = 0.33$) compared to the placebo group (Duggan et al., 2012).

Similarly, a trial was conducted among HIV-infected children (1 to 5 years old) in Uganda (Principal Investigator: Ndeezi) to examine the effects of multiple micronutrient supplementation at two times the RDA level (1.2 mg vitamin B$_1$, 1.2 mg vitamin B$_2$, 1.6 mg niacin, 1.2 mg vitamin B$_6$, 400 µg folate, 2.4 µg vitamin B$_{12}$, 800 µg vitamin A, 50 mg vitamin C, 400 IU vitamin D, 14 mg vitamin E, 60 µg selenium, 10 mg zinc, 800 µg copper, and 180 µg iodine) on child morbidity, weight gain, and mortality compared to multivitamins at the single RDA level (Ndeezi et al., 2010). Children who received the higher multivitamin dose daily for six months had no significant differences in the risk of mortality (5.90% vs. 6.70%; RR, 0.90; 95% CI, 0.50–1.50; $p > 0.05$) or mean survival time (10.7 vs. 10.6 months; $p = 0.64$) compared to children who received multivitamins at the single RDA level (Ndeezi et al., 2010).

Infections and Vaccine Response

Findings from randomized trials that examined the effects of maternal or child multivitamin supplementation on the risk of pediatric respiratory and diarrheal infections have been heterogeneous. In the TOV study, children born to HIV-infected mothers who received daily multivitamin supplementation (B-complex, C, and E vitamins at multiple RDA levels) had lower risks of all-cause diarrhea (≥3 watery stools/day; RR, 0.83; 95% CI, 0.71–0.98; $p = 0.03$) and acute diarrhea (duration <14 days; RR, 0.83; 95% CI, 0.71–0.98; $p = 0.03$) compared to no multivitamin supplementation (Fawzi et al., 2003). There were no differences in the occurrence of respiratory infections ($p > 0.05$), and findings did not vary by HIV status of the child ($p > 0.05$). In the same study, children born to HIV-infected women who received daily multivitamin supplementation also had a decreased risk of clinical malaria (parasitemia > 5000/μL and fever; RR, 0.29; 95% CI, 0.09–0.89; $p = 0.02$) compared to receiving no multivitamins (Villamor et al., 2007).

In two randomized trials (Principal Investigator: Bennish; Principal Investigator: Mda) of multivitamin supplementation among HIV-infected or HIV-exposed children, a daily multivitamin (containing B-complex, A, C, D, E, and K vitamins and minerals at multiple RDA levels) had no significant effects on the risks of diarrheal or respiratory infections ($p > 0.05$) compared to a placebo or standard of care (i.e., vitamin A supplementation) (Luabeya et al., 2007; Mda et al., 2010). However, in a randomized trial (Principal Investigator: Fawzi, Child1) of multivitamin supplementation in Tanzania among HIV-exposed children, daily multivitamin supplements including B-complex (0.5 mg thiamine, 0.6 mg riboflavin, 4 mg niacin, 0.6 mg vitamin B_6, 130 μg folic acid, and 1 mg vitamin B_{12}, with dose doubled at 6 months of age) decreased the risk of HIV-associated complications, including fever (RR, 0.79; 95% CI, 0.67–0.93; $p = 0.005$) and a combined endpoint of cough and fever (RR, 0.79; 95% CI, 0.65–0.96; $p = 0.019$) compared to the placebo (Duggan et al., 2012). The effects of daily multivitamin supplementation in children on measles vaccine response was also evaluated in this study; there were no significant effects of multivitamin supplementation on measles IgG seropositivity, IgG concentrations, or IgG avidity compared to the placebo ($p > 0.05$) (Sudfeld et al., 2013).

Anthropometry and Growth

Pediatric anthropometry and growth outcomes evaluated in randomized trials included weight, length, head circumference, and mid-upper arm circumference, including weight for age (WAZ), weight for length (WLZ), and length for age (LAZ) WHO z-scores (underweight, WAZ < –2; wasting, WLZ < –2; stunting, LAZ < –2). In the TOV study, daily maternal multivitamin supplementation during the pregnancy and postpartum periods significantly increased child weight (but not length) during follow-up (Villamor et al., 2005a). Children born to HIV-infected women who received multivitamin supplements had significantly greater weight gain from birth to 24 months of life (+459; 95% CI, 35–882 g; $p = 0.03$), greater weight for length (+0.38; 95% CI, 0.07–0.68; $p = 0.01$), and greater weight for age (+0.42; 95% CI, 0.07–0.77; $p = 0.01$) z-scores compared to children born to women who did not receive multivitamin supplements (Villamor et al., 2005a). There were no significant effects of maternal multivitamin supplementation on the risks of child wasting, stunting, or underweight from birth to 24 months of age (Villamor et al., 2005a).

In the randomized trial of multivitamin supplementation among HIV-exposed children in Tanzania, children born to HIV-infected women were randomized to receive a daily multivitamin supplement (0.5 mg thiamine, 0.6 mg riboflavin, 4 mg niacin, 0.6 mg vitamin B_6, 130 μg folic acid, and 1 mg vitamin B_{12}, with dose doubled at 6 months of age) or a placebo from 6 weeks to 24 months of age (Kupka et al., 2013). Child multivitamin supplementation had no significant effects on LAZ, WLZ, or WAZ or on the incidence of stunting (LAZ < –2), wasting (WLZ < –2), or underweight (WAZ < –2) at 104 weeks of follow-up compared to a placebo (Kupka et al., 2013). In a trial from Uganda, HIV-infected children were randomized to receive either a multivitamin supplement that included B-complex vitamins at two times the RDA level or a multivitamin supplement at the single RDA level (Principal Investigator: Ndeezi) (Ndeezi et al., 2010). The higher dose multivitamin had no significant effects on child WAZ or height for age (HAZ) at 12 months follow-up compared to the single RDA level (Ndeezi et al., 2010).

Cognitive and Psychomotor Development

Two randomized trials to date have been conducted to evaluate the effects of multivitamin supplementation administered to HIV-infected mothers or HIV-exposed infants on cognition and psychomotor development in children, as assessed using the Bayley Scales of Infant and Toddler Development (BSID, versions II and III). In the TOV study, the Bayley Scales of Infant and Toddler Development were administered to a subgroup of children to examine the effects of maternal multivitamin supplementation on cognitive and psychomotor development in offspring (McGrath et al., 2006). Children born to women who received multivitamin supplementation had significantly higher psychomotor development indices at 6 months of age (95.9 vs. 92.8; $p = 0.03$) and higher psychomotor indices (+2.6; 95% CI, 0.1–5.1; $p = 0.04$) and raw motor scores (+0.8; 95% CI, 0.002–1.6; $p = 0.04$) at 18 months of age compared to children born to women who did not receive multivitamins (McGrath et al., 2006).

In the aforementioned randomized trial among HIV-exposed children in Tanzania, daily multivitamin supplementation (0.5 mg thiamine, 0.6 mg riboflavin, 4 mg niacin, 0.6 mg vitamin B_6, 130 µg folic acid, and 1 mg vitamin B_{12}, with dose doubled at 6 months of age) was not associated with significantly improved fine motor skills (mean difference: 0.38; 95% CI, −0.01–0.78; $p = 0.06$) or cognition, expressive language, receptive language, or gross motor skills ($p > 0.05$) at 15 months of age compared to the placebo group (Manji et al., 2014).

Hematological Status

In an analysis in the TOV study, infants born to HIV-infected women who had received daily multivitamin supplements (20 mg vitamin B_1, 20 mg vitamin B_2, 25 mg vitamin B_6, 100 mg niacin, 50 µg vitamin B_{12}, and 0.8 mg folic acid) throughout pregnancy and lactation had significantly higher hemoglobin concentrations at 2 years ($p = 0.0009$) and 4 years ($p = 0.0001$) of age and lower risk of severe hypochromic microcytosis during follow-up (RR, 0.51; 95% CI, 0.31–0.84; $p = 0.004$) compared to no multivitamin supplementation (Fawzi et al., 2007). However, maternal multivitamin supplementation did not significantly reduce the risk of infant anemia (Hb < 11.0 g/dL), severe anemia (Hb < 8.5 g/dL), or macrocytosis compared to infants born to mothers who received no multivitamin supplementation ($p > 0.05$). In the randomized trial of micronutrient supplementation among HIV-exposed children in Tanzania, daily pediatric multivitamin supplementation decreased the risk of anemia (11.0 g/dL; RR, 0.88; 95% CI, 0.79–0.99; $p = 0.03$), severe anemia (Hb < 8.5 g/dL; RR, 0.79; 95% CI, 0.65–0.95; $p = 0.01$), and microcytic anemia (RR, 0.76; 95% CI, 0.61–0.93; $p = 0.009$) in children compared to the placebo group (Liu et al., 2013). In analyses of a subgroup of HIV-infected children, daily multivitamin supplementation did not significantly increase hemoglobin concentrations compared to the placebo (p-interaction HIV status = 0.08) (Liu et al., 2013).

FOLIC ACID AND VITAMIN-B$_{12}$ SUPPLEMENTATION

In another randomized trial, HIV-infected adults were randomized to receive (1) folinic acid* and vitamin B_{12} with zidovudine or (2) zidovudine alone (Principal Investigator: Falguera). There were no significant differences between the two groups with respect to their hemoglobin concentrations, hematocrit, or mean corpuscular volume during follow-up ($p > 0.05$). However, folinic acid and vitamin B_{12} supplementation with zidovudine significantly increased serum vitamin B_{12}, serum folate, and erythrocyte folate concentrations at 3, 6, 9, and 12 months follow-up ($p < 0.05$) compared to zidovudine alone (Falguera et al., 1995).

RANDOMIZED TRIALS OF SINGLE MICRONUTRIENT SUPPLEMENTATION

The majority of randomized trials of B-vitamin supplementation in HIV-infected populations have focused on B-complex vitamins in combination with other vitamins and minerals. To date, randomized trials of single micronutrient supplements in HIV-infected individuals have focused on folic

---

* Folinic acid is a vitamer of folic acid typically used in cancer therapy, but functionally it acts as a vitamin.

acid and niacin. These studies have examined the effects of folic acid or niacin on ART safety, efficacy, and failure; anemia and micronutrient status; and dyslipidemia, insulin resistance, and adverse vascular events. Findings from these randomized trials are summarized in detail in Table 2.3.

Folic Acid Supplementation

Findings regarding the effects of folic acid supplementation on hemoglobin concentrations and anemia in HIV-infected patients are conflicting. In a trial of patients with AIDS examining toxicity of trimethoprim–sulfamethoxazole (TMP–SMZ) treatment, patients were randomized to folic acid supplementation with TMP–SMZ or TMP–SMZ alone (Brossard et al., 1994). Folinic acid supplementation (7.5 mg/day) with TMP–SMZ had no significant effects on the incidence of anemia ($\geq 10\%$ decrease in hematocrit; $p = 0.40$) compared to TMP–SMZ alone (Safrin et al., 1994). However, in a study examining the potential benefit of folic acid supplementation for cytopenia in HIV-infected patients (WHO stages 2 and 3) receiving pyrimethamine, zidovudine, and pentamidine isothinonate aerosol, individuals who also received folic acid supplementation for 180 days (Group 1, 5 mg 3×/week; Group 2, 25 mg 3×/week) had significantly higher hemoglobin concentrations at 180 days of follow-up ($p < 0.05$) compared to the placebo (Brossard et al., 1994).

Folic acid supplementation (400 µg daily) is part of standard prenatal care for the prevention of neural tube defects and anemia (WHO, 2012). However, there are concerns that requirements could be higher in the context of HIV, particularly with the use of anti-folate medications. In individuals with HIV infection, anti-folinic drugs are often prescribed to treat bacterial and protozoan infections, and several malaria prophylactic medications are folate antagonists (e.g., sulfadoxine–pyrimethamine with its mechanism of action—dihydrofolate reductase), which impair folate status and increase the risk of anemia. Four randomized trials have been conducted to examine the effects of folic acid supplementation on anemia and cardiovascular outcomes in HIV-infected patients.

A cohort of patients with AIDS (95.7% ART-naïve) and pneumonia infection who were receiving trimethoprim–sulfamethoxazole (TMP–SMZ) was randomized to receive daily folic acid supplementation (7.5 mg/day) or a placebo throughout the duration of TMP–SMZ treatment. Folic acid supplementation significantly increased the risk of treatment failure ($p = 0.005$) and death ($p = 0.02$) compared to the placebo (Safrin et al., 1994). However, folic acid supplementation was not associated with risk of TMP–SMZ dose-limiting toxicity ($p = 0.40$), time of discontinuation of TMP–SMZ ($p = 0.70$), or adverse clinical symptoms ($p > 0.05$).

To date, one randomized trial has been conducted to examine the effects of folic acid supplementation on cardiovascular outcomes in HIV-infected individuals (Grigoletti et al., 2013). In a four-week randomized trial of folic acid (5 mg) supplementation or placebo among HIV-infected adults on HAART, folic acid had no effect on endothelium-independent vasodilation ($p = 0.834$) but significantly improved forearm reactive hyperemia ($p < 0.001$), an indicator of vascular reactivity (Grigoletti et al., 2013). Additional trials on folic acid supplementation are needed to determine the potential benefits on cardiovascular and cardiometabolic outcomes to expand upon these preliminary findings.

Niacin Supplementation

Niacin is commonly used to treat dyslipidemia and improve lipid profiles when supplemented in high doses. Extended-release (ER) niacin interventions have been examined for their potential benefits on cardiovascular outcomes in HIV-infected individuals, including dyslipidemia, insulin resistance, vasodilation changes, and safety of ER-niacin therapy. ER-niacin supplementation improved dyslipidemia and related outcomes in HIV-infected individuals in all randomized trials to date. In a study among 14 HIV-infected adults who were stable on HAART, treatment with ER-niacin (maximum 2000 mg/day for 14 weeks) significantly decreased total cholesterol (–14; 95% CI, –9 to –25 mg/dL; $p = 0.005$), triglycerides (–34; 95% CI, –17 to –42 mg/dL; $p = 0.019$), and non-HDL cholesterol (–19; 95% CI, –10 to –31 mg/dL; $p = 0.004$) from pretreatment to 14 weeks follow-up (Gerber et al., 2004). Similarly, in HIV-infected ART-stable adults with dyslip-idemia (HDL-C $\geq$ 4.66 nmol/L and triglycerides $\geq$ 2.26 mmol/L), 22% of participants reached their composite lipid goal, and 84% had lower triglycerides (<5.65 mmol/L) after 44 weeks of ER-niacin supplementation (maximum 2000 mg/day) (Dube et al., 2006). In a third intervention study examining ER-niacin tolerability in HIV-infected individuals, ER-niacin supplementation significantly decreased triglycerides ($p < 0.05$), but there were no significant changes in choles-terol, HDL or LDL levels during the 24-week follow-up period ($p > 0.05$) (Souza et al., 2010). However, in a randomized trial of the effects of niacin therapy in combination with a low-saturated fat diet on metabolic outcomes in HIV-infected adults with dyslipidemia, niacin supplementation (50 mg) increased HDL-C (43.3 $\pm$ 1.5 vs. 39.7 $\pm$ 1.3 mg/dL; $p = 0.03$) and decreased the total cho-lesterol-to-HDL-C ratio (4.3 $\pm$ 0.02 vs. 4.8 $\pm$ 0.2; $p = 0.01$) after 24 weeks compared to the placebo (Balasubramanyam et al., 2011). In another trial of HIV-infected patients with dyslipidemia who were stable on ART, ER-niacin supplementation (maximum 1500 mg/day) significantly increased median HDL-C concentrations after 12 weeks (44.0 vs. 30.5 mg/dL; $p = 0.03$) compared to the placebo, although there were no significant differences in total cholesterol, LDL, or triglycerides ($p > 0.05$) (Chow et al., 2010; Lin et al., 2013).

Few studies have been conducted to examine the effects of ER-niacin treatment on other car-diovascular outcomes in HIV-infected patients. In a randomized trial examining the effects of ER-niacin on endothelial function in HIV-infected, HAART-stable adults, ER-niacin supplementa-tion (maximum 1,500 mg/day) for 12 weeks did not result in any significant changes in flow-medi-ated vasodilation, an indicator of endothelial function ($p = 0.67$), compared to the placebo (Chow et al., 2010). However, flow-mediated vasodilation increased from baseline to 12 weeks follow-up in the ER-niacin treatment group, after adjusting for baseline flow-mediated dilatation (FMD) and HDL cholesterol levels ($p = 0.048$) (Chow et al., 2010).

Preliminary evidence from studies on ER-niacin therapy in HIV-infected individuals suggests adverse effects on insulin sensitivity. For example, a study among HIV-infected, HAART-stable adults taking high-dose ER-niacin (maximum 2000 mg/day) reported increased insulin resistance (homeostatic model assessment of insulin resistance [HOMA-IR], 1.54 to 3.36; $p = 0.05$) and a higher β-cell secretion rate (152 to 262 pmol/min; $p = 0.01$) after 14 weeks of ER-niacin treatment (Gerber et al., 2004). A randomized trial found that HIV-infected adults taking niacin supplementa-tion (50 mg) in combination with a diet and exercise regime had increased HOMA-IR (2.76 $\pm$ 0.75 vs. 1.38 $\pm$ 0.36; $p = 0.008$) and lower insulin sensitivity index (2.88 $\pm$ 0.67 vs. 4.95 $\pm$ 1.10; $p = 0.007$) at 24 weeks of follow-up compared to diet and exercise alone (Balasubramanyam et al., 2011). Participants in the same niacin-supplemented group also had higher mean plasma glucose (95.4 $\pm$ 3.2 vs. 88.7 $\pm$ 3.0 mg/dL; $p = 0.002$) and greater mean oral glucose tolerance test (OGTT) (18,113 $\pm$ 1110 vs. 17,207 $\pm$ 1022 mg/dL over 120 min; $p = 0.02$) compared to the group that received diet and exercise alone, suggesting impaired glucose control.

The safety of ER-niacin therapy has not been extensively evaluated in HIV-infected adults receiving antiretroviral therapy. Potential adverse effects evaluated with ER-niacin treatment include hepatotoxicity (i.e., elevated aminotransferases), glucose intolerance, flushing, and adverse events (grade 3 or higher). In a study among HIV-infected individuals receiving ART (90% protease inhibitor [PI]-based regimen, 30% efevirenz-based regimen) with ER-niacin supplementation for 24 weeks, there were no increased risks of adverse events (grade 3 or higher), greater hepatic ami-notransferases, or altered glucose metabolism ($p > 0.05$) from baseline to post-treatment (Souza et al., 2010). In another trial of 33 HIV-infected adults on ART (70% PI, 48% non-nucleoside reverse transcriptase inhibitor [NNRTI]) who received ER-niacin (maximum 2000 mg/day) for 44 weeks, four participants stopped ER-niacin therapy and another four participants did not reach the maxi-mum dosage for ER-niacin therapy or meet the composite lipid goal by the end of follow-up (Dube et al., 2006). Further studies are warranted to determine the safety, efficacy, and appropriate dose and administration of ER-niacin treatment in HIV-infected patients receiving ART.

DISCUSSION

B-vitamin deficiencies are prevalent in HIV-infected individuals and have been associated with increased risk of HIV disease progression and other adverse HIV-associated outcomes. To date, 21 randomized trials have been conducted to examine the effects of B-vitamins on health outcomes in HIV-infected populations: 13 randomized trials of B-complex vitamins with other micronutrients and 8 trials of individual B-vitamins, niacin, and folic acid. In randomized trials among HIV-infected pregnant and non-pregnant adults, B-vitamin supplementation has been found to decrease the risk of AIDS progression and AIDS-related mortality, decrease HIV RNA viral load, and improve CD4 T-cell counts, in addition to decreasing the risk of adverse pregnancy outcomes, including low birthweight, preterm birth, and fetal loss. Among HIV-exposed infants, B-vitamin supplementation in complex with other micronutrients has not been associated with mother-to-child transmission of HIV or weight gain, but improved psychomotor development. Randomized trials of multivitamins containing a B-vitamin complex at multiple RDA levels have not demonstrated a consistent additional benefit on HIV disease progression, immune function, or AIDS-related mortality compared to the single RDA level. In randomized trials of individual micronutrients in HIV-infected populations, extended-release niacin improved dyslipidemia, but the evidence of the effects of folic acid on hematological outcomes is conflicting. The safety and efficacy of B-vitamin supplementation for HIV-infected individuals have not been studied extensively in the context of antiretroviral therapy.

Randomized trials with B-vitamins in combination with other micronutrients have been reported to slow the progression of HIV and decrease the risk of mortality and AIDS-related mortality (Jiamton et al., 2003; Fawzi et al., 2004b), decrease HIV-1 RNA viral load (Fawzi et al., 2004b), lower the risk of tuberculosis recurrence (Villamor et al., 2008), and improve markers of immune status (Fawzi et al., 1998; Baum et al., 2013). B-vitamin supplementation in HIV-infected, ART-naïve pregnant women decreased the risk of adverse pregnancy outcomes, including low birthweight, small-for-gestational age, severe preterm birth, and fetal loss (Fawzi et al., 1998, 2000), and reduced the risk of MTCT of HIV among women who were nutritionally or immunologically compromised at baseline (Fawzi et al., 2002). Maternal prenatal B-vitamin supplementation also conferred benefit to pediatric outcomes in offspring, including reduced risk of AIDS-associated conditions and opportunistic infections (Fawzi et al., 2003; Villamor et al., 2007) and decreased risk of microcytosis (Fawzi et al., 2007). Among HIV-exposed infants, B-vitamin supplementation in complex with other micronutrients did not reduce the risk of AIDS-associated mortality (Ndeezi et al., 2010; Duggan et al., 2012) or childhood weight gain (Ndeezi et al., 2010; Kupka et al., 2013) but did improve psychomotor development (McGrath et al., 2006). The evidence to date on the safety and efficacy of micronutrient supplementation (including B-vitamins) in HIV-infected pregnant women (see Chapter 6 of this volume) and HIV-infected and HIV-exposed children (see Chapter 8 of this volume) are discussed in further detail in other chapters in this volume. Randomized trials comparing different doses of B-complex regimens (i.e., multiple vs. single RDA level) have not consistently demonstrated a benefit on HIV-related outcomes among ART-naïve pregnant women (Kawai et al., 2010a; Isanaka et al., 2012), adult men and women initiating HAART (Isanaka et al., 2012), or infants (Ndeezi et al., 2010).

Few randomized trials have been conducted to examine the effects of individual micronutrients on health outcomes in HIV-infected populations, and research to date has focused on folic acid and ER-niacin. Findings regarding the effects of folic acid supplementation on hemoglobin and anemia were conflicting (Brossard et al., 1994; Safrin et al., 1994). Extended-release niacin consistently improved lipid profile and reversed indicators of dyslipidemia among HIV-infected ART-stable individuals (Gerber et al., 2004; Dube et al., 2006; Chow et al., 2010; Souza et al., 2010; Balasubramanyam et al., 2011; Lin et al., 2013). However, interventions with ER-niacin also increased the risk of insulin resistance and elevated blood glucose concentrations (Gerber et al., 2004; Balasubramanyam et al., 2011).

RESEARCH GAPS

Study Design—B-Vitamin Supplementation

Despite findings from randomized trials to date, the role of specific B-vitamins (or potential mechanisms involved) in the etiology of HIV-related outcomes is unclear. Few trials to date have focused specifically on B-vitamins, such as B-complex vitamins alone or individual B-vitamins as compared to a placebo (or no B-vitamin supplementation). B-vitamin interventions have also been administered in combination with other micronutrients (e.g., B-complex, C, and E vitamins together with vitamin A or selenium). Supplementation with multiple micronutrients constrains causal inference regarding the specific effects of B-vitamins on HIV-related outcomes. Also, the variation in B-vitamin composition, dose, and administration and the co-administration with other micronutrients in these trials limit the ability to compare findings across studies. The potential effects of micronutrient supplementation of other B-vitamins on immune function, such as thiamin, riboflavin, vitamin B_6, folate, or vitamin B_{12}, warrant further investigation in single-supplementation trials.

B-Vitamin Biomarkers

Few studies in this review assessed biomarkers of B-vitamin status in study participants. The inclusion of multiple micronutrients in intervention regimes and lack of assessment of specific biomarkers constrain interpretation of findings of specific effects of B-vitamins on health outcomes. For example, studies measuring the role of B-vitamins either in complex with other micronutrients or as a single micronutrient (e.g., folic acid) on outcomes such as hemoglobin or anemia did not measure vitamin B_{12} and folate, deficiencies of which are known causes of anemia. Two studies that did measure vitamin B_{12} and folate status in participants assessed total vitamin B_{12} and serum/plasma folate as the only biomarkers of B-vitamin status (Baylin et al., 2005; Ndeezi et al., 2011). Total vitamin B_{12} is a circulating biomarker of vitamin B_{12} status that does not reflect the metabolic uptake of vitamin B_{12}. Inclusion of functional vitamin B_{12} biomarkers, such as MMA and erythrocyte folate concentrations, would improve the assessment of B-vitamin status (Yetley and Johnson, 2011; Yetley et al., 2011a,b,c). In addition to the limited assessment of B-vitamin biomarkers, these indicators were often assessed at a single time point, and few studies in this review used standardized cutoffs for deficiency or insufficiency of B-vitamins. Measurement of B-vitamin supplementation, adherence, and biomarkers of B-vitamin status are critical to elucidating mechanisms between B-vitamins and HIV-related outcomes.

Generalizability

Randomized trials from Tanzania (Principal Investigator: Fawzi) have reported that multivitamin supplementation with B-complex, C, and E vitamins significantly reduces the risk of various adverse HIV-related and perinatal outcomes among ART-naïve, HIV-infected pregnant women. However, few multivitamin trials have been conducted in other regions of the world. Also, some trials included individuals who were co-infected with tuberculosis or children who were both HIV-infected and HIV-exposed, which limits comparison with other studies. The limited evidence regarding the effects of B-vitamins in other settings constrains generalizability and interpretation of findings, particularly in the ART era.

MICRONUTRIENT SUPPLEMENTATION IN THE CONTEXT OF ANTIRETROVIRAL THERAPY

Randomized trials of B-vitamin supplementation and HIV-related outcomes to date have primarily been conducted in ART-naïve populations. Among trials in which HIV-infected individuals received B-vitamins in complex with other micronutrients, only one trial recruited participants initiating HAART (TOV3) (Isanaka et al., 2012); other trials of B-vitamins stratified participants by ART status or enrolled mothers and infants as ART became available during the course of the trial

(Luabeya et al., 2007; Ndeezi et al., 2010; Duggan et al., 2012). The variability in ART exposure and the ancillary focus on ART for these trials constrains causal inference of the effects of B-vitamins in the context of antiretroviral therapy. Further research is urgently needed to determine the efficacy and safety of B-vitamin supplementation as an adjunct to essential antiretroviral therapy.

Research to date on the effects of single B-vitamin nutrient supplements in ART-stable populations has focused on folic acid and extended-release niacin. Two trials of folic acid supplementation in ART-stable, HIV-infected individuals did not demonstrate significant effects on anemia or cardiovascular blood flow (Brossard et al., 1994; Grigoletti et al., 2013). In contrast, randomized trials of ER-niacin therapy among ART-stable, HIV-infected adults have demonstrated a consistent benefit of ER-niacin therapy for dyslipidemia (Gerber et al., 2004; Dube et al., 2006; Chow et al., 2010; Souza et al., 2010; Balasubramanyam et al., 2011).

IMPLICATIONS FOR CLINICAL CARE AND PUBLIC HEALTH PRACTICE

B-vitamin deficiencies are prevalent in HIV-infected individuals and have been associated with increased risk of adverse health outcomes. Randomized trials to date have demonstrated a consistent benefit of B-vitamin supplementation on HIV disease progression and HIV-related health outcomes in ART-naïve populations. Current evidence supports the use of B-vitamin supplementation at the single RDA level for HIV-infected individuals. There is, however, more limited evidence of the additional benefit of higher dose B-vitamin supplementation compared to the single RDA level. Improved dietary intake of B-vitamins using food fortification and dietary diversification approaches is needed, particularly in resource-limited settings where the burden of B-vitamin deficiencies is high.

Extended-release niacin has demonstrated consistent benefits for lipid profiles and dyslipidemia in HIV-infected adults who are stable on ART. ER-niacin therapy is a feasible method to maintain a normal lipid profile for HIV-infected individuals on ART. However, findings regarding the potential effects on insulin resistance and elevated blood glucose concentrations warrant caution, and individuals must be carefully monitored for insulin resistance and diabetes.

To date, there is limited evidence on the effects of B-vitamin supplementation among HIV-infected individuals on antiretroviral therapy. The importance of ensuring universal access to ART cannot be overemphasized. Further research is needed to examine the role of B-vitamin supplementation as an adjunct to essential ART and to elucidate potential micronutrient–ART interactions and their implications for health outcomes. The safety and efficacy of B-vitamin supplementation in HIV/AIDS urgently need to be examined as an adjunct to essential antiretroviral therapy.

REFERENCES

Abrams, B., D. Duncan, and I. Hertz-Picciotto. (1993). A prospective study of dietary intake and acquired immune deficiency syndrome in HIV-seropositive homosexual men. *Journal of Acquired Immune Deficiency Syndromes* 6(8): 949–58.

Addo, A. A., G. S. Marquis, A. A. Lartey, R. Pérez-Escamilla, R. E. Mazur, and K. B. Harding. (2011). Food insecurity and perceived stress but not HIV infection are independently associated with lower energy intakes among lactating Ghanaian women. *Maternal & Child Nutrition* 7(1): 80–91.

Allen, L. H. (2012). Vitamin B-12. *Advances in Nutrition* 3(1): 54–5.

Arsenault, J. E., S. Aboud, K. P. Manji, W. W. Fawzi, and E. Villamor. (2010). Vitamin supplementation increases risk of subclinical mastitis in HIV-infected women. *Journal of Nutrition* 140(10): 1788–92.

Balasubramanyam, A., I. Coraza, E. O. Smith et al. (2011). Combination of niacin and fenofibrate with lifestyle changes improves dyslipidemia and hypoadiponectinemia in HIV patients on antiretroviral therapy: results of "heart positive," a randomized, controlled trial. *Journal of Clinical Endocrinology & Metabolism* 96(7): 2236–47.

Baum, M. K., G. Shor-Posner, Y. Lu et al. (1995). Micronutrients and HIV-1 disease progression. *AIDS* 9(9): 1051–6.

Baum, M. K., A. Campa, S. Lai et al. (2013). Effect of micronutrient supplementation on disease progression in asymptomatic, antiretroviral-naive, HIV-infected adults in Botswana: a randomized clinical trial. *JAMA* 310(20): 2154–63.

Baylin, A., E. Villamor, N. Rifai, G. Msamanga, and W. W. Fawzi. (2005). Effect of vitamin supplementation to HIV-infected pregnant women on the micronutrient status of their infants. *European Journal of Clinical Nutrition* 59(8): 960–8.

Beach, R. S., E. Mantero-Atienza, G. Shor-Posner et al. (1992). Specific nutrient abnormalities in asymptomatic HIV-1 infection. *AIDS* 6(7): 701–8.

Brenchley, J. M. and D. C. Douek. (2007). HIV infection and the gastrointestinal immune system. *Mucosal Immunology* 1(1): 23–30.

Brossard, G., D. Neau, P. Barbeau, J. L. Pellegrin, and B. Leng. (1994). [Primary prophylaxis against cerebral toxoplasmosis. Efficacy of folinic acid in the prevention of hematologic toxicity of pyrimethamine]. *La Presse Médicale* 23(13): 613–5.

Chow, D. C., J. H. Stein, T. B. Seto et al. (2010). Short-term effects of extended-release niacin on endothelial function in HIV-infected patients on stable antiretroviral therapy. *AIDS* 24(7): 1019–23.

Christensen, M. H., E. K. Pedersen, Y. Nordbø et al. (2012). Vitamin B6 status and interferon-gamma-mediated immune activation in primary hyperparathyroidism. *Journal of Internal Medicine* 272(6): 583–91.

Combs, Jr., G. F. (2012). *The Vitamins: Fundamental Aspects in Nutrition and Health*. San Diego: Academic Press.

Coyle, T. E. (1997). Hematologic complications of human immunodeficiency virus infection and the acquired immunodeficiency syndrome. *Medical Clinics of North America* 81(2): 449–70.

Deminice, R., H. S. Vassimon, A. A. Machado, F. J. A. de Paula, J. P. Monteiro, and A. A. Jordao. (2013). Plasma homocysteine levels in HIV-infected men with and without lipodystrophy. *Nutrition* 29(11–12): 1326–30.

Dhur, A., P. Galan, and S. Hercberg. (1991). Folate status and the immune system. *Progress in Food & Nutrition Science* 15(1–2): 43–60.

Dube, M. P., J. W. Wu, J. A. Aberg et al.; AIDS Clinical Trials Group A5148 Study Team. (2006). Safety and efficacy of extended-release niacin for the treatment of dyslipidaemia in patients with HIV infection: AIDS Clinical Trials Group Study A5148. *Antiviral Therapy* 11(8): 1081–9.

Duggan, C., K. P. Manji, R. Kupka et al. (2012). Multiple micronutrients supplementation in Tanzanian infants born to HIV-infected mothers: a randomized, double-blind, placebo-controlled clinical trial. *American Journal of Clinical Nutrition* 96(6): 1437–46.

Erkurt, M. A., I. Aydogdu, M. Dikilitas et al. (2008). Effects of cyanocobalamin on immunity in patients with pernicious anemia. *Medical Principles and Practice* 17(2): 131–5.

Falguera, M., J. Perez-Mur, T. Puig, and G. Cao. (1995). Study of the role of vitamin B_{12} and folinic acid supplementation in preventing hematologic toxicity of zidovudine. *European Journal of Haematology* 55(2): 97–102.

Fawzi, W. W., G. I. Msamanga, D. Spiegelman et al. (1998). Randomised trial of effects of vitamin supplements on pregnancy outcomes and T cell counts in HIV-1-infected women in Tanzania. *The Lancet* 351(9114): 1477–82.

Fawzi, W. W., G. Msamanga, D. Hunter et al. (2000). Randomized trial of vitamin supplements in relation to vertical transmission of HIV-1 in Tanzania. *Journal of Acquired Immune Deficiency Syndromes* 23(3): 246–54.

Fawzi, W. W., G. I. Msamanga, D. Hunter et al. (2002). Randomized trial of vitamin supplements in relation to transmission of HIV-1 through breastfeeding and early child mortality. *AIDS* 16(14): 1935–44.

Fawzi, W. W., G. I. Msamanga, R. Wei et al. (2003). Effect of providing vitamin supplements to human immunodeficiency virus-infected, lactating mothers on the child's morbidity and CD4+ cell counts. *Clinical Infectious Diseases* 36(8): 1053–62.

Fawzi, W., G. Msamanga, G. Antelman et al. (2004a). Effect of prenatal vitamin supplementation on lower-genital levels of HIV type 1 and interleukin type 1 beta at 36 weeks of gestation. *Clinical Infectious Diseases* 38(5): 716–22.

Fawzi, W. W., G. I. Msamanga, D. Spiegelman et al. (2004b). A randomized trial of multivitamin supplements and HIV disease progression and mortality. *New England Journal of Medicine* 351(1): 23–32.

Fawzi, W. W., G. I. Msamanga, R. Kupka et al. (2007). Multivitamin supplementation improves hematologic status in HIV-infected women and their children in Tanzania. *American Journal of Clinical Nutrition* 85(5): 1335–43.

Finkelstein, J. L., A. J. Layden, and P. J. Stover. (2015). Vitamin B-12 and perinatal health. *Advances in Nutrition* 6(5): 552–63.

Friis, H., E. Gomo, N. Nyazema et al. (2004). Effect of multimicronutrient supplementation on gestational length and birth size: a randomized, placebo-controlled, double-blind effectiveness trial in Zimbabwe. *American Journal of Clinical Nutrition* 80(1): 178–84.

Gay, R. and S. N. Meydani. (2001). The effects of vitamin E, vitamin B_6, and vitamin B_{12} on immune function. *Nutrition in Clinical Care* 4(4): 188–98.

Gerber, M. T., K. E. Mondy, K. E. Yarasheski et al. (2004). Niacin in HIV-infected individuals with hyperlipidemia receiving potent antiretroviral therapy. *Clinical Infectious Diseases* 39(3): 419–25.

Goodgame, R. W., K. Kimball, C. N. Ou et al. (1995). Intestinal function and injury in acquired immunodeficiency syndrome-related cryptosporidiosis. *Gastroenterology* 108(4): 1075–82.

Grigoletti, S. S., G. Guindani, R. S. Moraes, J. P. Ribeiro, and E. Sprinz. (2013). Short-term folinic acid supplementation improves vascular reactivity in HIV-infected individuals: a randomized trial. *Nutrition* 29(6): 886–91.

Gross, R. L., J. V. Reid, P. M. Newberne, B. Burgess, R. Marston, and W. Hift. (1975). Depressed cell-mediated immunity in megaloblastic anemia due to folic acid deficiency. *American Journal of Clinical Nutrition* 28(3): 225–32.

Isanaka, S., F. Mugusi, C. Hawkins et al. (2012). Effect of high-dose vs. standard-dose multivitamin supplementation at the initiation of HAART on HIV disease progression and mortality in Tanzania: a randomized controlled trial. *JAMA* 308(15): 1535–44.

Jiamton, S., J. Pepin, R. Suttent et al. (2003). A randomized trial of the impact of multiple micronutrient supplementation on mortality among HIV-infected individuals living in Bangkok. *AIDS* 17(17): 2461–9.

Kamanna, V. S. and M. L. Kashyap. (2008). Mechanism of action of niacin. *American Journal of Cardiology* 101(8A): 20B–26B.

Kawai, K., R. Kupka, F. Mugusi et al. (2010a). A randomized trial to determine the optimal dosage of multivitamin supplements to reduce adverse pregnancy outcomes among HIV-infected women in Tanzania. *American Journal of Clinical Nutrition* 91(2): 391–7.

Kawai, K., G. Msamanga, K. Manji et al. (2010b). Sex differences in the effects of maternal vitamin supplements on mortality and morbidity among children born to HIV-infected women in Tanzania. *British Journal of Nutrition* 103(12): 1784–91.

Kawai, K., S. N. Meydani, W. Urassa et al. (2014). Micronutrient supplementation and T cell-mediated immune responses in patients with tuberculosis in Tanzania. *Epidemiology & Infection* 142(7): 1505–9.

Knox, T. A., D. Spiegelman, S. C. Skinner, and S. Gorbach. (2000). Diarrhea and abnormalities of gastrointestinal function in a cohort of men and women with HIV infection. *American Journal of Gastroenterology* 95(12): 3482–9.

Koka, P. S., B. D. Jamieson, D. G. Brooks, and J. A. Zack. (1999). Human immunodeficiency virus type 1-induced hematopoietic inhibition is independent of productive infection of progenitor cells in vivo. *Journal of Virology* 73(11): 9089–97.

Kreuzer, K. A. and J. K. Rockstroh. (1997). Pathogenesis and pathophysiology of anemia in HIV infection. *Annals of Hematology* 75(5–6): 179–87.

Kupka, R., K. P. Manji, R. J. Bosch et al. (2013). Multivitamin supplements have no effect on growth of Tanzanian children born to HIV-infected mothers. *Journal of Nutrition* 143(5): 722–7.

Kwak, H. K., C. M. Hansen, J. E. Leklem, K. Hardin, and T. D. Shultz. (2002). Improved vitamin B-6 status is positively related to lymphocyte proliferation in young women consuming a controlled diet. *Journal of Nutrition* 132(11): 3308–13.

Lin, C., A. Grandinetti, C. Shikuma et al. (2013). The effects of extended release niacin on lipoprotein sub-particle concentrations in HIV-infected patients. *Hawai'i Journal of Medicine & Public Health* 72(4): 123–7.

Liu, E., C. Duggan, K. P. Manji et al. (2013). Multivitamin supplementation improves haematologic status in children born to HIV-positive women in Tanzania. *Journal of the International AIDS Society* 16(1): 18022.

Luabeya, K. K., N. Mpontshane, M. Mackay et al. (2007). Zinc or multiple micronutrient supplementation to reduce diarrhea and respiratory disease in South African children: a randomized controlled trial. *PLOS One* 2(6): e541.

Lu'o'ng, K. v. q. and L. T. H. Nguyê~ n. (2013). The role of thiamine in HIV infection. *International Journal of Infectious Diseases* 17(4): e221–7.

Manji, K. P., C. M. McDonald, R. Kupka et al. (2014). Effect of multivitamin supplementation on the neurodevelopment of HIV-exposed Tanzanian infants: a randomized, double-blind, placebo-controlled clinical trial. *Journal of Tropical Pediatrics* 60(4): 279–86.

Masaisa, F., J. B. Gahutu, J. Mukiibi, J. Delanghe, and J. Philippé. (2011). Anemia in human immunodeficiency virus-infected and uninfected women in Rwanda. *American Journal of Tropical Medicine and Hygiene* 84(3): 456–60.

McClelland, R. S., J. M. Baeten, J. Overbaugh et al. (2004). Micronutrient supplementation increases genital tract shedding of HIV-1 in women: results of a randomized trial. *Journal of Acquired Immune Deficiency Syndromes* 37(5): 1657–63.

McCormick, D. B. and H. Chen. (1999). Update on interconversions of vitamin B-6 with its coenzyme. *Journal of Nutrition* 129(2): 325–7.

McGrath, N., D. Bellinger, J. Robins, G. I. Msamanga, E. Tronick, and W. W. Fawzi. (2006). Effect of maternal multivitamin supplementation on the mental and psychomotor development of children who are born to HIV-1-infected mothers in Tanzania. *Pediatrics* 117(2): e216–25.

Mda, S., J. M. van Raaij, F. P. de Villiers, U. E. MacIntyre, and F. J. Kok. (2010). Short-term micronutrient supplementation reduces the duration of pneumonia and diarrheal episodes in HIV-infected children. *Journal of Nutrition* 140(5): 969–74.

Merchant, A. T., G. Msamanga, E. Villamor et al. (2005). Multivitamin supplementation of HIV-positive women during pregnancy reduces hypertension. *Journal of Nutrition* 135(7): 1776–81.

Milman, N. (2012). Intestinal absorption of folic acid—new physiologic & molecular aspects. *Indian Journal of Medical Research* 136(5): 725–8.

Moses, A. V., S. Williams, M. L. Heneveld et al. (1996). Human immunodeficiency virus infection of bone marrow endothelium reduces induction of stromal hematopoietic growth factors. *Blood* 87(3): 919–25.

Ndeezi, G., T. Tylleskär, C. M. Ndugwa, and J. K. Tumwine. (2010). Effect of multiple micronutrient supplementation on survival of HIV-infected children in Uganda: a randomized, controlled trial. *Journal of the International AIDS Society* 13: 18.

Ndeezi, G., J. K. Tumwine, C. M. Ndugwa, B. J. Bolann, and T. Tylleskär. (2011). Multiple micronutrient supplementation improves vitamin B_{12} and folate concentrations of HIV infected children in Uganda: a randomized controlled trial. *Nutrition Journal* 10: 56.

Olofin, I. O., D. Spiegelman, S. Aboud, C. Duggan, G. Danaei, and W. W. Fawzi. (2014). Supplementation with multivitamins and vitamin A and incidence of malaria among HIV-infected Tanzanian women. *Journal of Acquired Immune Deficiency Syndromes* 67(Suppl. 4): S173–8.

Powers, H. J. (2003). Riboflavin (vitamin B-2) and health. *American Journal of Clinical Nutrition* 77(6): 1352–60.

Remacha, A. F., J. Cadafalch, P. Sardà, M. Barceló, and M. Fuster. (2003). Vitamin B-12 metabolism in HIV-infected patients in the age of highly active antiretroviral therapy: role of homocystreine in assessing vitamin B-12 status. *American Journal of Clinical Nutrition* 77(2): 420–4.

Safrin, S., B. L. Lee, and M. A. Sande. (1994). Adjunctive folinic acid with trimethoprim–sulfamethoxazole for *Pneumocystis carinii* pneumonia in AIDS patients is associated with an increased risk of therapeutic failure and death. *Journal of Infectious Diseases* 170(4): 912–7.

Smith Fawzi, M. C., S. F. Kaaya, J. Mbwambo et al. (2007). Multivitamin supplementation in HIV-positive pregnant women: impact on depression and quality of life in a resource-poor setting. *HIV Medicine* 8(4): 203–12.

Souza, S. A., D. C. Chow, E. J. Walsh, S. Ford, III, and C. Shikuma. (2010). Pilot study on the safety and tolerability of extended release niacin for HIV-infected patients with hypertriglyceridemia. *Hawaii Medical Journal* 69(5): 122–5.

Stover, P. J. (2009). One-carbon metabolism–genome interactions in folate-associated pathologies. *Journal of Nutrition* 139(12): 2402–5.

Sudfeld, C. R., C. Duggan, A. Histed et al. (2013). Effect of multivitamin supplementation on measles vaccine response among HIV-exposed uninfected Tanzanian infants. *Clinical Vaccine Immunology* 20(8): 1123–32.

Sullivan, P. S., D. L. Hanson, S. Y. Chu, J. L. Jones, and J. W. Ward. (1998). Epidemiology of anemia in human immunodeficiency virus (HIV)-infected persons: results from the multistate adult and adolescent spectrum of HIV disease surveillance project. *Blood* 91(1): 301–8.

Sundaram, U. (2000). Regulation of intestinal vitamin B2 absorption. Focus on 'Riboflavin uptake by human-derived colonic epithelial NCM460 cells.' *American Journal of Physiology—Cell Physiology* 278(2): C268–9.

Tamura, J., K. Kubota, H. Murakami et al. (1999). Immunomodulation by vitamin B_{12}: Augmentation of CD8+ T lymphocytes and natural killer (NK) cell activity in vitamin B_{12}-deficient patients by methyl-B_{12} treatment. *Clinical & Experimental Immunology* 116(1): 28–32.

Tang, A. M., N. M. Graham, A. J. Kirby, L. D. McCall, W. C. Willett, and A. J. Saah. (1993). Dietary micronutrient intake and risk of progression to acquired immunodeficiency syndrome (AIDS) in human immunodeficiency virus type 1 (HIV-1)-infected homosexual men. *American Journal of Epidemiology* 138(11): 937–51.

Tang, A. M., N. M. Graham, and A. J. Saah. (1996). Effects of micronutrient intake on survival in human immunodeficiency virus type 1 infection. *American Journal of Epidemiology* 143(12): 1244–56.

Tang, A. M., N. M. Graham, R. K. Chandra, and A. J. Saah. (1997). Low serum vitamin B-12 concentrations are associated with faster human immunodeficiency virus type 1 (HIV-1) disease progression. *Journal of Nutrition* 127(2): 345–51.

Theofylaktopoulou, D., A. Ulvik, Ø. Midttun et al. (2014). Vitamins B_2 and B_6 as determinants of kynurenines and related markers of interferon-gamma-mediated immune activation in the community-based Hordaland Health Study. *British Journal of Nutrition* 112(7): 1065–72.

Villamor, E., G. Msamanga, D. Spiegelman et al. (2002). Effect of multivitamin and vitamin A supplements on weight gain during pregnancy among HIV-1-infected women. *American Journal of Clinical Nutrition* 76(5): 1082–90.

Villamor, E., E. Saathoff, R. J. Bosch et al. (2005a). Vitamin supplementation of HIV-infected women improves postnatal child growth. *American Journal of Clinical Nutrition* 81: 880–8.

Villamor, E., E. Saathoff, K. Manji, G. Msamanga, D. J. Hunter, and W. W. Fawzi. (2005b). Vitamin supplements, socioeconomic status, and morbidity events as predictors of wasting in HIV-infected women from Tanzania. *American Journal of Clinical Nutrition* 82(4): 857–65.

Villamor, E., G. Msamanga, E. Saathoff, M. Fataki, K. Manji, and W. W. Fawzi. (2007). Effects of maternal vitamin supplements on malaria in children born to HIV-infected women. *American Journal of Tropical Medicine and Hygiene* 76(6): 1066–71.

Villamor, E., F. Mugusi, W. Urassa et al. (2008). A trial of the effect of micronutrient supplementation on treatment outcome, T cell counts, morbidity, and mortality in adults with pulmonary tuberculosis. *Journal of Infectious Diseases* 197(11): 1499–505.

Villamor, E., I. N. Koulinska, S. Aboud et al. (2010). Effect of vitamin supplements on HIV shedding in breast milk. *American Journal of Clinical Nutrition* 92(4): 881–6.

Webb, A. L., S. Aboud, J. Furtado et al. (2009). Effect of vitamin supplementation on breast milk concentrations of retinol, carotenoids and tocopherols in HIV-infected Tanzanian women. *European Journal of Clinical Nutrition* 63(3): 332–9.

WHO. (2012). *Guideline: Daily Iron and Folic Acid Supplementation in Pregnant Women.* Geneva: World Health Organization.

Woods, M. N., A. M. Tang, J. Forrester et al. (2003). Effect of dietary intake and protease inhibitors on serum vitamin B_{12} levels in a cohort of human immunodeficiency virus-positive patients. *Clinical Infectious Diseases* 37(Suppl. 2): S124–31.

Yetley, E. A. and C. L. Johnson. (2011). Folate and vitamin B-12 biomarkers in NHANES: history of their measurement and use. *American Journal of Clinical Nutrition* 94(1): 322S–331S.

Yetley, E. A., P. M. Coates, and C. L. Johnson. (2011a). Overview of a roundtable on NHANES monitoring of biomarkers of folate and vitamin B-12 status: Measurement procedure issues. *American Journal of Clinical Nutrition* 94(1): 297S–302S.

Yetley, E. A., C. M. Pfeiffer, K. W. Phinney et al. (2011b). Biomarkers of vitamin B-12 status in NHANES: A roundtable summary. *American Journal of Clinical Nutrition* 94(1): 313S–321S.

Yetley, E. A., C. M. Pfeiffer, K. W. Phinney et al. (2011c). Biomarkers of folate status in NHANES: a roundtable summary. *American Journal of Clinical Nutrition* 94(1): 303S–312S.

Ziegler, T. R., G. A. McComsey, J. K. Frediani, E. C. Millson, V. Tangpricha, and A. R. Eckard. (2014). Habitual nutrient intake in HIV-infected youth and associations with HIV-related factors. *AIDS Research and Human Retroviruses* 30(9): 888–95.

3 Iron and HIV/AIDS

Nabila R. Khondakar and Julia L. Finkelstein

CONTENTS

INTRODUCTION

IRON

Iron is a trace element required for essential physiological and cellular pathways in all life forms, including oxygen transport to tissues via hemoglobin, oxidative energy production, cell proliferation, and immune function (Camaschella, 2017). Iron is required for pathogen growth and is a key micronutrient in the context of immune function, with bidirectional associations between iron status and infection. Iron deficiency has been associated with impaired immune function, bactericidal macrophage activity, and T-cell function (Jonker and van Hensbroek, 2014). However, because pathogens also require iron for survival, host sequestration of iron is a defense mechanism and part of the innate immune response, and it has been associated with lower incidence of bacterial and viral infections (Murray et al., 1978; Weinberg, 1996; Berlim and Abeche, 2001). Findings from these studies have led to the use of iron deprivation to target some infections, such as *Mycobacterium tuberculosis* (Gomes, 1999; Pal et al., 2015).

IRON AND HIV

As with many infections, the associations between iron and HIV are complex and bidirectional. Whereas iron deficiency and anemia are common in HIV-infected individuals, higher iron status has also been associated with increased HIV infection and replication (Traoré and Meyer, 2004; Chang et al., 2015). Based on evidence that HIV utilizes iron to replicate, iron deprivation has been proposed as a potential strategy to target HIV-associated bacterial infections, as well as the course of HIV infection itself (Boelaert et al., 1996).

IRON AND HIV/AIDS: EVIDENCE FROM OBSERVATIONAL STUDIES

Anemia and Iron Deficiency Are Common in HIV-Infected Individuals

Iron deficiency is the most common micronutrient deficiency worldwide, resulting in poor health outcomes, impaired development, and increased susceptibility to infectious diseases and often coexisting with infection, including HIV (WHO, 2017). Iron deficiency is also a leading cause of anemia, accounting for approximately 50% of cases of anemia worldwide (50%; 95% CI, 47–53) (WHO, 2015). Anemia is one of the most common conditions in patients with HIV (Fuchs, 1993; Dikshit et al., 2009; Ogbe et al., 2012; Redig and Berliner, 2013). Epidemiological studies have noted a high prevalence of anemia in HIV-infected populations, ranging from 42.5% to 73% in HIV-infected adults in varying regions (Dikshit et al., 2009; Omoregie et al., 2009; Meidani et al., 2012; Petraro et al., 2016): HIV-infected pregnant women in southwestern Nigeria (Ezechi et al., 2013), injection drug users in Maryland (Semba et al., 2002), and children in Cape Town (Eley et al., 2002), in Thailand and Cambodia (Kosalaraksa et al., 2012), and in Italy (Castaldo 1996). Observational studies have also noted a higher prevalence of anemia and iron deficiency among HIV-infected individuals compared to HIV-uninfected individuals (Meda, 1999; Friis et al., 2001; Silva et al., 2001; Dairo et al., 2005; Lewis et al., 2007) and lower hemoglobin concentrations in HIV-infected individuals compared to HIV-uninfected individuals in the same setting (Friis et al., 2001; Dairo et al., 2005; Masaisa et al., 2011; Ogbe et al., 2012; Mugisha et al., 2013; Swetha et al., 2015).

Anemia and Iron Deficiency Have Been Associated with Adverse Health Outcomes in HIV-Infected Individuals

Iron deficiency has been associated with adverse health outcomes in HIV-infected populations, including lower CD4 T-cell counts, increased HIV disease progression, and increased risk of opportunistic infections (Gordeuk et al., 2001; Malvoisin et al., 2014). Anemia has also been associated with poorer prognoses in HIV-infected patients, including lower CD4 T-cell counts (Antelman et al., 2000; Eley et al., 2002; Salomé and Grotto, 2002; Dikshit et al., 2009; Chatterjee et al., 2010; Finkelstein et al., 2012; Petraro et al., 2013; Shen et al., 2013) and HIV-related mortality (O'Brien et al., 2005; Finkelstein et al., 2012; Shen et al., 2013; Porter et al., 2015). For example, in a study of HIV-infected patients in Mskutfi, Nigeria, 55.2% of patients with lower CD4 T-cell counts (<200 cells/mm^3) were anemic compared to 32.5% of patients with higher CD4 T-cell count (≥200 cells/mm^3) (Ogbe et al., 2012).

Elevated Iron Status

In contrast, elevated iron status (e.g., serum ferritin) has also been associated with adverse health outcomes in observational studies in HIV-infected populations. For example, in a study among 571 asymptomatic HIV-infected patients in Spain (86.2% on ART and 36.3% diagnosed with AIDS), iron overload (i.e., serum ferritin ≥ 200 µg/L in women and > 300 µg/L in men) was associated with lower CD4 T-cell counts (<350 cells/µL) and greater prevalence of AIDS cases (with iron overload, 49.2% diagnosed with AIDS; without iron overload, 34.6%; $p = 0.02$) (López-Calderón et al., 2015). Among 168 HIV-infected individuals in Spain, individuals with lower CD4 T-cell counts (<300 × 10^6/L) had significantly higher ferritin levels compared to those with higher CD4 T-cell counts (mean, 330 vs. 261–418 µg/L; $p < 0.001$) (Riera et al., 1994). Observational studies have also noted associations between higher serum ferritin concentrations and increased HIV disease progression (Tohill et al., 2007; Rawat et al., 2009), lower CD4 T-cell counts (Dikshit et al., 2009), and higher HIV RNA viral load (Friis et al., 2003). However, some of these studies did not assess or adjust for inflammation, such as C-reactive protein (CRP), which constrains the interpretation of findings.

IRON SUPPLEMENTATION IN THE CONTEXT OF HIV: A DOUBLE-EDGED SWORD?

Iron is required for survival by both the host and virus, and iron supplementation is the standard of care for prevention and treatment of anemia (WHO, 2012). However, associations between elevated iron stores and increased HIV disease progression and mortality raise concern regarding the safety and efficacy of iron supplementation in the context of HIV, particularly in iron-replete individuals. Iron may be a "double-edged sword"—that is, because HIV also utilizes iron for growth and replication, iron interventions (i.e., additional iron in circulation) may be harmful in the context of HIV infection (Sunder-Plassmann et al., 1999; Clark and Semba, 2001; Gordeuk et al., 2001).

RESEARCH GAPS

Findings from observational studies to date suggest that the associations between iron and HIV are complex and likely bidirectional. Emerging evidence regarding the associations between higher iron status and advanced HIV disease progression and mortality have raised concerns regarding the use of iron supplementation in the context of HIV. However, current World Health Organization (WHO) guidelines do not differ according to HIV status, and there are no specific guidelines for iron supplementation in HIV-infected populations. Further research is needed regarding iron supplementation in the context of antiretroviral therapy (ART). Antiretroviral therapy regimens have had varying effects on iron status in different HIV-infected populations. Whereas prenatally administered zidovudine has been associated with maternal and infant anemia postpartum, highly active antiretroviral therapy (HAART) has also been associated with increased hemoglobin concentrations in non-pregnant HIV-infected adults (Widen et al., 2015; Dryden-Peterson et al., 2011). Cotrimoxazole, recommended as prophylaxis for infants born to HIV-infected mothers, has been associated with increased risk of anemia (Makubi et al., 2015). Conflicting findings on the efficacy of iron supplementation, as well as uncertainty regarding the role of antiretroviral therapy, highlight the need for future studies to elucidate the multifactorial etiology of anemia in HIV-infected populations. Further research is necessary to evaluate the role of iron status in HIV infection and to establish the efficacy and safety of iron supplementation in HIV-infected populations, particularly in the context of antiretroviral therapy.

OBJECTIVES

The objective of this review was to examine the role of iron in the context of HIV/AIDS, with an emphasis on evidence from randomized clinical trials and prospective cohort studies. We examine the efficacy and safety of iron supplementation on health outcomes among HIV-infected individuals, including HIV disease progression, mortality, and hematological status, and adverse maternal and child health outcomes. We also examine the directionality of association between HIV and iron. First, we evaluate the association between HIV and hematologic outcomes, such as iron status and anemia. Second, we review the association between anemia and poor iron status and HIV-related outcomes. We then discuss research gaps and the implications of findings for clinical care and public health practice, with an emphasis on resource-limited settings.

METHODS

A structured literature search was conducted using MEDLINE® electronic databases. Relevant Medical Subject Heading (MeSH®) terms were used to identify published studies through November 18, 2015. The MeSH terms and search strategy are presented in Figure 3.1. Initial inclusion criteria for this review were the availability of an abstract and the availability of data on iron (intake, status, or supplementation) and HIV. Abstracts of all studies were searched, and full-text articles were retrieved, indexed, and assessed for data on iron and HIV. The following iron biomarkers were

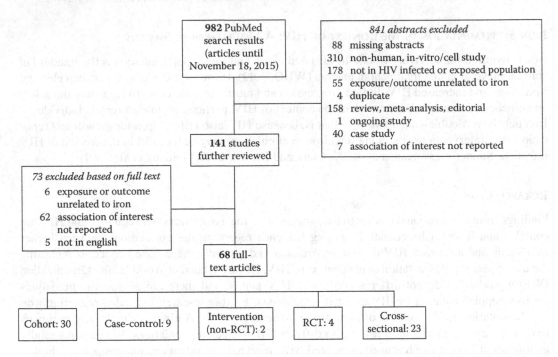

FIGURE 3.1 Search strategy (search date closed November 18, 2015; last updated July 11, 2016). Randomized controlled trials (RCTs) are RCTs with intervention as iron and RCTs with intervention as HAART or HAART/iron. Search terms: (HIV Infections[MeSH] OR HIV[MeSH] OR hiv[tw] OR hiv-1*[tw] OR hiv-2*[tw] OR hiv1[tw] OR hiv2[tw] OR hiv infect*[tw] OR human immunodeficiency virus[tw] OR human immunedeficiency virus[tw] OR human immuno-deficiency virus[tw] OR human immune-deficiency virus[tw] OR ((human immun*) AND (deficiency virus)) OR acquired immunedeficiency syndrome[tw] OR aids[tw] OR acquired immunodeficiency syndrome[tw] OR acquired immunodeficiency syndrome[MeSH] OR acquired immune-deficiency syndrome[tw] OR acquired immuno-deficiency syndrome[tw] OR ((acquired immun*) AND (deficiency syndrome[tw])) OR "sexually transmitted diseases, viral"[MESH:NoExp]) AND (ferrous OR iron OR ferric OR iron compounds[mh]).

included in this review: hemoglobin, serum ferritin (SF), soluble transferrin receptor (sTfR), and total body iron (TBI); hepcidin concentrations; and indicators of inflammation, including C-reactive protein (CRP) and α-1-acid glycoprotein (AGP). The following HIV-related data were included in this review: all-cause mortality, AIDS-related mortality, WHO-defined HIV disease stage, HIV disease progression, opportunistic infections, CD4 and CD8 T-cell counts, neopterin, HIV RNA viral load, HIV RNA viral shedding, and antiretroviral therapy, including HAART and combination ART therapy (cART). For studies among HIV-infected pregnant women, we evaluated the following:

- *Maternal outcomes*—Maternal weight gain during pregnancy, anemia, and hematological status
- *Pregnancy outcomes*—Miscarriage (<28 weeks gestation), stillbirth (≥28 weeks gestation), fetal loss (miscarriage or stillbirth), gestational age at delivery, preterm birth (<37 weeks gestation), birthweight, low birthweight (<2500 g), small for gestational age (SGA; birthweight < 10th percentile for gestational age), mother-to-child transmission of HIV, and breast milk composition
- *Infant outcomes*—HIV infection; other infections (e.g., malaria, tuberculosis); anthropometry and growth (i.e., weight, length, head circumference, mid-upper arm circumference), including weight for age (WAZ), weight for length (WLZ), and length for age (LAZ) WHO z-scores (underweight, WAZ < –2; wasting, WLZ < –2; stunting, LAZ < –2); anemia; and iron biomarkers.

Available abstracts of all studies were searched, full-text articles were extracted and reviewed, and the following inclusion criteria were applied: (1) human studies, (2) HIV-infected individuals, and (3) availability of data on iron status, intake, or supplementation and HIV-related outcomes. All observational cross-sectional, cohort, and case-control studies, as well as randomized trials and interventions and quasi-randomized and uncontrolled trials meeting participant and methodological criteria, were included in supplementary tables. However, the main focus of this chapter is on evidence from randomized trials ($n = 4$), interventions ($n = 2$), and prospective cohort studies ($n = 30$). Sources were retrieved, collected, indexed, and assessed for iron and HIV-related data. Bibliographies of published studies and manual searches of related articles were used to identify additional sources. An additional search was conducted to find review articles, which were examined to cross-reference other relevant studies. A standardized data table was used to extract and summarize key information from all studies that met the aforementioned inclusion criteria. As part of this protocol, publication date, authors, study design, setting, target population, definitions of exposures and outcomes, main findings, and study limitations were recorded.

RESULTS

SEARCH STRATEGY RESULTS

The structured literature search resulted in 982 abstracts. After 841 articles were excluded ($n = 88$ missing abstracts, $n = 310$ non-human/laboratory studies, $n = 178$ not in HIV-infected populations, $n = 55$ exposure or outcome not related to iron, $n = 4$ duplicates, $n = 158$ reviews/meta-analyses/ editorials, $n = 1$ ongoing study, $n = 40$ case studies, $n = 7$ missing data on the associations between iron and HIV), 141 full-text articles were extracted for further review (Figure 3.1). After excluding 73 additional articles that did not meet inclusion criteria ($n = 6$ exposure or outcome not related to iron, $n = 62$ missing data on the associations between iron and HIV, $n = 4$ not in English), a total of 68 studies were included in this review: 23 cross-sectional, 9 case-control, 30 cohort studies, 4 randomized controlled trials (RCTs) (i.e., 3 RCTs with iron supplementation as the intervention and 1 RCT with ART as the intervention), and 2 non-RCT intervention studies of iron supplementation. Findings from these studies are summarized in Tables 3.1 to 3.5.

TABLE 3.1
Randomized Controlled Trials

Study	Sample	Location	Enrollment	Methods	Exposure	Outcomes	Main Findings
Esan et al. (2013)	196 HIV-infected children (6–59 months) with moderate anemia (Hb 7.0–9.9 g/dL)	Southern Malawi	Study was conducted from January 2009 to August 2010. Participants were seen 1, 2, 3, and 6 months after recruitment during 6-month follow-up.	Participants were randomized to one of two arms for 3 months: (1) iron + multivitamins ($n = 100$), or (2) multivitamins alone ($n = 96$). Blood samples were taken at enrollment. Participants were followed for 6 months. All participants received routine cotrimoxazole prophylaxis.	*Treatment*: 3 mg/kg/day of elemental iron and multivitamins (1500 IU/mL vitamin A, 35 mg/mL vitamin C, and 400 IU/mL vitamin D) *Control*: Placebo and multivitamins for 3 months	Anemia (Hb <11 g/dL) Moderate anemia (Hb 7.0–9.9 g/dL) AIDS (CD4 T-cell percentage <20%) Iron deficiency (SF levels <30 µg/dL for CRP level of ≥5.0 mg/L and <12 µg/dL for CRP level of <5.0 mg/L) Malaria (asexual *Plasmodium falciparum* parasites on Giemsa-stained thick blood smear microscopy) Parasite density (number of parasites per 200 white blood cells in thick smear)	Participants receiving iron supplementation + multivitamins compared to placebo + multivitamins: • Had greater CD4 T-cell % response (AMD, 6.00; 95% CI, 1.84–10.16; $p = 0.005$) at 3 months • Had increased risk of malaria at 3 months (IR, 78.1 vs. 36.0; AIRR, 2.68; 95% CI, 1.08–6.63; $p = 0.03$) and 6 months (IR, 120.2 vs. 71.7; AIRR, 1.81; 95% CI, 1.04–3.16; $p = 0.04$) • Had reduced risk of progression to AIDS only in iron-deficient children (IRR, 0.25; 95% CI, 0.08–0.83; $p = 0.02$, p-interaction = 0.07)
Semba et al. (2007)	458 female injection drug users with HCV (320 HIV negative, 138 HIV positive)	Baltimore, MD	Trial commenced enrollment on September 1, 2002, and follow-up ended on September 30, 2005.	Phase 3 double-blind, randomized clinical trial randomized participants to one of two arms for 12 months: (1) iron and micronutrients ($n = 149$), or (2) micronutrients alone ($n = 159$).	*Treatment*: Micronutrients (5000 IU vitamin A, 400 IU vitamin D, 30 IU vitamin E, 60 mg vitamin C, 1.5 mg thiamin, 1.7 mg riboflavin, 20 mg niacin, 2 mg vitamin B₆, 400 mg folate, 10 mg pantothenic acid,	Anemia (Hb <12 g/dL) Iron deficiency anemia (Hb <12 g/dL and plasma ferritin <30 ng/mL) Iron deficiency (plasma ferritin <30 ng/mL and transferrin saturation <16%) CD4 T-cell differences CD8 T-cell differences	Among HIV-infected women only, there were no significant differences between the groups in plasma viral load (HIV or HCV) at enrollment, 6 months, or 12 months: • Mean log₁₀ HIV RNA at 6 months for the iron group was 3.8 copies/mL (SD, 1.1); for the no-iron group, 3.7 copies/mL (SD, 1.0) ($p = 0.75$). • Mean log₁₀ HIV RNA at 12 months for the iron group was 3.7 copies/mL (SD, 1.2); for the no-iron group, 4.1 copies/mL (SD, 1.0) ($p = 0.19$).

Participants were screened for HIV-1 using ELISA, confirmed by western blot.

Participants were eligible if not pregnant and SF < 200 ng/mL at time of screening.

6 mg vitamin B_{12}, 15 mg zinc, and 20 mg selenium plus 18 mg iron daily)

Control: Micronutrients without iron daily

Among HIV-infected women only, there were no significant differences in CD8 T-cell count. Participants receiving iron and micronutrients compared to micronutrients alone had higher CD4 T-cell counts at 6 months: iron group mean was 388 cells/μL (SD, 277); no-iron group mean was 260 (SD, 151) (p = 0.01).

Among all women, both HIV positive and negative, participants receiving iron and micronutrients compared to micronutrients alone

- Had significantly higher Hb at 3 months, 6 months, and 9 months (p = 0.005, p = 0.003, p = 0.058, respectively)

- Had a significantly lower proportion of women with anemia at 3 months (p = 0.026) and 6 months (p = 0.008) but not at 9 months (p = 0.18) or 12 months (p = 0.5)

- Had a significantly lower proportion of women with iron deficiency anemia at 6 months (p = 0.003) but not at 12 months (p = 0.18)

- Had a significantly lower proportion of women with ferritin < 30 ng/mL at 6 months (p = 0.0001) and at 12 months (p = 0.0018)

(continued)

TABLE 3.1 (continued)
Randomized Controlled Trials

Study	Sample	Location	Enrollment	Methods	Exposure	Outcomes	Main Findings
Olsen et al. (2004)	45 HIV-infected adults	Western Kenya	Study was conducted from November 1994 to January 1996. Data are based on historical iron trial from November 1994 to January 1996 (see Olsen et al., 2000).	Participants randomized to one of two groups for 4 months: (1) iron (60 mg) twice weekly ($n = 22$), or (2) placebo twice weekly ($n = 23$) Original historical iron trial assessed effects of iron supplementation on helminth reinfections. HIV status was tested on repository samples from original trial. Participants with Hb ≤ 80 g/dL were excluded.	*Treatment*: 60 mg ferrous dextran twice weekly *Control*: Placebo tablets twice weekly	Viral load (geq/mL)	Participants receiving iron compared to placebo had higher viral load at baseline (5.57 geq/mL vs. 4.93 geq/mL; $p = 0.02$). There were no differences in viral load at 4 months (0.6 vs. 0.8 log geq/mL; $p = 0.31$).
Widen et al. (2015)	537 HIV-infected mothers (gestational age ≤ 30 weeks; CD4 > 200 cells/μL) and their infants	Lilongwe, Malawi	Breastfeeding, Antiretrovirals, and Nutrition (BAN) study was conducted 2004–2010 (NCT00164736).	2 × 3 factorial design in which HIV-infected mother and infant pairs were randomized at delivery to one of 6 groups for 28 weeks (only 2 of which are currently relevant). Of 537 mothers and infants for whom additional iron marker data were available (BAN "subsample"), 262 belonged to the following groups: (1) maternal ARV (initially	*Treatment:* Maternal ARV without LNS ($n = 85^a$) for 28 weeks *Control:* No ARV and no LNS ($n = 177^a$) for 28 weeks	Maternal anemia (Hb < 120 g/L) Maternal iron deficiency (ferritin < 15 ng/mL and sTfR > 8.3 mg/L) Tissue iron depletion (sTfR >8.3 mg/L) Depleted iron stores (ferritin < 15 ng/mL) Changes in maternal and infant Hb, ferritin, and transferrin receptors Infant anemia (inflammation-adjusted Hb <105 g/L)	Maternal HAART alone, without LNS, compared to control at 24 weeks postpartum: • Was associated with increased risk of tissue iron depletion (RR, 3.1; 95% CI, 1.32–7.32; $p = 0.01$) • Was not associated with increased risk of depleted iron stores (RR, 0.99; 95% CI, 0.68–1.44; $p = 0.94$) • Was not associated with risk of anemia (RR, 1.14; 95% CI, 0.78–1.68; $p = 0.49$) No differences in any iron status outcomes among infants born to mothers on HAART compared to controls

Infant iron deficiency (inflammation-adjusted ferritin = 12 ng/mL; TfR > 8.3 mg/L)

zidovudine, lamivudine, nevirapine; after the first 39 women were randomized, nelfinavir replaced nevirapine, and lopinavir + ritonavir replaced nelfinavir) (n = 85), or (2) control (n = 177).

Maternal and infant Hb was measured at birth and at 2, 6, 12, 18, and 24 weeks postpartum. In the first week after delivery, all mothers and infants were given single doses of nevirapine and twice daily lamivudine and zidovudine.

ª See Table 4 of Widen et al. (2015).

Note: AIRR, adjusted incidence rate ratio; AMD, average mean difference; CI, confidence interval; CRP, c-reactive protein; geq/mL, genome equivalents per milliliter; Hb, hemoglobin; HCV, hepatitis C virus; IR, incidence rate; IRR, incidence rate ratio; RR, risk ratio; SD, standard deviation; SF, serum ferritin; sTfR, soluble transferrin receptor; ZDV, zidovudine.

TABLE 3.2

Intervention Studies

Study	Sample	Location	Period	Methods	Exposure	Outcomes	Main Findings
van Eijk et al. (2007)	3108 post-partum women with known HIV status	Western Kenya	Before intervention but during pregnancy (June 1996 to September 1997) After iron supplementation but before implementation of IPTp–SP (September 1997 to March 1999) After implementation of IPTp–SP—March 1999 to June 2000 (not relevant)	Women were stratified by 3 periods of enrollment (of which 2 are relevant), each period lasting the duration of pregnancy: (1) control (n = 1172) or (2) routine iron supplementation (60 mg, 3× per day) plus 5 mg folic acid per day (n = 1140). Malaria status was assessed using placental and peripheral thick blood films stained with 10% Giemsa. HIV status was assessed using initial SeroStrip HIV-1/2 and Capillus HIV-1/HIV-2; western blot on discordant samples.	HIV infection Group 1: Control (no iron supplementation) (n = 308 HIV-infected, n = 864 HIV-uninfected) Group 2: Routine iron supplementation (60 mg elemental iron, 3× daily) and 5 mg folic acid once daily (n = 257 HIV-infected, n = 883 HIV-uninfected)	Maternal anemia (Hb < 11g/dL) Severe anemia (Hb < 8 g/dL) Placental malaria (presence of asexual parasites in thick smear) Whether above outcomes differed by HIV status	Regression model—Iron supplementation was associated with increase in postpartum Hb over time, with the greatest increase being observed in HIV-uninfected women, but the difference was not significant (p = 0.3 interaction between HIV and period). During third trimester—Overall, 76.7% of women were anemic: 86.1% of the HIV-seroinfected women vs. 73.8% of the HIV-seronegative women (OR, 2.21; 95% CI, 1.76–2.77). At delivery—There was a significant difference in the proportion of anemia between HIV-infected and HIV-uninfected women: 63.7% vs. 50.4% (OR, 1.72; 95% CI, 1.46–2.04).

Salmon-Ceron et al. (1995) and Jacobus (1999) informed main findings and exposure	200 patients with AIDS as defined by 1987 CDC criteria	Multiple	Enrolled between February 1989 and August 1991	Inadvertent randomized intervention study	Group 1: Iron protoxolate–dapsone (30 mg/day soluble iron and 50 mg/day dapsone) ($n = 93$)	Mortality	Mortality in patients who received iron protoxolate–dapsone was 42% compared to 21% in patients who received aerosolized pentamidine.
				Patients with AIDS were inadvertently randomized to two groups for secondary prophylaxis of pneumocystosis: (1) dapsone (50 mg/day) plus 30 mg soluble iron, or (2) aerosolized pentaidine (300 mg every month).	Group 2: Aerosolized pentamidine (300 mg administered over a 30-minute period through jet nebulizer once a month) ($n = 103$)		In iron–dapsone group, the relative risk of mortality was 2.18 (95% CI, 1.27–3.74; $p < 0.003$), adjusted for age, time since diagnosis of AIDS, and CD4 cell count.
				Study was prematurely closed due to excess mortality in the dapsone group.			The estimated mortality rates at 18 months for the two groups were 53.1% and 24.6%, respectively ($p < 0.003$; log rank test).

Note: CDC, Centers for Disease Control and Prevention; CI, confidence interval; IPTp, intermittent preventive treatment in pregnancy; OR, odds ratio; SP, sulfadoxine–pyrimethamine.

TABLE 3.3
Cohort Studies

Study	Sample	Location	Methods	Exposure	Outcomes	Main Findings
Shet et al. (2015)	240 HIV perinatally infected children (2–12 years old); ART exposed and ART naive included; excluded if had blood transfusion within 6 weeks of enroll-ment	Bangalore and Chennai, India	Iron was given for 3 months based on WHO guidelines for iron therapy; if subjects remained anemic, iron continued for 6 months. Subjects were enrolled at 3 sites, followed for 1 year (mean age, 7.7 years), and assessed every 3 months. Iron biomarkers (ferritin, soluble transferrin receptors) and micronutrient levels (vitamins A and B_{12}, folate) were measured. 24-hour dietary recall was compared to RDA at enrollment.	Subjects received colloidal form of iron-containing ferric hydroxide with elemental iron; 53% were prescribed a dose of 3 mg/kg body weight, according to WHO criteria; 43.3% were on antiretroviral therapy (ZDV or stavudine, with lamivudine and nevirapine, efavirenz, or lopinaivr/ritonavir) at baseline. Dietary intake (%RDA)	Anemia: 6–59 months (Hb < 11.0 g/dL), 5–11 years (Hb < 11.5 g/dL), >12 years (Hb < 12.0 g/dL); Severe anemia: 6–59 months (Hb < 7.0 g/dL), 5 years and older (Hb < 8.0 g/dL); Iron deficiency: soluble transferring receptor-log ferritin index > 1.5; Low CD4 T-cell count defined as <25%; Inflammation CRP > 1.0 mg/dL; Anemia of inflammation: sTfR/lf ≥ 1.5 plus CRP > 1.0 mg/dL; Advanced WHO clinical defined as stages 3 or 4	Low CD4 T-cell independent risk factor for anemia: anemic (66.4%) vs. non-anemic (41%) (OR, 3.2; 95% CI, 1.8–5.7). Viral load ≥ 400 copies/mL independent risk factor for anemia: anemic (82.4%) vs. non-anemic (52.8%) (OR, 2.4; 95% CI, 1.1–5.4; $p = 0.035$). Iron intake was associated with decreased trend in clinical severity; severe WHO clinical stage (3, 4) was 25.7% at baseline and 10.9% at 1-year follow up. A similar, but smaller, decrease was observed in children who did not receive iron (16.7% at baseline to 12.5% at 1-year follow-up). In iron group vs. no-iron group: • Number of hospitalizations for concurrent infections (pneumonia, TB, other) was 3 in iron group and 2 in non-iron group. • No malaria was reported in either group. • No difference was observed in CD4 T-cell percent after 1 year (iron, 26.5% vs. no-iron, 26.0%; $p = 0.7$). • At baseline, there was a significant difference in prevalence of advanced WHO clinical stage: (iron, 25.7% vs. non-iron, 16.7%; $p = 0.04$). • At 1 year, there was no difference in prevalence of advanced WHO clinical stage (iron, 10.9 vs. non-iron, 12.5%; $p = 1.0$)

Study	Location	Population	Study description	Definitions	Results
Flax et al. (2015)	Lilongwe, Malawi	690 pregnant women with HIV	BAN study (see Table 3.1) HAART combination regimen (protease inhibitor-based triple therapy): (1) combination of lamivudine and ZDV, (2) nelfinavir, or (3) lopinavir/ritonavir. Iron–folic acid (40 mg elemental iron, 0.25 mg folic acid, daily) was given to all mothers from the first visit during pregnancy through 1-week postpartum.	Anemia: Hb < 120 g/L at baseline and 24 weeks CRP > 5 mg/L at 24 weeks AGP > 1 g/L at 24 weeks CD4 < 250 cells/mm³ at 24 weeks Concentrations of Hb, sTfR, folate, ferritin at 24 weeks	HAART was not associated with ferritin or Hb concentrations but was associated with greater sTfR concentrations (suggesting poorer iron status) and lower plasma folate concentrations (−12%; $p = 0.04$). There was no difference in proportion of women in the four groups with anemia at 24 weeks (control, 19% vs. HAART, 18% vs. LNS, 16% vs. LNS + HAART, 14%; $p = 0.69$).
Minchella et al. (2015)	The Gambia	196 HIV-infected antiretroviral-naïve (age ≥ 18 years; existing plasma aliquot within 3 months of first HIV diagnosis)	Retrospective cohort study with 10-year follow up Patients received free clinical care at Medical Research Council Unit in The Gambia. Baseline plasma hepcidin was measured by competitive enzyme immunoassay within 3 months of HIV diagnosis. CD4 T-cell counts were obtained by FACScan. All-cause mortality was ascertained every 3 months. Cotrimoxazole prophylaxis was the standard of care.	HIV infection Hepcidin levels (by tertile): lowest tertile (≤7.8 µg/L), intermediate (>7.8 to <57.6 µg/L), or elevated (≥57.6 µg/L) Anemia in men: Hb < 13 g/dL Anemia in women: Hb < 12 g/dL Inflammation, as measured by alpha-1-antichymotrypsin (ACT) levels (in g/L): elevated (>0.6), normal (0.2–0.6), lower (<0.2) CD4 T-cell count: low (<200 cells/µg), normal (200–500 cells/µg), elevated (>500 cells/µg)	Elevated hepcidin was associated with greater all-cause mortality in a dose-dependent manner: intermediate vs. lowest tertile (unadjusted HR, 1.95; 95% CI, 1.22– 3.10), upper vs. lowest tertile (unadjusted HR, 3.02; 95% CI, 1.91– 4.78). Anemia was associated with lower absolute CD4 T-cell count at HIV diagnosis: anemia (233 cells/µL; 77,498); no anemia (408 cells/µL; 243,699) ($p = 0.003$). Anemia was associated with higher hepcidin at HIV diagnosis ($p = 0.06$). Increasing hepcidin was associated with iron homeostasis biomarkers (higher ferritin and lower transferrin, Hb, and sTfR), inflammation (higher ACT), and lower CD4 T-cell count, BMI, advancing age, and male gender ($p < 0.001$ for all, except $p = 0.021$ for Hb).

(continued)

TABLE 3.3 (continued)
Cohort Studies

Study	Sample	Location	Methods	Exposure	Outcomes	Main Findings
Armitage et al. (2014)	Multiple cohorts: (1) 12 initially HIV-seronegative plasma donors who acquired acute HIV infection; (2) 17 men who have sex with men; (3) 20 healthy male controls	—	Multiple measurements of plasma concentrations of hepcidin, SAA, C-CRP, IFN-alpha, ferritin, IL-10, IL-18, TNF-alpha, IL-6, IL-22, and plasma iron were taken.	HIV infection Setpoint viral load: mean $\log_{10}$ plasma viral loads measured between 3 and 12 months after infection	Changes in hepcidin levels	Acute infection was observed in 12 initially seronegative plasma donors; within 15 days of infection, the increase in hepcidin levels was significant ($p < 0.01$). Among 17 men who have sex with men, hepcidin elevation occurred early in infection and later stabilized at setpoint viremia: geometric mean hepcidin for days 0–60 was 47.8 ng/mL (95% CI, 34.1–66.8; 42 samples measured); for days 89–366, it was 33.9 ng/mL (95% CI, 22.7–50.8; 36 samples measured) ($p = 0.0378$, paired t-test, $n = 17$ pairs). In the chronic stage of infection, HIV-infected individuals ($n = 31$) compared to uninfected individuals: • Had significantly higher hepcidin levels (19.13 vs. 8.35 ng/mL; $p = 0.0089$) • Had higher acute-phase proteins CRP, SAA, and cytokines IL-10, IL-18, and TNF-alpha • Had no difference in IL-6 There was no significant association between hepcidin and plasma viral load ($r = 0.195$, $p = 0.312$) in any cohort. Changes in hepcidin were associated with changes in SAA in every cohort.

Study	Population	Location	Methods	Variables	Measures	Results
Minchella et al. (2014)	196 HIV-infected antiretroviral-naïve (age ≥ 18 years; existing plasma aliquot within 3 months of first HIV diagnosis)	The Gambia	See above; participants were followed for 496 person-years (median follow-up, 1.8 years; IQR, 1.3–2.3).	Hepcidin levels (by quartiles): lowest (<3.4 ng/mL); second (3.4–22.1 ng/mL); third (22.1–85.9 ng/mL); highest (>85.9 ng/mL)	TB incidence rate per 1000 person-years	Elevated hepcidin was associated with greater incident TB: 32 incident cases of TB Dose–response association: upper hepcidin quartile accounted for 40% of all incident TB cases; for upper hepcidin quartile vs. lower three quartiles combined, twofold increase in the incidence of TB (unadjusted IRR, 2.05; 95% CI, 1.01–4.16); in adjusted models, only the model with hepcidin adjusted for HIV type was statistically significant (adjusted IRR, 2.10; 95% CI, 1.03–4.26)
Wisaksana et al. (2013)	127 HIV-infected patients	Bandung, Indonesia	Nested case-control study Group 1: 42 HIV-infected patients starting TB treatment > 30 days after enrollment Group 2: 42 HIV-infected patients matched for age, gender, CD4 count to case group (matched controls) Group 3: 43 HIV-infected patients with CD4 greater than 200 cells/mm³ (unmatched controls) Iron biomarkers, including hepcidin, were compared using samples collected at enrollment with serum hepcidin reference values. ART was begun if (1) HIV stage 4, (2) HIV stage 3 with CD4 < 350 cells/mm³, or (3) HIV stage 1 or 2 with CD4 < 200 cells/mm³.	HIV infection stage Anemia: mild (Hb 10.5–12.99 g/dL for men and 10.5–11.99 g/dL for women), moderate (Hb 8.0–10.49 g/dL), severe (Hb < 8.0 g/dL) ART status: CD4 count and hepatitis C co-infection	Serum hepcidin levels Iron parameters	Advanced HIV infection was associated with elevated serum hepcidin and elevated ferritin. Inverse relationship was observed between hepcidin and CD4 count and between hepcidin and Hb.

(continued)

TABLE 3.3 (continued)
Cohort Studies

Study	Sample	Location	Methods	Exposure	Outcomes	Main Findings
Kruger et al. (2013)	58 HIV-infected children	South Africa	Prospective (2-year) cohort study in children who attended outpatient Harriet Shezi Children's Clinic, Chris Hani Barahwanath Hospital, Soweto HIV/AIDS outcomes were compared in iron-deficient and iron-sufficient children after 18 months on HAART; no children were previously exposed to ART. Data (Hb, CD4 T-cell cell counts, viral load, anthropometric measurements) were collected at baseline before HAART began and at 6, 12, and 18 months. STfR was measured at baseline and at 18 months.	At baseline, multivitamin syrup (not containing iron) was provided to all children. Children < 6 years were given vitamin A every 6 months (as part of national vitamin A program). Dietary iron was assessed in all subjects. HAART was given to all subjects.	Iron deficiency: sTfR > 9.4 mg/L Mild anemia: children <5 years (Hb 100–109 g/L), children 5–11 years (Hb 110–114 g/L), children 12–24 years (Hb 110–119 g/L) Moderate anemia: children <5 years (Hb 70–99 g/L), children 5–14 years (Hb 80–109 g/L) CD4 T-cell count (%) Log viral load (copies/mL) Anthropometric measurements	At baseline, 15.5% were iron deficient and had marginally significantly higher viral load compared to iron sufficient ($p = 0.05$). In univariate regression analysis, CD4 T-cell% was not associated with ID (CD4 T-cell% > 25% vs. CD4 T-cell% ≤ 25%; OR, 0.80; 95% CI, 0.42–1.58; $p = 0.53$). After 18 months on HAART: • Log viral load (copies/mL) were not significantly different (iron deficient, 1.6 ± 0.9 vs. iron sufficient, 1.4 ± 0.04; $p = 0.99$). • No difference was observed in CD4 T-cell% (iron deficient, 29.0 ± 7.2 vs. iron sufficient, 29.9 ± 8.2; $p = 0.7$). • No difference was observed in Hb (g/L) (iron deficient, 122 ± 10 vs. iron sufficient, 126 ± 8; $p = 0.18$). • Proportion of anemic children decreased (baseline, 31.7% vs. 18 months, 3.8%), but proportion of iron-deficient children increased (baseline, 15.2% vs. 18 months, 37.2%). • Incidence of iron deficiency increased from 15.2% to 37.2% after 18 months.

Study	Sample	Country	Study design	Definitions	Results
Isanaka et al., (2012)	840 HIV-infected women (subset of 1078 HIV-infected women) and their children (808 with known HIV status)	Tanzania	Nested prospective cohort study as part of TOV Child health was studied from ages 2–5 years. Repeated measures of maternal anemia and hypochromic microcytosis were made over time. Hypochromic microcytosis was used as proxy for iron deficiency.	Maternal anemia: severe (<8.5 g/dL), moderate (8.5–11.0 g/dL), absent (≥11.0 g/dL) Iron deficiency (hypochromasia): severe (≥25% and microcytic cells observed), moderate (< 2% and microcytic cells observed), mild (any hypochromasia without microcytosis), absent (no hypochromasia)	Maternal anemia was associated with greater risk of child mortality (severe anemia HR, 2.58; 95% CI, 1.66–4.01; p-trend < 0.0001). Maternal hypochromic microcytosis was associated with child mortality (severe hypochromic microcytosis HR, 2.36; 95% CI, 1.27–4.38; p-trend = 0.001). Maternal anemia was not associated with greater risk of child HIV infection (severe anemia HR, 1.46; 95% CI, 0.91–2.33; p-trend = 0.08). Maternal anemia predicted lower CD4 T-cell counts among HIV-uninfected children; the difference in CD4 T-cell count per μL for severe anemia was −93 (95% CI, −204–17; p-trend = 0.02).
Shet et al. (2012)	80 HIV-infected children	India	Prospective cohort study enrolled from St. John's Pediatric Clinic and Freedom Foundation Children were followed for 6 months after enrollment. Biomarkers were measured prospectively for 6 months and at 12- and 24-week post- enrollment. Anemic children were given iron supplementation (250 mg/mL elemental iron). ART was given as part of Indian national guidelines.	Anemia: children 6–59 months (Hb <11.0 g/dL), children 5–11 years (Hb <11.5 g/dL), children 12–14 years (Hb <12.0 g/dL) Red-cell folate deficiency: <140 ng/mL Iron-deficiency: sTfR/f > 0.75 and CRP ≤ 1.0 mg/dL Iron-deficiency anemia: ferritin ≤ 12 ng/mL in presence of CRP < 1.0 mg/dL and ferritin ≤ 30 ng/mL in presence of CRP > 1.0 mg/dL Anemia of inflammation: sTfR/f ≤ 0.75 and CRP > 1.0 mg/dL	Hb status after taking ART was higher than baseline (baseline, 11.6 g/dL vs. 6 months, 12.2 g/dL; p = 0.03). Taking ART and iron increased Hb more than not taking ART or iron (mean change in Hb, 1.5 g/dL; p < 0.01). Taking ART and iron increased Hb more than not taking ART alone: • Compared to no treatment, ART + Fe mean = 5.45, SE = 1.76 (p < 0.01) • Compared to no treatment, ART alone mean = 2.54, SE = 1.49 (p = 0.09) • ART showed a protective effect on anemia (OR, 5.3; 95% CI, 1.7–16.3; p = 0.002) Compared to non-anemic children, anemic children were more likely to have lower CD4 T-cell counts (18% vs. 24%; p < 0.01) and higher log viral load (11.1 vs. 7.1; p < 0.01).

(continued)

TABLE 3.3 (continued)
Cohort Studies

Study	Sample	Location	Methods	Exposure	Outcomes	Main Findings
Johannessen et al. (2011)	102 non-pregnant patients, as part of a larger study including 838 HIV-infected adults	Tanzania	Hb concentrations were assessed before and after ART initiation. Follow-up was 12 months after ART initiation.	Pre-/post-ART: zidovudine/stavudine + lamivudine + efavirenz/ nevirapine Of 102 patients in substudy, 62 took stavudine + lamivudine + nevirapine, 17 took stavudine + lamivudine + efavirenz, 16 took ZDV + lamivudine + nevirapine, and 7 took ZDV + lamivudine + efavirenz.	Changes in Hb concentrations Persistent anemia (anemia after 12 months of ART): <12 g/dL (women), < 13 g/dL (men) Low mean cell volume: <76.0 fL	One year after ART initiation, mean Hb: • For all patients, increased by 2.5 g/dL ($p <$ 0.001) • For patients with severe anemia at ART initiation, increased by 4.6 g/dL • For patients with moderate anemia, increased by 3.0 g/dL • For patients with mild anemia, increased by 1.8 g/dL One year after ART initiation, 38.2% of patients were still anemic. Zidovudine use associated with persistent anemia (OR, 2.91; 95% CI, 1.03–8.19; $p =$ 0.043). Compared to patients who received ART, patients who did not receive ART had greater odds of persistent anemia (OR, 5.99; 95% CI, 1.82–19.8; $p =$ 0.003).
Dryden-Peterson et al. (2011)	1719 HIV-uninfected but exposed infants	Botswana	Infants of HIV-infected mothers were categorized into 3 groups based on exposure to maternal HAART (components not stated in paper)	Three categories of infant exposures to HAART Group 1 ($n =$ 691): HAART *in utero* and during breastfeeding (BF), and 1 month postnatal ZDV (HAART–BF)	Severe infant anemia: Grade 3 or 4, Division of AIDS 2004 Toxicity Table	Group 1 (HAART–BF) infants had significantly increased odds of severe anemia compared to group 2 (ZDV–BF) and group 3 (ZDV–FF). Severe anemia outcomes were mostly asymptomatic. Halting ZDV exposure or providing multivitamin and iron supplementation resolved most episodes of severe anemia.

				Group 2 ($n = 503$): maternal ZDV *in utero*, 6 months postnatal ZDV, and BF (ZDV–BF) Group 3 ($n = 525$): maternal ZDV *in utero*, 1 month postnatal ZDV, formula feeding (ZDV–FF)		
Pinnetti et al. (2011)	119 HIV-infected pregnant women on HAART and neonates	Italy	Women were recruited from the National Program on Surveillance on Antiretroviral Treatment in Pregnancy. Women were categorized into 3 groups based on timing/type of HAART (see exposure).	HAART defined as at least two nucleoside analogs plus protease inhibitor or nevirapine Group 1 ($n = 60$): Women who started ZDV–lamivudine (3TC)–based HAART during pregnancy and continued until delivery (ZDVs) Group 2 ($n = 18$): Women on ZDV–3TC-based HAART from conception and continued until delivery (ZDVc) Group 3 ($n = 41$): Women on ZDV-free HAART from conception to delivery (ZDVf)	Maternal and infant Hb Anemia in pregnancy: Hb < 11 g/dL Anemia at birth: Hb < 13 g/dL	*Maternal outcomes:* Compared to baseline, at 36 weeks there was a significantly greater decline in Hb in women belonging to the ZDVf group compared to the ZDVs group (ZDVf, 2.03 g/dL vs. ZDVs, 1.36 g/dL; $p = 0.036$). ZDV-free regimen was associated with maternal anemia (50% of ZDVf women had anemia at end of pregnancy). *Newborn outcomes:* ZDVf regimen (newborns *not* exposed to ZDV) had significantly higher Hb levels at birth compared to newborns exposed to ZDV (ZDVf, 16.1 ±1.4 g/dL; ZDVs, 14.3 ±2.0 g/dL; ZDVc, 14.6 ± 2.4 g/dL; $p = 0.044$ and 0.003, respectively) ZDV was associated with lower Hb in newborns.

(continued)

TABLE 3.3 (continued)
Cohort Studies

Study	Sample	Location	Methods	Exposure	Outcomes	Main Findings
Wisaksana et al. (2011)	869 HIV-infected adults (≥ 14 years); 70.3% ART-naïve, 29.7% on ART	West Java, Indonesia	Prospective cohort study conducted at Hasan Saidkin Hospital, referral hospital for HIV in West Java. Factors associated with survival, including anemia, in patients with HIV were studied. Patient characteristics, ART history, and iron biomarkers were recorded and analyzed for associations with high ferritin concentration.	Anemia: mild (Hb 10.5–12.99 g/dL for men and 10.5–11.99 g/dL for women), moderate (Hb 8.0–10.49 g/dL), severe (Hb < 8.0 g/dL). ART status	Stage of HIV disease: HIV clinical stage 4 (ART), clinical stage 3 (CD4 T-cell count < 350/mm³), clinical stage 1 or 2 (CD4 T-cell count < 200/mm³). SF: 30–400 ng/mL for men and 35–150 ng/mL for women. High SF: >400 ng/mL for men and >150 ng/mL for women. Low ferritin: <30 mg/mL. sTfR: 1870–2,450 U/mL. Low CD4 T-cell count: <200/mm³	*ART-naïve patients:* Anemia prevalence was 30.4% mild, 14.1% moderate, and 4.6% severe. Anemia was associated with low CD4 T-cell count ($p < 0.001$) and TB treatment ($p < 0.001$). Significant negative correlation was observed between ferritin concentration and CD4 T-cell count in patients without ART ($r^2 = 0.48$; $p < 0.0001$). SF concentrations were elevated in patients with anemia ($p = 0.07$) and/or low CD4 T-cell counts ($p < 0.0001$). No difference was observed in HCV prevalence among patients with or without anemia (56.9% vs. 59.6%; $p = 0.54$). Excluding patients with TB co-infection, the only factor associated with hyperferritinemia was low CD4 T-cell count. Beside CD4 T-cell count < 50/mm³ (HR, 5.7; IQR, 1.6–17.8; $p = 0.003$), only moderate to severe anemia was independently associated with an increased risk of death (HR, 6.5; IQR, 2.0–21.2; $p = 0.002$). Survival rates (Kaplan–Meier) at 6 months were 98.6% (95% CI, 97.3–99.9%) for patients without anemia, 95.1% (95% CI, 92.0–98.5%) for patients with mild anemia, and 82.5% (95% CI, 75.5–89.4%) for patients with moderate or severe anemia ($p < 0.001$).

Reference	Sample	Country	Study design	Definitions	Results
Chatterjee et al. (2010)	829 children of HIV-infected mothers	Tanzania	Prospective cohort study. Maternal characteristics were collected during pregnancy and Hb measurements taken at 3-month intervals from birth. Information about malaria and HIV infection was collected in children up to 24 months after birth.	Child HIV diagnosed on basis of infected peripheral mononuclear cell specimen by PCR before 18 months. Anemia: Hb < 8.5 g/dL. Anemia suggesting Fe deficiency: Hb < 8.5g/dL and hypochromic microcytic erythroctye morphology with >75% cells showing hypochromasia and microcytosis	*ART patients:* Of the 62.8% of patients on ZDV-containing regimes, 14.3% had mild anemia and 1.9% had moderate anemia; no patient had severe anemia ($p < 0.001$). ZDV was associated with anemia: with ZDV, 20.3% anemia; without ZDV, 7.4% anemia ($p = 0.01$). No significant negative correlation was found between ferritin and CD4 T-cell counts in patients with ART ($r^2 = 0.004$; $p = 0.70$). SF was lower but not significantly different between ART and ART-naïve patients ($p = 0.12$). Duration of ART was not associated with plasma concentrations of ferritin or sTfR. Advanced maternal clinical HIV disease (RR, 1.31; 95% CI, 1.14–1.51) and low CD4 T-cell counts during pregnancy (RR, 1.58; 95% CI, 1.05–2.37) were associated with increased risk of anemia among children. Maternal WHO HIV clinical disease stage ≥2 compared to stage 1 during pregnancy was associated with anemia risk up to 1 year (RR, 1.31; 95% CI, 1.14–1.51). Child HIV infection was independently associated with anemia risk (RR, 1.61; 95% CI, 1.40–1.85). Maternal CD4 T-cell count < 350 cells/mm³ during pregnancy was associated with risk of anemia suggestive of iron deficiency (RR, 1.58; 95% CI, 1.05–2.37). Child anemia (Hb < 8.5 g/dL) was not associated with mortality (HR, 1.38; 95% CI, 0.95–2.01) nor with risk of death in the HIV-uninfected subgroup (HR, 1.86; 95% CI, 0.96–3.61; $p = 0.07$).

(continued)

TABLE 3.3 (continued)
Cohort Studies

Study	Sample	Location	Methods	Exposure	Outcomes	Main Findings
Rawat et al. (2009)	643 HIV-infected women	Zimbabwe	Prospective cohort and cross-sectional study (nested part of ZVITAMBO clinical trial of postpartum vitamin A supplementation) to find associations among postpartum iron status, viral load, and HIV-related mortality	SF categorized into three groups: (1) <15 µg/L, (2) 15–45 µg/L, or (3) >45 µg/L Viral load: CD4 T-cell count categories (cells × 10^9/L): (1) ≤100, (2) 101–200, (3) 201–400, or (4) ≥401 Mortality Alpha-1-acid glycoprotein	—	Log$_{10}$ increase in SF was associated with 2.27-fold increase in viral load (β = 0.356; p = 0.019) in non-anemic women; no association in anemic women was found. Log$_{10}$ increase in SF was associated with fourfold increase in mortality by 12 months (p = 0.002). Hb was negatively associated with viral load (p = 0.001) and mortality (p = 0.047). Hb was lower among women with CD4 T-cell count ≤ 100 (mean, 105 g/L; SD, 20) vs. CD4 T-cell count ≥ 401 (mean, 112 g/L; SD, 19) (p < 0.05). SF was higher among women with CD4 T-cell count ≤ 100 vs. CD4 T-cell count ≥ 401: mean 40.1 (95% CI, 30.9–52.1) vs. 19.3 (95% CI, 16.9–21.9) (p < 0.05) When controlling for AGP and CD4 T-cell count, anemic women had higher viral loads than non-anemic women if SF < 15 µg/L (p = 0.003) or SF = 15–45 µg/L (p = 0.033), but not if SF > 45 µg/L.

| McDermid et al. (2009) | 1362 HIV-infected adults | The Gambia | Prospective cohort study (11.5 years) that collected baseline plasma, DNA, clinical data

Iron biomarkers: plasma iron, sTfR, ferritin, transferrin, transferrin index, log(sTfR/ferritin)

Haptoglobin HP and 5 SLC11A1 (NRAMP1) polymorphisms genotyped | Iron-related genes SLC11A1-SLC3 and CAAA polymorphisms and HP genotypes

Iron (μmol/L): low (<8.6), normal (8.6–30.0), elevated (>30.0)

STfR (nmol/L): low (<29.9), normal (10.6–29.9), elevated (>10.6)

Transferrin (g/L): low (<2.0), normal (2.0–3.6), elevated (>3.6)

Ferritin for women ≤ 44 years (μg/L): low (<12), normal (12–150), elevated (>150)

Ferritin for men ≤ 44 years (μg/L): low (<12), normal (12–200), elevated (>200)

Ferritin for women > 44 years (μg/L): low (<12), normal (12–200), elevated (>200)

Ferritin for men > 44 years (μg/L): low (<12), normal (12–300), elevated (>300)

TfR: low (<−1.45), normal (−1.45–0.40), elevated (>0.40)

Anemia (g/L): normal (Hb ≥100), anemia (Hb 80–100), severe anemia (Hb <80) | All-cause mortality | Mortality was significantly lower in HIV-2 than in HIV-1 infection in the presence of abnormal (low or elevated) iron status.

Gene–iron interaction was detected (likelihood-ratio test $p = 0.018$).

LC11A1-SLC3 and CAAA polymorphisms were best independent genetic predictors of mortality (adjusted mortality rate ratio, 95% CI): SLC3:G/C = 0.59 (95% CI, 0.45–0.85), CAAA:indel = 1.51 (95% CI, 1.10–2.07).

Adjusting for all polymorphisms, SLC1: 199/199, SLC1: other/other, SLC6a: A/A, and CAAA:indels were associated with significantly greater mortality, whereas Hp 2–1 and SLC3:G/C were protective. |

(continued)

TABLE 3.3 (continued)
Cohort Studies

Study	Sample	Location	Methods	Exposure	Outcomes	Main Findings
Gordeuk et al. (2009)	32 HIV-infected, ART-naïve patients with TB (subset of total 49 subjects with TB)	Zimbabwe	Patients were treated for TB for 2 months. No one received ART. Blood samples could not be attained weekly: they were grouped by weeks 1, 3, 4–6, 7–9, and month 3. Neopterin concentrations were measured using radioimmunoassay.	High dietary iron intake: life consumption of traditional beer > 1000 L ($n = 7$) Low dietary iron ($n = 25$)	Neopterin	HIV-infected patients who had high dietary iron intake had lower neopterin levels than HIV-infected patients with lower dietary iron intake ($p < 0.0001$).
Mlisana et al. (2008)	57 HIV-infected women	South Africa	Prospective cohort study as part of Centre for the AIDS Programme of Research in South Africa (CAPRISA) Acute Infection Study Baseline evaluation included physical exam and blood collection. Women who presented with new HIV-1 infection were enrolled in acute HIV infection phase; patients were followed weekly for 3 weeks, fortnightly until 3 months, monthly until 1 year post-enrollment, and 3 months thereafter.	Seroconverters defined as positive HIV antibody test result within 3 months of negative test result Acute infection: infected HIV RNA PCR with absence of HIV-1 antibodies ("pre"-seroconversion) or detection of HIV-1 antibodies within 3 months of previously negative antibody result	Anemia: Hb < 12 g/dL Measured serum iron, vitamin B_{12}, folate, ferritin, total iron	57 women had acute HIV-1 infection (28 from HIV-uninfected cohort and 29 from other seroincidence studies). Of the 28 from the HIV-uninfected cohort, mean pre-infection Hb = 12.7 g/dL (SD 1.40), 11 were anemic (39.3%). Decline in Hb from pre-infection to first post-infection study visit had mean = 0.46 g/dL (SD, 1.09). Decline in Hb between identification of acute infection and 3 months post-infection had mean = 0.55 g/dL (SD, 1.05). Prevalence of anemia increased in first 6 months following acute infection (for 26 participants with available data at 12 months): 61.1% at 6 months compared to initially 25.0%. At 12 months, the prevalence of anemia was 51.4%. Mean serum iron, vitamin B_{12}, and folate did not change significantly at acute infection identification over next 12 months.

					HIV-progression: stage 4 (CD4 T-cells < 200 cells/μL)	
Mlisana et al. (2008)			If CD4 T-cell count < 350 cells/mm^3 at more than one study visit, patients were referred to ART program ($n = 0$).	Time of infection = 14 days < positive RNA PCR assay result in absence of HIV-1 antibodies or as midpoint between last HIV seronegative test and first HIV seroinfected test		Mean iron level (μmol/L) at pre-infection was 10.79 (5.82); at acute infection, 9.64 (5.56); at 12 months, 7.58 (6.10). Mean ferritin (ng/mL) at pre-infection was 64.13 (55.82); at acute infection, 79.09 (87.73); at 12 months post-infection, 38.09 (42.35). Viral load and Hb relationship: Pearson's correlation between Hb at 3 months and viral load closest to time of infection was significant at −0.2731 ($p = 0.0398$); correlations between Hb level closest to time of infection and Hb rate of decline and viral load at different time points were not significant.
Kupka et al. (2007)	Tanzania	584 HIV-infected women	Nested cohort study (part of RCT on multivitamins and maternal/child health) All women received 400 mg ferrous sulfate (120 mg ferrous iron) and folate (5 mg) as well as weekly doses of 500 mg chloroquine phosphate. No ART was available. Women were followed during and after pregnancy monthly. Baseline was gestational age 12–27 weeks.	Anemia: Hb <110 g/L Elevated sTfR: >4.4 mg/L Elevated CRP: >10 mg/L Low SF: <12.0 μg/L in absence of inflammation (CRP ≤ 10.0 mg/L) and SF < 20.0 μg/L in presence of inflammation (CRP > 10.0 mg/L) IDA: Anemia and either low SF or elevated sTfR, or both Low iron stores: <12.0 μg/L and 12.0–29.0 μg/L Adequate iron stores: 30.0–89.9 and 90.0–150.0 μg/L High iron stores: >150/0 μg/L		Cox proportional hazards regression models adjusted for age and vitamin regimen group, SF > 150 μg/L compared with 12.0 μg/L marginally associated with progression to stage 4 ($p = 0.08$) and associated with composite endpoint AIDS-related death or progression to stage 4 ($p = 0.01$). Adjustment for Hb and CRP: SF > 150.0 μg/L was associated with greater risk of progression to stage 4 compared to SF < 12.0 μg/L (RR, 1.75); composite endpoint: RR = 1.40 (95% CI, 0.83–2.39; $p = 0.21$). Adjustment for markers of HIV disease progression and wasting: RR = 1.78 (95% CI, 0.68–4.64; $p = 0.24$). SF was inversely correlated with HIV disease progression and positively related to viral load (stronger among women with CRP > 10.0 mg/L).

(continued)

TABLE 3.3 (continued)
Cohort Studies

Study	Sample	Location	Methods	Exposure	Outcomes	Main Findings
McDermid et al. (2007)	1362 Gambian adults	The Gambia	Prospective cohort study that assessed all-cause mortality from HIV over 11.5 years. Baseline iron status, age, gender, Hb, BMI, HIV type, absolute CD4 T-cell count, malaria status, and alpha-1-antichymotrypsin were measured.	HIV infection exposed Standard of care: Symptomatic, opportunistic infections were treated and prophylactic treatment of opportunistic infections, including TB, was initiated in 1999 when people with absolute CD4 T-cell count < 500 cells/mm^3 got prophylactic cotrimoxazole.	Main outcome: Time from the first HIV-seroinfected diagnosis to all-cause mortality	Mortality rate: 25.9/100 person-years. Elevated iron universally predicted greater mortality compared to normal iron status, with the exception of sTfR in unadjusted models. Significant predictors of mortality for full adjusted models: • Transferrin (elevated vs. normal) HR = 1.77 (95% CI, 1.30–2.42; p = 0.001) • Ferritin (elevated vs. normal) HR = 1.40 (95% CI, 1.07–1.83; p = 0.014) • Combined iron status index (highly elevated vs. normal) HR = 2.20 (95% CI, 1.16–4.18; p = 0.016) Hb concentration and CD4 T-cell counts were inversely associated with mortality.
Boom et al. (2007)	138 initially HAART-naïve, HIV-infected adults	Thailand	STACCATO HAART nested cohort study that examined stored plasma samples. Low baselines ferritin	HAART interruption	Time to meeting HAART interruption criteria (CD4 T-cells ≥ 350 cells/µL)	Low baseline serum ferritin (<30.0 µg/L) was associated with a shorter time to meet criteria for HAART interruption.
Sinha et al. (2007)	467 HIV-infected pregnant women, nested in PMTCT	Pune, India	PMTCT HIV-infected pregnant women taking ZDV. Between August 16, 2002, and January 30, 2006, pregnant women presenting for antenatal care at Sassoon General Hospital	ZDV: 300 mg twice daily, beginning at 36 weeks gestation; duration ≥ 2 weeks	Maternal anemia (Hb < 10 g/dL), severe anemia (Hb < 8 g/dL), mild anemia (Hb = 8 to 10 g/dL). Preterm birth (gestational age < 37 weeks). Low birthweight (<2500 g)	Children born to women who took ZDV had significantly lower Hb concentrations at birth and 4 weeks of age compared to infants of mothers who did not take ZDV: • Birth—with ZDV, Hb = 16.5 g/dL (95% CI, 16.2–16.9); no ZDV, Hb = 17.2 g/dL (95% CI, 16.9–17.5) (p = 0.02) • 4-weeks—with ZDV, Hb = 11.6 g/dL (95% CI, 11.4–11.9); no ZDV, Hb = 12.1 g/dL (95% CI, 11.19–12.3) (p = 0.03)

Reference	Sample	Country	Methods	Groups	Definitions	Results
Miller et al. (2006)	136 infants born to HIV-uninfected mothers, 575 infants born to HIV-infected mothers	Zimbabwe	Nested longitudinal cohort study within ZVITAMBO. Measured Hb, EPO, sTfR, SF at ages 6 weeks and 3 and 6 months in randomly selected infants (136 born to HIV-uninfected mothers, 99 to HIV-infected mothers, and 324 born to HIV-infected mothers but who did not become infected in 6 months following birth)	Group 1 ($n = 136$): HIV-uninfected mother, HIV-uninfected infant Group 2 ($n = 324$): HIV-infected mother, HIV-uninfected infant Group 3 ($n = 99$): HIV-infected mother, HIV-uninfected baby	Anemia: Hb = 105 g/L Did not define anemia in infants < 3 months age Absent or depleted iron stores: 12 μg/L SF	Maternal ZDV was associated with lower mean corpuscular volume in infants at 4 weeks of age. *Infant outcomes (no ZDV vs. ZDV):* • No infants had clinical anemia at any time-point. • No difference was observed in low birthweight, still birth, small for gestational age, or intrauterine growth restriction. • There was a significant difference in mean gestational age at delivery ($p < 0.01$), with smaller age babies born to no-ZDV mothers: no ZDV, 38.0 months (95% CI, 37.7–38.3) vs. ZDV, 38.6 months (95% CI, 38.4–38.8). • There was a significant difference in preterm birth: no ZDV, 21.2% ($n = 44$) vs. ZDV, 5.8% ($n = 11$) ($p < 0.01$). HIV-infected infants were more likely to be anemic than HIV-uninfected infants (adjusted OR, 5.26; $p < 0.001$).

(continued)

TABLE 3.3 (continued)
Cohort Studies

Study	Sample	Location	Methods	Exposure	Outcomes	Main Findings
Phiri et al. (2006)	135 HIV-infected, lactating women	Lusaka, Zambia	Longitudinal cohort investigating breast milk HIV RNA viral load in lactating women Maternal blood was collected during pregnancy and at 6 weeks postpartum. Milk was collected 10 days and 6 weeks postpartum.	Analyses for iron supplements, which were given in the first 2 weeks postpartum, were conducted only for women with Hb ≤ 100 g/L at either day 3 or day 7. Hemoglobin levels in the groups with and without supplementation were significantly different ($p < 0.001$).	Breast milk viral load	Maternal Hb or receiving iron supplements was not associated with milk viral load. Maternal health was the only factor contributing to milk viral load. Women given iron supplements did not have higher viral loads than women with moderate anemia who were not supplemented for day 10 and week 6 milk viral load. Iron supplements vs. no iron supplements: regression coefficient, 0.08 (95% CI, −0.54–0.70; $n = 56$; $p = 0.80$) Week 6 plasma viral load: regression coefficient, 0.09 (95% CI, −0.42–0.59; $n = 54$; $p = 0.74$) Day 10 and week 6 milk viral load: regression coefficient, 0.08 (95% CI, −0.17–0.01); regression coefficient, 0.06 (95% CI, −0.16–0.04; $n = 121$; $p = 0.25$) Day 7 Hb = 114 g/dL ($p = 0.08$)
Dairo et al. (2005)	—	Ibadan, Nigeria, clinics	Prospective case-control study to find contribution of HIV/AIDS to anemia in pregnancy HIV-infected and -uninfected mothers were followed until delivery to obtain iron, folate, vitamin B, and daraprium use information Cases: anemic pregnant women; control: non-anemic women	HIV infection	Anemia: Hb < 11 g/dL or packed cell volume 33%	Iron use ($p < 0.006$) significantly reduced risk of anemia, but use of daraprium and HIV seropositive increased risk of anemia in pregnancy, although not significantly. HIV prevalence: 13.3% in cases (anemic) vs. 3.3% in controls ($p < 0.026$) Adjusted odds ratio for anemia in pregnancy if HIV-infected: 1.00 (95% CI, 0.51–0.93; $p < 0.015$)

Reference	Population	Location	Study design	Anemia definition	Outcomes	Results
O'Brien et al. (2005)	1062 HIV-infected women (subset of 1078 enrolled in TOV)	Tanzania	Nested cohort study (women enrolled in TOV); adjusted analysis by intervention arm Study was conducted to investigate effect of anemia on HIV/AIDS disease progression and AIDS-related mortality.	Normal Hb ≥ 11.0 g/dL Moderate anemia: Hb 8.5–10.9 g/dL Severe anemia: Hb < 8.5 g/dL	Time to all-cause death AIDS-related death 50% decrease in CD4 T-cell count	Low Hb was associated with increased risk of mortality, independent of CD4 T-cell count or stage of disease, age, treatment arm, or BMI. Risk of death was higher for patients with anemia than without anemia: moderate anemia (RH, 2.06; 95% CI, 1.52 to 2.79), severe anemia (RH, 3.19; 95% CI, 2.23–4.56). Each 1-g/dL decrease in Hb was associated with a 25% increased risk of death due to any cause (RH, 1.25; 95% CI, 1.17–1.33) and a 28% increased risk of AIDS- related death (RH, 1.28; 95% CI, 1.19–1.38). The risk of AIDS-related mortality was also more than doubled for patients with anemia compared with patients without anemia: moderate anemia (RH, 2.21; 95% CI, 1.53–3.19); severe anemia (RH, 3.47; 95% CI, 2.25–5.33). Anemia—moderate (RH, 1.79; 95% CI, 1.38–2.33) and severe (RH, 1.59; 95% CI, 1.02–2.49), compared with normal—was associated with time with a 50% decrease in CD4 T-cell count from baseline (with adjustment for baseline CD4 T-cell count, WHO stage of disease, age, pregnancy, treatment arm in vitamin study, and BMI). Compared with normal Hb (<11.0 g/dL), risk of AIDS-related death was twice as great for patients with moderate anemia and three times as great if they had severe anemia.

(continued)

TABLE 3.3 (continued)
Cohort Studies

Study	Sample	Location	Methods	Exposure	Outcomes	Main Findings
Miller et al. (2003)	2314 infants born to HIV-infected mothers, 535 infants born to HIV-uninfected mothers	Zimbabwe	Measured total body iron (TBI) in infants of HIV-uninfected and HIV-infected mothers	Total body iron at birth (TBI) Quantity of circulating iron at birth in the form of Hb (HbI) Quantity of body storage iron at birth (BSI) TBI = HbI + BSI (mg)	Defined infantile anemia as Hb < 105 g/L at ages 3 and 6 months and Hb < 100 g/L at ages 9 and 12 months Low birthweight (<2500 g), preterm birth (gestational age < 38 weeks), parity (1, 2– 4, 5), and low maternal mid-upper arm circumference (<23 cm)	Maternal and infant HIV infection, especially among girls, was associated with apparently greater TBI. TBI increased with maternal and infant HIV infection, with a greater effect in females . Further examination of the components of TBI demonstrated that the differences in TBI by HIV status could be explained by differences in the BSI component. SF, an acute-phase protein, was used to estimate BSI, and HIV-infected female babies, compared with males, had an odds ratio of 4.3 (95% CI, 1.8–10.2) for an elevated ferritin concentration (>500 µg/L). HIV-exposed, but not infected, girls were also more likely than boys to have an elevated ferritin with an odds ratio of 1.5 (95% CI, 1.1–2.1).
Sarcletti et al. (2003)	35 HIV-infected men	Austria	HIV initially ART-naïve patients enrolled between November 1996 and December 1998 Follow-up: 6 months Neopterin was measured from frozen plasma.	ART	Neopterin	An inverse relationship was found between Hb and neopterin; decreasing neopterin levels were associated with increased Hb between start of ART and at 3 and 6 months.

| Canani et al. (1999) | Naples, Italy | 10 HIV-infected children (clinical class B or C and immuno-logical class 3 according to CDC) | Prospective study to assess intestinal function All children received combination therapy (see Exposure). Viral load and CD4 cell counts were assessed at 3 and 6 months after enrollment. Serum iron was assessed at 3 and 6 months by HIV-1 RNA PCR and immunofluorescence imaging (how serum iron measured not indicated) | Combination therapy Ritonavir and two HIV reverse transcriptase inhibitors: 400 mg/m^2 of ritonavir every 12 hours, starting at 50% full dose, escalating to full dose in 1 week; IRTs (5 children given stavudine and lamivudine, 3 given ZDV and lamivudine, and 2 given stavudine and didanosine) | Difference in serum iron levels between baseline and 3 and 6 months | Mean serum iron levels increased significantly at 3 months and 6 months on treatment ($p < 0.05$). |
| de Monyé et al. (1999) | Washington, DC | — | Retrospective cohort of adults grouped by macrophage iron grades; survival and infections noted | Macrophage iron grades (0–5) Grade 0 ($n = 9$): no iron granules, absent iron stores Grade 1 ($n = 27$): rare iron granules by oil immersion indicating low iron stores Grade 2 ($n = 94$): small iron granules by low power indicating normal iron stores | Infections caused by Candida spp., Pneumocystis carinii, and Mycobacterium spp. Mortality rates | Adjusted estimated rate of death (hazards ratio) was higher in patients with high iron stores compared with patients with low iron stores from baseline bone marrow study (HR, 2.1; 95% CI, 1.3–3.5; $p = 0.003$). Infections caused by Candida spp., Pneumocystis carinii, and Mycobacterium spp. were more common in patients with high macrophage iron grades than those with low or normal iron grades ($p \leq 0.006$). Compared with subjects with bone marrow macrophage iron grades of 0 to 2, patients with iron grades of 4 to 5 were less likely to have a history of hemophilia ($p = 0.013$) and were more likely to have histories of blood transfusions ($p = 0.002$) and of infections with Candida spp., Pneumocystis carinii, and Mycobacterium spp. ($p \leq 0.006$). They also had lower CD4 T-cell counts ($p = 0.027$), absolute lymphocyte counts ($p \leq 0.001$), and hemoglobin concentrations ($p < 0.001$). |

(continued)

TABLE 3.3 (continued)
Cohort Studies

Study	Sample	Location	Methods	Exposure	Outcomes	Main Findings
				Grade 3 ($n = 30$): numerous iron granules in all bone marrow spicules (high to increased iron stores) Grade 4 ($n = 178$): large granules in small clumps indicating markedly increased iron stores Grade 5 ($n = 10$): large clumps of granules indicating massively increased iron stores		Cox proportional hazards models confirmed that iron grades of 4 to 5 were associated with higher mortality rates than iron grades of 0 to 2, both from the time of the bone marrow aspiration and from the time of the determination of HIV seropositivity. The estimated rate of death (hazards ratio) after the diagnosis of HIV seropositivity in subjects with bone marrow iron grades of 4 to 5 was 2.8-fold higher than the rate in patients with iron grades of 0 to 2 (95% CI, 1.5–4.9; $p = 0.001$), after adjustment for the year of the bone marrow study. *Mycobacterium tuberculosis* (MTb) was significantly different among patients with iron grades 0 to 2 (MTb 0) and 4 to 5 (MTb 8) ($p = 0.023$). *Mycobacterium avium intracellulare* was significantly greater in patients with iron grades 4 to 5 than 0 to 2. *Mycobacterium* infections were significantly greater in patients with iron grades 4 to 5 than 0 to 2.

Note: 3TC, lamivudine; ACT, activated clotting time; AGP, alpha-1-acid glycoprotein; AOR, adjusted odds ratio; ART, antiretroviral therapy; BF, breastfeeding; BMI, body mass index; CI, confidence interval; CRP, c-reactive protein; EPO, erythropoietin; FF, formula feeding; HAART, highly active antiretroviral therapy; Hb, hemoglobin; HR, hazard ratio; ID, iron deficiency; IQR, interquartile range; IRR, incidence rate ratio; IUGR, intrautertine growth restriction; LNS, lipid-based nutrient supplements; MTb, *Mycobacterium tuberculosis*;; OR, odds ratio; PMTCT, prevention of mother-to-child transmission trial; RDA, recommended dietary allowance; RH, relative hazard; RR, risk ratio; SAA, serum amyloid A; SD, standard deviation; SF, serum ferritin; sTfR, soluble transferrin receptor; TB, tuberculosis; TBI, total body iron; WHO, World Health Organization; ZDV, zidovudine; ZVITAMBO, Zimbabwe Vitamins for Mothers and Babies Project.

TABLE 3.4

Case-Control Studies

Study	Sample	Location	Methods	Exposure	Outcomes	Main Findings
Selvam et al. (2015)	87 pregnant women (45 HIV-infected, 42 HIV-uninfected)	Pretoria, South Africa	Maternal venous blood and cord blood sampled at delivery (see Outcomes)	HIV	Levels of serum iron, ferritin, and transferrin concentrations; transferrin saturation; sTfR concentration; sTfR/log ferritin index	Women with HIV, compared to women without HIV, had lower white blood cell counts and higher concentration of serum ferritin. There were no differences between the two groups in other iron indicators, including Hb at enrollment (HIV-infected vs. HIV-uninfected: 11.4 ± 0.3 vs. 11.4 ± 0.2 g/dL; $p = 0.974$) and delivery (HIV-infected vs. HIV-uninfected: 11.9 ± 0.3 vs. 11.6 ± 0.3 g/dL; $p = 0.393$). Cord blood findings: • Compared to maternal blood, cord blood ferritin was significantly higher ($p < 0.001$). • Cord blood ferritin was significantly higher in HIV-exposed infants ($p = 0.044$).
Malvoisin et al. (2014)	227 women (182 HIV-infected on HAART, 45 HIV-uninfected)	Lyon, France	Hepcidin concentrations measured by commercial RIA Serum iron and serum ferritin concentrations measured by Dimension Vista® 500 Intelligent Lab System analyzer (Siemens Healthcare Diagnostics) Blood samples collected from 2002 to 2006 and from 2008 to 2013	HIV High viral load (>150,000 copies/mL)	Hepcidin levels (nmol/L) Serum iron concentration (µmol/L)	Compared to healthy controls, HIV-infected women on HAART had lower levels of hepcidin (3.20 ± 2.06 vs. 5.68 ± 3.66 nmol/L; $p = 0.009$). Among HIV-infected women, plasma viral levels were significantly associated with hepcidin ($p = 0.004$). Patients with undetectable viral load had significantly higher iron concentration compared to patients with high viral load (undetectable viral load: 15.79 ± 4.4 µmol/L vs. high viral load: 10.56 ± 5.45 µmol/L; $p = 0.008$).

(continued)

TABLE 3.4 (continued)
Case-Control Studies

Study	Sample	Location	Methods	Exposure	Outcomes	Main Findings
Banjoko et al. (2012)	130 adults with known HIV status (80 HIV-infected, 50 HIV-uninfected)	Ile Ife, Nigeria	Serum iron concentration using Garcic method Serum TIBC measured by spectrophotometry Transferrin saturation formula: (serum iron/TIBC) × 100%	HIV CD4 T-cell count	Iron indicator levels: serum total iron, transferrin, TIBC, CD4-T cells, transferrin saturation	CD4 T-cell count was inversely associated with serum iron levels ($r = -0.572$, $p < 0.001$). Compared to controls, cases had significantly higher serum iron concentration (mean ± SD: 35.3 ± 0.8 vs. 11.8 ± 0.9 µmol/L; $p < 0.001$).
Ogbe et al. (2012)	312 adults (207 HIV-infected, 105 HIV-uninfected)	Makurdi, Nigeria	CD4 T-cells counted using CyFlow® SL machine HIV screened using rapid screening (Uni-Gold™ Recombigen® HIV-1/2 and Alere Determine™ HIV-1/2 assay kits); confirmed using western blots Hb, RBC, and MCV measured using Sysmex KX-21 Hematology Analyzer Serum iron concentration and UIBC measured using Forrozine method and iron/TIBC reagent set by colometric method TIBC = Iron level × UIBC	HIV High CD4 T-cell count (≥200 cells/mm³) Low CD4 T-cell count (<200 cells/mm³)	Hb (g/dL)	Compared to controls, cases had significantly lower mean Hb (HIV-infected: 10.95 ± 1.69 g/dL vs. HIV-uninfected 13.84 ± 1.01 g/dL; $p < 0.001$). Patients with lower CD4 T-cell counts were more likely to be anemic than patients with higher CD4 T-cell counts (55.2% vs. 32.5%).
Gordeuk et al. (2006)	312 women (158 HIV-infected and HAART-naïve, 154 HIV-uninfected)	Washington, DC	Retrospective case-control study in which cases died before July 1996 HAART-naïve patients from Women's Interagency HIV Study (women enrolled between October 1994 and November 1995) Cases individually matched by CD4 T-cell count (within ±50 cells/µL)	HIV	Iron indicators: Hb, serum ferritin, transferrin receptor concentrations Odds of death	Compared to controls, cases had: • Higher serum ferritin levels (median: 392 vs. 330 µg/L; $p = 0.027$) • Higher serum TfR concentrations (6.5 vs. 5.5 mg/L, $p = 0.048$) • Lower Hb concentrations (10.8 [95% CI, 9.8–11.8] vs. 11.7 [95% CI, 10.7–12.6]; $p < 0.001$)

Reference	Location	Sample	Study details	Definitions/Measurements	Group	Outcomes
			and HIV RNA level (within ± 0.5 $\log_{10}$ copies/mL) to controls			• $\log_{10}$ increase in serum ferritin associated with 1.67-fold increase in odds of death (95% CI, 0.98–2.86); (logistic regression model adjusted for self-reported antiretroviral therapy use, age, smoking status, ethnicity, Hb, C-reactive protein, and aspartate amino transferase)
Totin et al. (2002)	Kampala, Uganda	204 infants (165 HIV-infected, 39 HIV-uninfected)	9-month-old infants; Study conducted between January 1995 and June 1998; Infants screened at 3–5 months of age for HIV-1 using qualitative HIV-1 RNA PCR and quantitative HIV-1 RNA PCR; Hb measured at 9 months by automated Beckman/Coulter T540 hematology analyzer; Plasma HIV load at 9 months measured by HIV-1 RNA PCR	Underweight: weight-for-age z-score (WAZ) < -2 SD; Wasting: weight for-length z-score (WLZ) < -2 SD; Stunting: length-for-age z-score (LAZ) < -2 SD; Anemia: <110 g/L; Moderate to severe anemia: Hb < 90 g/L; Iron deficiency: plasma ferritin < 12 µg/L	HIV; More severe HIV disease defined as viral load > 1,119,000 copies/mL	Prevalence of anemia was higher in cases than controls (90.9% vs. 76.9%; $p = 0.015$). There was no difference in iron deficiency between cases and controls ($p = 0.29$). Birth outcomes: • No difference in birthweight between cases and control • Higher prevalence of underweight and wasting in cases compared to controls (WAZ < -2 SD, 42.4% vs. 25.6%, $p = 0.054$; WLZ < -2 SD, 12.7% vs. 0%, $p = 0.02$).
Silva et al. (2001)	São Paolo, Brazil	79 children of HIV-infected mothers (26 HIV-infected, 53 seroreverters [non-infected])	Longitudinal study of HIV-infected children and seroreverters; included children taking antiretrovirals; Used ELISA, western blot, PCR–DNA for diagnosis of infection; clinical and lab protocols carried out at 3-month intervals until age 18 months and afterward at 6-month intervals; Follow-up period: March 1996 to November 1997; Age at beginning of follow-up: 20 days to 7 years and 9 months; >75% children infected with HIV at delivery	Anemia: reference measurements defined (see Silva et al., 1999)	Group 1: HIV-infected children with clinical symptoms and positive lab exams; Group 2: HIV-uninfected (seroreverters)	Compared to seroreverters, anemia in HIV-infected children was more frequent (73.1% vs. 41.5%; $p = 0.008$).

(continued)

TABLE 3.4 (continued)
Case-Control Studies

Study	Sample	Location	Methods	Exposure	Outcomes	Main Findings
Gangaidzo et al. (2001)	98 patients with pulmonary TB (68 HIV-infected), 98 controls (15 HIV-infected)	Zimbabwe	Subjects matched by age, sex, and residence location Patient treatment: isoniazid, rifampicin, ethambutol, streptomycin for 2 months, then isoniazid and rifampcin continued for 4 months outpatient; patients followed monthly Follow-up from 1 week to 9 months after start of treatment Assessments of iron status performed between 1 and 3 weeks of treatment	HIV TB Increased dietary iron estimated by lifetime consumption of traditional beer (>1000 L)	Differences in indicators: SF, Hb	HIV patients had similar levels of SF compared to HIV-uninfected patients at all time-points. HIV patients had significantly lower Hb concentrations. HIV infection was associated with a 17.3-fold increase in the estimated odds of developing tuberculosis (95% CI, 7.4–40.6; $p < 0.001$). Increased dietary iron was associated with a 3.5-fold increase in the odds of developing TB (95% CI, 1.4–8.9; $p = 0.009$).
Camacho et al. (1992)	42 anemic, HIV-infected patients (30 with AIDS and 12 with AIDS-related conditions) and 93 uninfected but anemic individuals	Madrid, Spain	Reference (control) population: 36 patients with ACD and 57 individuals with IDA Blood samples taken after 12-hour fast	HIV-infected (advanced disease) ($n = 42$) HIV-uninfected: ACD ($n = 36$); IDA ($n = 57$)	Differences in iron indicators: serum iron, transferrin, ferritin, Hb Serum EPO response	Compared to controls, cases had higher SF levels. In subjects with IDA, there was a significant linear relationship between log serum EPO and Hb, whereas in case subjects (subjects with advanced HIV disease), the serum EPO response was weaker ($p < 0.001$). There was no difference in Hb or SF levels between patients with HIV vs. patients without HIV.

Note: ACD, anemia of chronic disease; EPO, erythropoietin; HAART, highly active antiretroviral therapy; Hb, hemoglobin; IDA, iron-deficiency anemia; MCV, mean corpuscular value; RBC, red blood cell; TIBC, total iron-binding capacity; UIBC, unsaturated iron-binding capacity; SF, serum ferritin; sTfR, soluble transferring receptor; TB, tuberculosis.

TABLE 3.5
Cross-Sectional Studies

Study	Sample	Location	Methods	Exposure	Outcome	Main Findings
López-Calderón et al. (2015)	571 asymptomatic HIV outpatients (86.2% on ART, 74.8% undetectable viral load, 78.1% men)	Malaga, Spain	Physical exam and 12-hour fasting blood analysis	HIV Immunosuppression (CD4 T-cell count <350 cells/uL) Chronic HCV infection	High ferritin (HF) (plasma ferritin >200 µg/L in women, >300 µg/L in men) Iron overload: increased iron reserves independent of tissue damage	Associations with high ferritin: • Median CD4 T-cell count with HF (369 cells/µL) vs. CD4 T-cell without HF (483 cells/µL) ($p < 0.0001$) • Multivariate analysis: CD4 T-cell count <350 cells/µL (OR, 2.37; 95% CI, 1.3–4.1; $p = 0.0003$), CRP >3 mg/L (OR, 2.67; 95% CI, 1.5–4.7; $p = 0.001$), chronic HCV infection (OR 2.77; 95% CI, 1.5–4.9; $p = 0.001$) • Prevalence of CD4 T-cell <350 cells/µL (HF, 46.0% vs. not HF, 25.3%; $p = 0.0001$) • AIDS cases (HF, 49.2% vs. not HF, 34.6%; $p = 0.02$) • Undetectable viral load (HF, 77.5% vs. not HF, 87.3%; $p = 0.04$) Duration of HIV ($p > 0.05$)
Swetha et al. (2015)	77 HIV-infected children (1.5–15 years old) 45.5% anemic 44 on ART, 33 ART-naïve	Hyderabad, India	Assessed nutritional status over 1 year Opportunistic infections assessed at baseline and monthly Followed from July 2009 to February 2011 Blood samples collected at baseline, 6 months, and 1 year	Viral load	Anemia (Hb < 11 g/dL) Iron deficiency: undefined	Prevalence of anemia (mean, over 12 months): 45.5% No differences in anemia or iron deficiency depending on viral load (data not reported in tables or text)

(continued)

TABLE 3.5 (continued)
Cross-Sectional Studies

Study	Sample	Location	Methods	Exposure	Outcome	Main Findings
Mugisha et al. (2013)	1449 adults with known HIV status; median age, 62 years. Men: 8.0% HIV-infected Women: 5.5% HIV-infected	Entebbe, Uganda	Cross-sectional survey of anemia HIV rapid testing used to assess HIV status	HIV	Anemia (Hb < 12.0 g/dL for women, Hb < 13.0 g/dL for men)	Association with anemia: HIV infection independently associated (AOR, 2.17; 95% CI, 1.32–3.57; $p = 0.003$) Adjusted for age group, sex, and their interaction, all independent predictors of anemia including marital status, alcohol, fruit, blood pressure, hookworm intensity, and malaria
Visser and Mostert (2013)	180 HIV-infected, 140 HIV-uninfected	Pretoria, South Africa	Patients admitted between May 2005 and September 2010 if SF exceeded 1500 µg/L Retrospectively determined causes of possible hyper-ferritinaemia	HIV-1 status TB status	Elevated iron stores (SF ≥ 1500 µg/L)	Association with elevated iron stores: • In HIV-infected patients, TB infection was more likely to cause elevated iron stores compared to HIV-uninfected patients (OR, 17.98; 95% CI, 8.31–38.88). • Among HIV-uninfected patients, chronic renal failure was more likely to cause elevated iron stores. • Mean SF among HIV-infected patients was higher than for HIV-uninfected (4079 vs. 2348 µg/L).
Kosalaraksa et al. (2012)	296 HIV-infected, ART-naïve children (1–12 years old)	Thailand and Cambodia	Prevalence study of anemia, iron status, and thalassemia Parent trial: Pediatric Randomized to Early versus Deferred Antiretroviral Initiation in Cambodia and Thailand (PREDICT) study	HIV	Anemia (Hb < 11.0 g/dL for children <5 years; Hb < 11.5 g/dL for children 5–12 years)	Prevalence of anemia: 50% Prevalence of IDA: 2.7% Prevalence of thalassemia trait: 46.6%

Reference	Location	Sample	Methods	Exposure/intervention	Anemia definition	Findings
Masaisa et al. (2011)	Butare, Rwanda	250 women (200 HIV-infected, 50 HIV-uninfected)	Performed clinical exams, iron assays, CBC, serum folic acid, and CD4 T-cell count	HIV First-line HAART regimen: ZDV or stavudine plus lamivudine plus nevirapine or efavirenz	Anemia (Hb < 12.0 g/dL for women, Hb < 13.0 g/dL for men)	No differences in SF and folic acid between HIV-infected and uninfected groups. Associations with anemia: • Lack of HAART (OR, 1.44; 95% CI, 1.21–1.67) • ZDV use (OR, 1.14; 95% CI, 1.01–1.29) • HIV infection (HIV-infected, 29% vs. HIV-uninfected, 8%; $p <0.0001$) • CD4 T-cell count < 200 cells/μL (OR, 2.41; 95% CI, 2.01–3.07)
Dikshit et al. (2009)	Chandigarh, India	200 HIV-infected (65.5% anemic, 67.5% male, 33% on ART)	Patients screened for hematological abnormalities, blood culture, urine analysis, bone marrow evaluation	Group 1: CD4 T-cell <200 cells/μL Group 2: CD4 T-cell >200 cells/μL	Anemia (Hb < 12 g/dL in women, Hb < 13 g/dL in men)	Prevalence of anemia: 65.6%. Associations with CD4 T-cell: • SF (Pearson correlation, −0.213; $p = 0.016$) • Hb (Pearson correlation, 0.069; $p < 0.001$) • Packed cell volume % (Pearson correlation, 0.531; $p < 0.001$) • Mean corpuscular volume (Pearson correlation, 0.409; $p < 0.001$) • Serum iron (Pearson correlation, −0.076; $p = 0.399$) • TIBC (Pearson correlation, 0.126; $p = 0.16$) • Cumulative incidence of anemia greater in Group 1 patients vs. Group 2 patients ($p < 0.001$)
Shet et al. (2009)	India	248 HIV-infected children (1–12 years old)	Retrospective analysis of children attending 3 outpatient clinics	ART	Anemia (Hb < 11 g/dL) Severe anemia (Hb < 7 g/dL)	Associations with anemia: • Use of ART: (OR, 0.29; 95% CI, 0.16–0.53; $p < 0.01$) • ART type (ZDV or stavudine) not associated with anemia
Kagu et al. (2007)	Maiduguri, Borno State, Nigeria	50 anemic, HIV-infected adults (20 with AIDS-associated Kaposi's sarcoma) Median age: 37 years	Bone marrow evaluation	AIDS-associated Kaposi's sarcoma	Macrophage hemosiderin iron stores, graded from 0 to 6	Positive correlation between iron stores and opportunistic infection ($p = 0.001$)

(continued)

TABLE 3.5 (continued)
Cross-Sectional Studies

Study	Sample	Location	Methods	Exposure	Outcome	Main Findings
Lewis et al. (2007)	81 adults with Hb < 7 g/dL (79% HIV-infected, 25% iron deficient)	Blantyre, Malawi	Case-control design using bone marrow aspirates to compare against measurement of ferritin, TfR, MCH, MCV via biochemical assays	Presence of HIV infection	Iron deficiency (bone marrow aspirates with no iron or trace of iron)	Associations with iron status: • Presence of HIV infection (HIV-infected, 59% vs. HIV-uninfected, 16%; $p < 0.001$)
Tohill et al. (2007)	553 women (369 HIV-infected, 184 HIV-uninfected)	4 US communities (Boston, New York, Detroit, MI, and Providence, RI)	Nested case-control study part of the HIV Epidemiology Research Study (HERS)	Presence of HIV infection	Measurements of serum micronutrients (ferritin, iron, TIBC, Hb, MCV)	Associations with iron status: • Hb by HIV status (HIV-infected, 12.6 g/dL vs. HIV-uninfected, 13.3 g/dL; $p < 0.01$) • Mean corpuscular volume (HIV-infected, 100 mm^3 vs. HIV-uninfected, 90 mm^3; $p < 0.01$) • SF (ng/mL), median SE (HIV-infected, 70.0 ± 5.8 vs. HIV-uninfected, 43.0 ± 4.1; $p < 0.001$) • Serum iron (µg/dL), median SE (HIV-infected, 74.9 ± 2.3 vs. HIV-uninfected, 78.0 ± 4.5; $p = 0.60$) • Serum TIBC (µg/dL), median SE (HIV-infected, 334.3 ± 3.6 vs. HIV-uninfected, 351.5 ± 5.8; $p < 0.001$)
Friis et al. (2003)	526 HIV-infected pregnant women	Harare, Zimbabwe	Multiple linear regression analysis of cross-sectional study Viral load (geq/mL) Study conducted between 1996 and 1997 Enrolled between 22- and 35-weeks gestation	HIV Storage iron: SF	Viral load ($\log_{10}$ geq/mL)	Low SF associated with low viral load (SF < 6 µg/L, log viral load 3.63; 95% CI, 3.41–3.85; $p = 0.02$) All independent predictors of viral load: storage iron, haptoglobin 2-2, elevated ACT

Study	Population	Location	Study design	HIV/clinical classification	Anemia/iron definition	Results
Eley et al. (2002)	60 ART-naïve, HIV-infected children	Cape Town, South Africa	Prospective, cross-sectional analysis. Children took nutritional and micronutrient supplementation. Diagnosed according to 1994 revised CDC criteria	Clinical features of HIV defined according to CDC 1994 revised criteria: category A (mild), category B (moderate), category C (severe). Immunosuppression: category 1 (no immunosuppression), category 2 (moderately immunosuppressed), category 3 (severely immunosuppressed)	Iron depletion (ferritin < 10 µg/L)	Prevalence of anemia: 73%. Associations with HIV status: • Hb (median) by HIV status (Hb = 96 g/L vs. Hb = 104 g/L vs. Hb = 112 g/L); severe vs. mild (p = 0.006); moderate vs. mild (p = 0.04) • Anemia by HIV status: severe, 92% vs. mild, 58% (p = 0.04), moderate, 76% vs. mild, 58% (p = 0.2) • sTfR (median) by HIV status (severe 35.5 vs. 26.0 nmol/L; p = 0.01) No association of sTfR with immunological categories
Salomé and Grotto (2002)	111 HIV-infected (19 with anemia of chronic disease, 50 with other forms of anemia, 42 without anemia)	São Paulo, Brazil	All patients, except 3 without anemia, received AZT, DDI, lamivudine (3TC) and treatment of opportunistic infections	CDC classification of CD4 T-Cell number and clinical conditions	Anemia of chronic disease (decreased serum iron, reduced or normal Tfr, increased SF; no values given) Anemia (Hb < 12.0 g/dL for women, Hb < 14.0 g/dL for men)	Association with anemia of chronic disease: • CD4 T-cell/CD8 T-cell count lower in ACD group: median ACD, 0.13 (0.01–3.30) vs. non-anemic, 0.47 (0.06–1.56) (p = 0.0057)
Semba et al. (2002)	197 female injection drug users (136 HIV-infected, 61 HIV-uninfected)	Baltimore, MD	Participants seen in clinic every 6 months	HIV	Anemia (Hb < 120 g/L) Iron deficiency (plasma ferritin < 30 µg/L)	Prevalence of anemia among individuals with HIV higher than in individuals without HIV: 44.1% vs. 26.2%

(continued)

TABLE 3.5 (continued)
Cross-Sectional Studies

Study	Sample	Location	Methods	Exposure	Outcome	Main Findings
Friis et al. (2001)	1669 pregnant women with known HIV status (22- to 34-week gestation) 31.5% HIV-infected	Harare, Zimbabwe	Multiple linear regression of HIV infection and iron biomarkers	Presence of HIV infection	Depleted iron stores (SF < 12 μg/L) Normal iron stores (SF ≥ 12 μg/L) Hb	Regression coefficient for predictors of SF (μg/L); $\log_{10}$ transformed HIV infection (0.93; 95% CI, 0.86–0.99; $p = 0.03$) HIV associated with lower Hb
Antelman et al. (2000)	1064 HIV-infected pregnant women (<27 weeks gestation) 80% stage 1 HIV, 18% in stage 2, <1% in stage 3 of HIV	Dar es Salaam, Tanzania	Biomarkers analyzed from women previously in an RCT for vitamin supplementation on perinatal transmission of HIV Examined red blood cells, looking at Hb for T-cell count and infectious diseases Absolute T lymphocyte subset counting of CD4 T-cell, CD8 T-cell, and CD3+ cells done by FACS count system	CD4 and CD8 T-cell count Higher CD4 T-cell count ≥ 500 cells/μL Lower CD4 T-cell count < 200 cells/μL	Anemia (Hb ≤ 110 g/L) Severe anemia (Hb ≤ 85 g/L)	Compared to women with higher CD4 T-cell count, women with lower CD4 T-cell count more likely to be anemic (36.5% vs. 23.0%; OR, 2.70; 95% CI, 1.42–5.12; $p = 0.002$) CD4 T-cell count/μL: Hb < 85 g/L, 398 ± 192; Hb 85–109, 433 ± 209; Hb ≥ 110, 458 ± 207 ($p = 0.014$)

Reference	Subjects	Location	Study design	Variable	Results
Meda et al. (1999)	2308 pregnant women (9.7% HIV-infected)	Bobo-Dioulasso, Burkina Faso	Women from previous study (Fawzi et al., 1999) were in 1 of 4 groups: (1) vitamin A, (2) multivitamin with vitamin A, (3) multivitamin without vitamin A, or (4) placebo. Study conducted between 1995 and 1996. Women attending two prenatal clinics were enrolled as part of clinical trial of ZDV in pregnancy. Study assessed prevalence and risk factors of maternal anemia	Presence of HIV infection. Anemia (Hb < 11 g/dL)	HIV infection significantly and independently associated with anemia ($p < 0.001$). Prevalence of anemia HIV-infected, 78.4% vs. HIV seronegative, 64.7% ($p < 0.001$). Relative risk of HIV increased with severity of anemia. No association between severity of anemia and HIV status
Castaldo et al. (1996)	71 HIV-infected children	Italy	Cross-sectional analysis	HIV. Anemia	Prevalence of anemia: 66%

(continued)

TABLE 3.5 (continued)
Cross-Sectional Studies

Study	Sample	Location	Methods	Exposure	Outcome	Main Findings
Riera et al. (1994)	168 HIV-infected patients	Barcelona, Spain	Evaluated liver type SF in patients with HIV infection	Group 1: Asymptomatic HIV-infected patients ($n = 86$) Group 2: Asymptomatic patients who met CDC criteria for AIDS ($n = 22$) Group 3: AIDS patients with an acute complication requiring hospitalization ($n = 60$)	SF levels	Lower CD4 T-cell count and clinical worsening of HIV infection associated with increasing levels of SF ($p < 0.001$)
Fuchs et al. (1993)	63 HIV-infected individuals (15–66 years old)	Innsbruck, Austria	Compared immune activation markers (interferon-γ, serum and urine neopterin, and B_2-microglobulin) to iron metabolism in order to identify causes of anemia in HIV-infected patients	HIV and immune activation markers: neopterin, interferon-γ, B_2-microglobulin Iron markers: serum iron, transferrin, free iron-binding capacity, ferritin	HIV and immune activation markers: neopterin, interferon-γ, B_2-microglobulin Iron markers: serum iron, transferrin, free iron-binding capacity, ferritin	Associations between HIV and immune markers and iron markers: • Low Hb was associated with greater immune activation as measured by interferon-γ, neopterin, and B_2-microglobulin

| Castella et al. (1985) | 49 patients with CDC-defined AIDS (55 bone marrow biopsies; 44 male, 5 female) | New York, NY | Cross-sectional analysis of bone marrow biopsies Biopsies conducted from January 1983–January 1984 | AIDS | Anemia | 85% of patients anemic |

Note: 3TC, lamivudine ACD, anemia with chronic disease AOR, adjusted odds ratio ART, antiretroviral therapy AZT, azidothymidine CDC, Centers for Disease Control and Prevention CRP, c-reactive protein DDI, didanosine geq/mL, genome equivalents/milliliter Hb, hemoglobin HF, high ferritin IDA, iron-deficiency anemia MCH, mean cell hemoglobin MCV, mean cell volume OR, odds ratio RCT, randomized controlled trial TB, tuberculosis TfR, transferrin receptor TIBC, total iron-binding capacity ZDV, zidovudine.

The main focus of this chapter is on evidence from cohort studies ($n = 30$), randomized controlled trials ($n = 4$), and intervention studies ($n = 2$). Of these included studies, most were conducted as part of 4 parent randomized clinical trials: 5 studies came from the Trial of Vitamins (TOV) conducted in Tanzania; 3 studies were conducted as part of the Zimbabwe Vitamins for Mothers and Babies Project (ZVITAMBO); 2 studies were part of the Breastfeeding, Antiretrovirals, and Nutrition (BAN) study conducted in Malawi; and 1 study was part of the Centre for the AIDS Programme of Research in South Africa (CAPRISA) Acute Infection Study. Few randomized clinical trials have been conducted to date to examine the effects of iron supplementation on health outcomes in HIV-infected populations.

Although all of the eligible studies were assessed for data for all *a priori* outcomes (see Methods section), most studies included data on a narrow subset of these outcomes. For example, most studies included data on the following HIV-related outcomes: all-cause mortality, AIDS-related mortality, WHO HIV disease stage, HIV disease progression, opportunistic infections, CD4 and CD8 T-cell counts, and HIV RNA viral load. Although most studies focused on hemoglobin concentrations or anemia, iron status biomarkers assessed included SF, sTfR, CRP, and AGP. Finally, studies conducted among HIV-infected pregnant women focused on a subset of perinatal outcomes: mother-to-child transmission of HIV, gestational age at delivery, preterm birth, birthweight, low birthweight, small-for-gestational age, and infant iron status.

IRON AND HIV-RELATED HEALTH OUTCOMES

Mortality Outcomes

Iron Supplementation and Mortality

To date, no randomized clinical trials have been conducted to examine the effects of iron supplementation on mortality in HIV-infected individuals. An unblinded trial was conducted to examine the effects of different treatment options on health outcomes in adult patients diagnosed with AIDS: iron protoxalate–dapsone (30 mg/day soluble iron and 50 mg/day dapsone) plus aerosolized pentamidine (300 mg administered over a 30-minute period through a jet nebulizer one time per month) compared to aerosolized pentamidine regimen alone (Salmon-Ceron et al., 1995). After 31 months (i.e., at the time the trial was terminated early), patients in the iron protoxalate–dapsone group had a significant twofold higher risk of mortality compared to the control group, after adjusting for age, time since diagnosis of AIDS, and CD4 T-cell count (42% vs. 21%; risk ratio [RR], 2.18; 95% CI, 1.27–3.74; $p < 0.003$). Similarly, the mortality rate at 18 months was significantly higher in the iron protoxalate–dapsone group compared to the control (53.1% vs. 24.6%; $p < 0.003$; log-rank test). There were no significant differences between groups for cause-specific mortality.

Anemia and Mortality

Anemia is common in HIV-infected individuals and has been associated with increased risk of mortality. Several prospective observational analyses have been conducted as part of the Trial of Vitamins (TOV), a randomized trial in Dar es Salaam, Tanzania, in which 1078 HIV-infected, ART-naïve pregnant women were randomized to receive vitamin A, multivitamins and vitamin A, multivitamins without vitamin A, or placebo in a 2×2 factorial design. In this trial, all HIV-infected, pregnant women also received daily supplementation of 400 mg ferrous sulfate (i.e., equivalent to 120 mg ferrous iron) and 5 mg folic acid, along with weekly chloroquine (500 mg) as malaria prophylaxis. In an observational analysis within the TOV, moderate anemia (hemoglobin [Hb] = 8.5 to 10.9 g/dL) at baseline was associated with a twofold greater risk of AIDS-related mortality (hazard ratio [HR], 2.21; 95% CI, 1.53–3.19; $p < 0.001$) and all-cause mortality (HR, 2.06; 95% CI, 1.52–2.79; $p < 0.001$) compared to women who were not anemic at baseline (Hb ≥ 11.0 g/dL) in analyses adjusted for CD4 T-cell counts, WHO HIV disease stage, pregnancy, age, treatment arm, and body mass index (BMI) (O'Brien et al., 2005). The risks of these outcomes were even higher among individuals with severe anemia (Hb < 8.5 g/dL) at baseline—AIDS-related mortality

HR = 3.47 (95% CI, 2.25–5.33; $p < 0.001$) vs. all-cause mortality HR = 3.19 (95% CI, 2.23–4.56; $p < 0.001$)—compared to women who were not anemic at baseline in multivariate analyses (O'Brien et al., 2005).

In a prospective analysis conducted among 829 children born to HIV-infected women who were enrolled in the TOV study, iron deficiency anemia (IDA; defined as Hb < 8.5 g/dL with hypochromasia and microcytosis) was associated with a twofold increase in the hazards of mortality in the first 24 months of life (HR, 1.99; 95% CI, 1.06–3.72; $p < 0.03$) in analyses adjusting for maternal characteristics, including CD4 T-cell counts taken every three months during pregnancy, education, and daily per-capita money spent on food, as well as for child's birthweight, child's age at the introduction of semisolid foods, time-varying CD4 T-cell counts, malaria parasitemia, and HIV infection status (Chatterjee et al., 2010). In multivariate analyses, severe anemia without indicators of iron deficiency (e.g., Hb < 8.5 g/dL but not exhibiting hypochromasia and microcytosis) was not associated with the hazards of overall child mortality during the first two years of life (HR, 1.38; 95% CI, 0.95–2.01; $p = 0.10$).

In a cohort study conducted in Indonesia among 869 HIV-infected ART-naïve patients (≥14 years), moderate anemia (Hb = 8.0 to 10.5 g/dL) and severe anemia (Hb < 8.0 g/dL) were associated with increased hazards of mortality at six months of follow-up (HR, 6.5; interquartile range [IQR], 2.0–21.2; $p = 0.002$) (Wisaksana et al., 2011). In analyses at six months of follow-up, individuals with moderate to severe anemia had significantly lower survival compared to individuals without anemia: 82.5% anemic (95% CI, 75.5–89.4%) vs. 98.6% non-anemic (95% CI, 97.3–99.9%; $p < 0.001$) (Wisaksana et al., 2011).

Serum Ferritin and Mortality

Several prospective analyses have been conducted to examine the associations between serum ferritin concentrations and risk of mortality in HIV-infected individuals. In a prospective analysis as part of the TOV study among 584 HIV-infected pregnant women, higher serum ferritin (SF >150 µg/L) was not associated with increased risk of AIDS-related mortality compared to women with low serum ferritin (SF < 12.0 µg/L) in multivariate analyses adjusted for maternal age, HIV disease progression, wasting, Hb, and CRP (composite endpoint rate ratio, 1.29; 95% CI, 0.75–2.21; $p = 0.36$) (Kupka et al., 2007). In a prospective analysis conducted as part of ZVITAMBO, among 643 HIV-infected, postpartum women, higher SF concentrations at baseline (within 96 hours of delivery) were associated with increased hazards of death in the first 12 months after delivery, after adjusting for AGP ($\log_{10}$ SF HR, 4.10; 95% CI, 1.64–10.23; $p = 0.002$), and individuals with elevated SF (>45.0 µg/L) at baseline had significantly increased risk of death in the first year compared to iron-deficient individuals (SF < 15.0 µ/L) or iron-replete individuals (SF, 15–45 µg/L) ($p < 0.001$) (Rawat et al., 2009). There were no significant differences in the hazards of mortality between iron-deficient and iron-replete individuals ($p = 0.57$). Findings did not vary by anemia status at baseline (p-interaction = 0.18) (Rawat et al., 2009).

Other Hematological Factors and Mortality

In other prospective analyses conducted as part of ZVITAMBO, sTfR concentrations were not associated with risk of mortality (Rawat et al., 2009). In a retrospective cohort study conducted in The Gambia among HIV-infected, ART-naïve adults, elevated baseline hepcidin concentrations were associated with increased risk of all-cause mortality: highest vs. lowest tertile HR = 3.02 (95% CI, 1.91–4.78; $p < 0.05$) and middle vs. lowest tertile HR = 1.95 (95% CI, 1.22–3.10; $p < 0.05$) (Minchella et al., 2015). In another cohort study conducted in The Gambia among 1362 HIV-infected adults, a higher combined iron status index, which included transferrin, ferritin, and Hb (elevated vs. normal), predicted increased risk of all-cause mortality (HR, 11.26; 95% CI, 7.36–17.24; $p < 0.001$) compared to normal iron status for all iron biomarkers measured (McDermid et al., 2007). Of the iron biomarkers measured in this study, only sTfR was not associated with significantly increased risk of all-cause mortality in multivariate analyses. In a case-control study that examined the bone marrow macrophage iron grades of 348 HIV-infected patients, those patients with higher iron grades (4–5) had significantly increased risk of mortality from the time of HIV diagnosis compared to those with lower iron grades (0–2) (HR, 2.80; 95% CI, 1.4–4.9; $p = 0.001$) (de Monyé et al., 1999).

HIV Disease Progression Outcomes

Measures of HIV disease progression-related outcomes, as they relate to iron and hematologic status, were categorized as follows: WHO HIV disease stage, CD4 T-cell counts, HIV RNA viral load, inflammatory markers, and co-infections and other clinical morbidities. The latter (co-infections and other clinical morbidities) makes reference specifically to malaria and tuberculosis (TB). Finally, other relevant maternal and child health outcomes among HIV-infected groups, as they relate to hematologic status, were considered.

WHO HIV Disease Stage

The association between iron and HIV disease progression has been investigated in several studies. In a randomized, placebo-controlled trial in Malawi among 209 HIV-infected children (36% taking ART at baseline) with moderate anemia (Hb = 7.0 to 9.9 g/dL), children were randomized to receive either daily iron supplementation (3 mg/kg/day ferrous sulfate) with multivitamins (vitamins A, C, and D) or multivitamins alone (Esan et al., 2013). Iron supplementation was associated with reduced risk of progression to AIDS (incidence rate ratio [IRR], 0.25; 95% CI, 0.08–0.83; $p = 0.02$; p-interaction = 0.07), but only in analyses among iron-deficient children (SF < 12.0 µg/dL if CRP < 5.0 mg/L, or SF < 30.0 µg/dL if CRP > 5.0 mg/L). According to the authors, this subgroup analysis was not adjusted for the following potential confounders: HAART use at recruitment, baseline Hb, bed net use, CD4 T-cell percentage at baseline, or blood transfusion before recruitment (Esan et al., 2013).

In a cohort study conducted in Bangalore, India, among 240 children who were HIV-infected at birth, iron supplementation (therapeutic iron supplementation based on WHO criteria, prescribed for three months at a 3-mg/kg/day dose) was not significantly associated with HIV disease stage after one year of follow-up compared to no iron supplementation. The prevalence of WHO HIV stage 3 or 4 at baseline among the iron group was 25.7% vs. 16.7% for the no-iron group ($p = 0.04$), and the prevalence of WHO HIV stage 3 or 4 after one year among the iron group was 10.9% vs. 12.5% for the no-iron group ($p > 0.05$) (Shet et al., 2015).

In an aforementioned observational analysis conducted as part of the TOV study, the association of iron status with HIV disease progression was assessed during follow-up (Kupka et al., 2007). Elevated SF (>150.0 µg/L) concentrations were not associated with risk of HIV disease progression to WHO stage 4 (RR, 1.78; 95% CI, 0.68–4.64; $p = 0.24$) compared to low SF (<12.0 µg/L) in models adjusted for Hb, CRP, wasting, and other markers of HIV disease progression.

CD4 T-Cell Counts

In the previously mentioned randomized trial in Malawi, children who received iron supplementation had significantly greater change in the percentage of CD4 T-cells from baseline to three months of follow-up compared to children in the placebo group (3.86 ± 12.15 iron vs. −1.45 ± 14.28 placebo; adjusted mean difference/prevalence ratio, 6.00; 95% CI, 1.84–10.16; $p = 0.005$), adjusted for baseline Hb, bed nets, HAART status, CD4 T-cell counts at baseline, and history of prior blood transfusion (Esan et al., 2013). As mentioned above, this randomized trial conducted in Malawi is the only RCT to date that investigates iron supplementation alone among HIV-infected individuals. In the aforementioned randomized uncontrolled (unblinded) trial among HIV-infected adults treated with iron–dapsone vs. pentamidine (Salmon-Ceron et al., 1995), there was no significant difference in mean CD4 T-cell count between treatment groups at baseline. Patients who received iron–dapsone showed no increase in CD4 T-cell counts during the first three months after initiation of treatment compared to patients who received only pentamidine (Jacobus, 1996). After a mean follow-up period of 13 ± 6.4 months, the mean CD4 cell count during the study was lower in the iron–dapsone treatment group (49 ± 61/mm^3) than in the pentamidine group (83 ± 88/mm^3; $p < 0.002$, t-test).

In a case-control study among 80 ART-naïve, HIV-infected and 50 HIV-uninfected individuals, in Ile Ife, Nigeria, CD4 T-cell count was inversely associated with serum iron levels ($r = -0.572$; $p < 0.001$) (Banjoko et al., 2012). In the aforementioned cohort study conducted among HIV-infected adults in The Gambia, higher hepcidin concentrations correlated with lower absolute CD4 cell counts. Log_{10}-transformed median hepcidin concentrations varied significantly across CD4 T-cell count categories ($p < 0.001$) (Minchella et al., 2015):

- CD4 T-cell count < 200 cells/μL—62.8 ng/mL hepcidin (IQR, 18.5–175.9 ng/mL)
- CD4 T-cell count 200–500 cells/μL—46.5 ng/mL hepcidin (IQR, 3.9–87.3 ng/mL
- CD4 T-cell count > 500 cells/μL—20.2 ng/mL hepcidin (IQR, 1.7–44.8 ng/mL)

Anemia was also associated with lower CD4 T-cell counts at baseline, time of HIV diagnosis, with anemia prevalence by CD4 T-cell count as follows: >500 cells/μL, 68%; 200–500 cells/μL, 73%; <200 cells/μL, 89% ($p = 0.032$) (Minchella et al., 2015). Similar relationships among hepcidin, anemia, and CD4 T-cell counts were also reported for an Indonesian population in which serum hepcidin (nM) was inversely correlated with both absolute log CD4 T-cell counts (cells/mm³) ($p < 0.001$) and Hb concentration (g/dL) ($p = 0.003$) (Wisaksana et al., 2013).

In the previously noted study conducted among HIV-infected children in Bangalore, shorter term (defined as three months) receipt of iron supplementation was not significantly associated with changes in CD4 T-cell counts compared to no iron supplementation from baseline to one year: iron group at baseline, 21.0% CD4; at one year, 26.5% vs. no-iron group at baseline, 20.5%; at one year, 26.0% ($p > 0.05$) (Shet et al., 2015). However, in analyses stratified by baseline anemia status, anemic children (based on WHO criteria, children ages 6–59 months, Hb < 11.0 g/dL; 5–11 years, Hb < 11.5 g/dL; ≥12 years, Hb < 12.0 g/dL) were significantly more likely to have low CD4 T-cell counts (<25%) compared to non-anemic children (anemic, 66.4%; non-anemic, 32.3%; adjusted odds ratio [AOR], 3.20; 95% CI, 1.80–5.70; $p < 0.001$) in analyses adjusted for stunting (height for age z-score < –2), antiretroviral therapy, low CD4 T-cell percent (<25%), viral load ≥ 400 copies/mL, and vitamin A deficiency (retinol binding protein < 0.7 μ moles/L).

In an analysis of HIV-infected, ART-naïve pregnant women in the TOV study, O'Brien et al. (2005) found that both moderate (Hb = 8.5 to 10.9 g/dL) and severe (Hb < 8.5 g/dL) anemia were significantly associated with time to a 50% decline in CD4 T-cell count in multivariate Cox proportional hazards models, adjusted for baseline CD4 T-cell counts, WHO HIV disease stage, age, pregnancy, treatment arm, and BMI: moderate anemia vs. no anemia (HR, 1.79; 95% CI, 1.38–2.33; $p < 0.001$) and severe anemia vs. no anemia (HR, 1.59; 95% CI, 1.02–2.49; $p = 0.04$). Participants with hypochromasia, with or without microcytosis, had significantly greater hazards of a 50% decline in CD4 T-cell counts, compared to individuals without hypochromasia or microcytosis (O'Brien et al., 2005).

In an analysis of the TOV study, Isanaka et al. (2012) found that severe maternal anemia (Hb < 8.5 g/dL), measured at six weeks postpartum and every six months thereafter, predicted lower CD4 T-cell counts among their children (difference in CD4 T-cell count/μL for severe anemia was –93; 95% CI, –204–17; p-trend = 0.02). Analyses were adjusted for maternal age, BMI, HIV RNA viral load, CD4 T-cell counts, WHO HIV disease stage, malaria, number of previous births, adherence with iron and folic acid supplementation, intervention arm in the vitamin study, and child's time-varying HIV-infection status.

HIV RNA Viral Load

Olsen et al. (2004) described data from a historical iron supplementation trial in western Kenya, where 181 adults received 60 mg iron supplementation or placebo. The historical trial assessed the effects of iron on helminth reinfection rates four months after baseline but did not publish data, and current data were based on respository samples. After randomization of HIV-infected subjects ($n = 45$) between placebo and iron groups, baseline viral load was higher in the iron group compared to the placebo group (log_{10} [geq/mL] 5.57 for iron vs. 4.93 for placebo; $p = 0.02$), despite no significant differences among the groups in levels of Hb, SF, or presence of infections. However, no significant difference in viral load was found among the groups after four months of receiving 60 mg supplementary iron (4.71 for iron vs. 4.21 for placebo; p-value not given) (Olsen et al., 2004).

In prospective analyses of various cohorts of HIV-infected individuals among 12 individuals who became HIV-infected after plasma donation, a rapid increase in plasma HIV-1 RNA levels in the acute phase of infection was associated with a significant increase in hepcidin (Armitage et al., 2014). As part of the same study, among 17 HIV-infected men who have sex with men, hepcidin levels during chronic HIV infection peaked in acute infection before stabilizing at setpoint viremia: geometric mean hepcidin for day 0–60 was 47.8 ng/mL (95% CI, 34.1–66.8; 42 samples measured), and for day 89–366 was 33.9 ng/mL (95% CI, 22.7–50.8; 36 samples measured; $p = 0.0378$; paired t-test; $n = 17$ pairs). Compared to HIV-uninfected individuals, HIV-infected individuals had approximately twofold higher hepcidin levels throughout the chronic stage of infection (19.13 vs. 8.35 ng/mL; $p = 0.0089$). Within this cohort, acute-phase proteins CRP and serum amyloid A (SAA) and cytokines IL-10, IL-18, and TNF-alpha were higher in the HIV-infected group, whereas no difference in IL-6 was observed (Armitage et al., 2014).

In a prospective analysis in the TOV study, SF concentrations (µg/L), measured approximately 30 weeks after delivery, were directly associated with viral load measurements (copies/mm^3) available from samples collected within four weeks of when the SF sample was collected (Spearman rank correlation, 0.288; $p < 0.01$) (Kupka et al., 2007). After controlling for AGP and CD4 count, Rawat et al. (2009) found that high SF (>45 µg/L) was associated with a two- to threefold increase in viral load in non-anemic, HIV-infected women as compared to the low-SF group (<15 µg/L). Relative HIV viral load in the high-SF group was 2.9 times that of the low-SF group (95% CI, 1.44–5.83). In an attempt to further control for elevated ferritin due to the presence of inflammation, the authors re-ran analyses excluding all women with elevated AGP values entirely, yielding a greater than 2.5 times higher viral load among non-anemic women with high ferritin as compared to the low-ferritin group ($p = 0.023$). These same results (increased SF associated with greater viral load) were not apparent among anemic women; the authors speculated that this could have been due to prioritization of iron for Hb formation and not for viral replication (Rawat et al., 2009).

In a cohort study assessing the health of women of reproductive age with pre- and post-HIV infection in South Africa, as part of the CAPRISA Acute Infection Study, Hb concentrations at three months post-infection were correlated with HIV viral load ($p = 0.04$), although the Hb concentrations were not significantly associated at other time-points during follow-up (at infection, 6-month, and 12-month follow-up) ($p > 0.05$) (Mlisana et al., 2008). Findings did not vary by anemia status.

Inflammatory Markers

Shet et al. (2015) found that there was no significant change in chronic inflammation among people who received iron. Kupka et al. (2007) found that the correlation between SF and viral load (VL) was stronger among women with elevated CRP (>10.0 mg/L). Rawat et al. (2009) found that the associations between SF and VL were attenuated when controlling for AGP, but SF and VL were still significantly correlated. In women with elevated AGP (>1 g/L), there was no association between SF and VL ($\beta = 0.191$; $p = 0.148$). Similarly, Gordeuk et al. (2009) reported that HIV-infected individuals with high dietary iron intake (defined as estimated life consumption of traditional beer > 1000 L) had lower neopterin levels than HIV-infected individuals with low dietary iron ($p < 0.0001$). In another study, Sarcletti et al. (2003) longitudinally assessed Hb levels in individuals taking ART over six months and found an inverse relationship between Hb changes and neopterin, with decreasing neopterin levels associated with increased Hb between start of ART and three and six months.

Co-infections and Other Clinical Morbidities

Several cross-sectional and case-control studies have been conducted to examine the links between iron status and the occurrence of co-infections in HIV-infected populations; however, to date, only one randomized controlled trial and four cohort studies have investigated the associations of iron supplementation with the risk of co-infections in HIV-infected individuals. One of these studies examined hospitalizations for intercurrent infections as an outcome (Shet et al., 2015). In the afore-mentioned cohort study conducted among children infected perinatally with HIV in Bangalore, India, children provided with iron supplements for three months (3-mg/kg/day dose) and followed for one year exhibited no significant difference in the absolute number of hospitalizations for inter-current infections as compared to those who were not supplemented (Shet et al., 2015). The total number of children (i.e, percent) in each group was not given. The remaining studies considered iron supplementation in the context of co-infections involving either malaria or tuberculosis.

Malaria

In the aforementioned randomized trial among HIV-infected children in Malawi, iron supplemen-tation was associated with increased risk of malaria at six months of follow-up (IR, 120.2 vs. 71.7; adjusted IRR, 1.81; 95% CI, 1.04–3.16; $p = 0.04$) and at three months of follow-up (IR, 78.1 vs. 36.0; adjusted IRR, 2.68; 95% CI, 1.08–6.63; $p = 0.03$) (Esan et al., 2013). In a cohort study conducted in western Kenya among multiple cohorts of HIV-uninfected and HIV-infected pregnant women over time, one enrollment period included provision of iron (200 mg ferrous sulfate three times daily for the duration of the pregnancy) per the recommendations of the Ministry of Health. When compared to an earlier enrollment period of no intervention at all, there was a similar prevalence of placental malaria (adjusted odds ratio, 1.07; 95% CI, 0.86–1.32), adjusted for maternal HIV status, gravity, interaction between HIV and gravity, age, place of residence (urban, semi-urban/rural), ethnicity, and socioeconomic status (presence of electricity in the house). The authors did not moni-tor viral load changes over the course of the supplementation during pregnancy. The effect of the intervention did not differ by HIV status, with an HIV-infected adjusted odds ratio of 1.21 (95% CI, 0.67–2.19) and an HIV-uninfected adjusted odds ratio of 1.01 (95% CI, 0.78–1.31; p for interaction term $= 0.2$), adjusted for the same variables, in addition to an interaction term between maternal HIV status and period of enrollment equal to whether supplemented or not (van Eijk et al., 2007).

Tuberculosis

In the retrospective cohort study conducted in The Gambia among 196 patients (60.2% HIV-infected), hepcidin in the highest quartile (>85.9 ng/mL) at HIV diagnosis was associated with greater inci-dence of tuberculosis (TB) compared to the three lowest quartiles of hepcidin (<3.4, 3.4–22.1, and 22.1–85.9 ng/mL). The only significant predictors of TB incidence were hepcidin (IRR, 2.05; 95% CI, 1.01–4.16) and HIV type (IRR, 2.10; 95% CI, 1.03–4.26) (Minchella et al., 2014). In the retro-spective cohort study in Washington, DC, which examined the associations between iron grades in bone macrophages and survival outcomes, HIV-infected individuals with higher iron grades (4–5) in bone macrophages had significantly increased risk of TB infection and *Mycobacterium avium* infection compared to lower iron grades (0–2) (de Monyé et al., 1999).

Maternal/Infant Hematologic Status and Child Health Outcomes

This review would not be complete without consideration of the relationships among maternal iron/hematologic status, child iron/hematological status, and child health outcomes. Two studies examined the associations between maternal iron status and pediatric outcomes, including infant mortality, child growth, infection, breast milk viral load, and child CD4 T-cell counts. One study examined the association between child iron status and HIV-related health outcomes. In an analysis of the TOV study, Isanaka et al. (2012) found that severe maternal anemia (<8.5 g/dL) in HIV-infected women was associated with a twofold increase in the risk of child mortality (adjusted HR, 2.58; 95% CI, 1.66–4.01; p-trend < 0.0001), as compared to HIV-infected mothers with no anemia. Severe hypochromic microcytosis (hypochromasia ≥ 25% and microcytic cells observed), as com-pared to absent hypochromic microcytosis, was also associated with increased risk of child mortal-ity (adjusted HR, 2.36; 95% CI, 1.27–4.38; p-trend = 0.001) (Isanaka et al., 2012). These analyses were adjusted for maternal age, BMI at baseline (kg/m^2), viral load at baseline (copies/mm^3), CD4 at baseline (cells/mL), WHO clinical stage at baseline (1, 2–4), malarial infection at baseline, parity, prenatal compliance with iron and folic acid supplementation based on attendance, treatment arm in the vitamin study, and child time-varying HIV infection status. However, maternal anemia was not associated with risk of child total HIV transmission (defined as HIV transmission *in utero*, intrapartum, or during breastfeeding), compared to mothers without anemia. Severe anemia had an adjusted HR of 1.46 (95% CI, 0.91–2.33; p-trend = 0.08), and mild anemia had an adjusted HR of 1.43 (95% CI, 1.0–2.04; p-trend = 0.08) compared to no anemia. These two analyses were adjusted for maternal age, BMI at baseline (kg/m^2), viral load at baseline (copies/mm^3), CD4 at baseline (cells/mL), WHO clinical stage at baseline (1, 2–4), malarial infection at baseline, parity, prenatal compliance with iron and folic acid supplementation based on attendance, and treatment arm in the vitamin study.

In a cohort study conducted in Lusaka, Zambia, among 135 HIV-infected and lactating women participating in the ZVITAMBO study, neither iron supplementation nor maternal Hb concentrations was associated with breast milk HIV viral load (Phiri et al., 2006). In the study of perinatally HIV-infected children 2 to 12 years of age in Bangalore, India, Shet et al. (2015) found no association between iron supplementation of the children and child growth from baseline to one year of follow-up. Improvements in WAZ and height for age (HAZ) were observed in groups that both did and did not receive iron supplements. As previously reviewed, no difference in the number of hospitalizations for intercurrent infections was observed between children who received and did not receive iron. However, iron supplementation did decrease the prevalence of advanced WHO clinical stages of HIV (defined as stages 3 and 4). In the iron-supplemented group, prevalence of advanced WHO clinical stage decreased from 25.7% at baseline to 10.9% after one year of follow-up. In the non-supplemented group, prevalence of advanced WHO clinical stage decreased from 16.7% to 12.5% after one year of follow-up (Shet et al., 2015).

Post-ART Era: Associations between Iron/Hematological Status with HIV-Related Health Outcomes in the Context of ART and HAART

The role of iron in HIV-related health outcomes must be considered within the context of antiretroviral therapy, since antiretrovirals (ARVs) are known to differentially influence both iron metabolism and HIV disease progression; for example, anemia is a known side effect of zidovudine (ZDV). However, several observational studies have found ART to be associated with reduced risk of anemia (Shet et al., 2009, 2012; Kruger et al., 2013). Longitudinal studies have also observed resolution of anemia upon treatment with ARVs in adults (Kerkhoff et al., 2014) and pregnant women (Odhiambo et al., 2016). It has been hypothesized that reducing viral load with ART reduces cytokine activity, allowing erythroid progenitor cells to proliferate and thereby reducing anemia (Sarcletti et al., 2003). In a nested cohort study among 852 HIV-infected patients (161 on ZDV, 628 on stavudine [d4T], and 63 on tenofovir [TDF]), ZDV was associated with severe anemia, and the greatest increase in Hb was associated with stavudine (Parkes-Ratanshi et al., 2015). Different classes of ARVs are known to also have different obstetric impacts on HIV-infected pregnant women. In this population, additional health outcomes must be taken into account; for example, ZDV continues to be widely given to HIV-infected pregnant women both alone (excluding in labor, when single-dose nevirapine is used) and in combination with other ARVs (Sebitloane and Moodley, 2017). No trials have been conducted to date to investigate the effects of iron supplementation on HIV-related outcomes in the context of ART.

In the cohort study in Bangalore, India, among perinatally HIV-infected children (43.3% on ART at baseline), iron supplementation and ART were associated with lower prevalence of HIV disease progression to WHO stages 3 or 4 during 12 months of follow-up compared to ART alone: WHO stages 3 or 4 at baseline 25.7% with iron vs. 16.7% with no iron (p = 0.04); at one year, 10.9% with iron vs. 12.5% with no iron (p > 0.05) (Shet et al., 2015). Iron supplementation was not associated with improvement in growth or CD4 T-cell counts in analyses adjusting for ART (p > 0.05). Children who were taking iron supplementation and ART also had greater increases in Hb concentrations during follow-up compared to those taking ART alone (Hb change, 1.3 vs. 0.4 g/dL; p = 0.009).

In a cohort study conducted among 58 HIV-infected children in Johannesburg, South Africa, after 18 months on HAART (i.e., lamivudine, stavudine, efavirenz), no differences were seen in CD4 T-cell counts, HAZ scores, BMI z-scores, or log viral load between iron-deficient (sTfR > 9.4 mg/L) and iron-sufficient children ($p > 0.05$) (Kruger et al., 2013). HAART duration was associated with increased Hb concentrations during the follow-up period: baseline, 106 ± 14 g/L; 6 months, 129 ± 12 g/L; 12 months, 129 ± 11 g/L; 18 months, 129 ± 9 g/L ($p < 0.01$ for baseline vs. 18 months; $p > 0.05$ for all other comparisons). Although the prevalence of anemia declined from 31.7% to 3.8% from baseline to 18 months of follow-up, the prevalence of iron deficiency (sTfR > 9.4 mg/L) increased from 15.2% to 37.2% ($p < 0.01$) during the same time period. Hemoglobin concentrations and dietary iron intake were not significantly different between iron-deficient and iron-sufficient children after 18 months on HAART.

A cohort study in 80 HIV-infected children (2 to 12 years old) in Bangalore, India, found that children who did not initiate ART had significantly lower mean Hb concentrations (11.2 vs. 9.8 g/dL; $p < 0.001$) and greater odds of developing anemia (OR, 5.3; 95% CI, 1.7–16.3; $p = 0.002$) compared to children who initiated ART and continued for at least six months (Shet et al., 2012). The four comparison groups were (1) no treatment, (2) ART + iron, (3) ART alone, and (4) iron alone. There was no statistically significant difference in CD4 percent or CD4 T-cell count when comparing ART + iron to ART alone (p not given; 95% CI not given). However, the mean change in percentage of CD4 T-cells (CD4%, according to study) among children taking ART + iron was significant (mean, 5.45%; SE, 1.76; $p < 0.01$) compared to that of the no-treatment group. The mean change among children taking ART alone was not significant (mean, 2.54%; SE, 1.79; $p = 0.09$) compared to that of the no-treatment group. Among children taking iron alone, the mean change in percent CD4 T-cell counts was not significant (mean, −0.73%; SE, 4.59; $p = 0.87$) compared to that of the no-treatment group.

HIV/AIDS AND HEMATOLOGICAL OUTCOMES

HIV disease may contribute to the etiology of anemia and iron deficiency through a number of mechanisms, such as infection of marrow stromal cells (Koka et al., 1999), impaired hematopoietic progenitor cell growth (Moses et al., 1996), bone marrow pathologies, autoimmune hemolysis, and intestinal blood loss (Coyle, 1997; Kreuzer and Rockstroh, 1997; Sullivan, 1998). Several case-control and cross-sectional studies have noted an association between HIV and adverse hematological outcomes; however, few prospective studies have been conducted to examine the associations of HIV and iron status over time. The search strategy presented in this chapter, which resulted in 68 studies overall, yielded one cohort study among adults and three cohort studies among mothers and infants that examined the association of HIV infection and hematological status. Additionally, four studies were found that assessed associations of antiretroviral therapy with hematological outcomes. In the aforementioned CAPRISA Acute Infection Study prospectively examining iron biomarkers in women at high risk of HIV infection, development of HIV infection was associated with a decline in Hb concentrations and an increase in the prevalence of anemia post-infection (mean decline in Hb, 0.46 g/dL; SD, 1.09; anemia prevalence pre-infection, 25.0%; 3 months post, 52.6%; 6 months post, 61.1%; 12 months post, 51.4%) (Mlisana et al., 2008). A similar decline in mean corpuscular volume (MCV) was noted from pre- to post-HIV infection (decline in MCV, 1.78 fL; SD, 2.74), although mean SF concentrations increased from 65.13 µg/L to 79.09 µg/L during the same time period.

HIV/AIDS and Maternal/Child Hematological and Other Relevant Outcomes

In a cohort study conducted among infants born to HIV-infected ($n = 575$) and HIV-uninfected ($n = 136$) mothers participating in the ZVITAMBO study (i.e., only mothers, both HIV-infected and HIV-uninfected, and infants assigned to the placebo group were included), the infants were categorized into the following groups: (1) mother HIV-uninfected, baby HIV-uninfected (Nn); (2)

mother HIV-infected, baby HIV-uninfected (Pn); and (3) mother HIV-infected, baby HIV-infected (Pp) (Miller et al., 2006). Gestational age at delivery was similar among the three groups; however, birthweight was slightly higher in HIV-uninfected infants born to HIV-infected mothers compared to HIV-uninfected infants born to HIV-uninfected mothers: Pn birthweight 2969 g (SD, 464) vs. Nn birthweight 2917 g (SD, 454) ($p < 0.05$). HIV-infected infants who were born to HIV-infected mothers had the lowest mean birthweight: Pp birthweight 2830 g (SD, 462) vs. Pn birthweight 2969 g (SD, 464) vs. Nn birthweight 2917 g (SD, 454) ($p = 0.03$). There were no significant differences in the proportion of low-birthweight infants among these groups. The prevalence of anemia (Hb < 105 g/L) was significantly higher in HIV-infected infants at 6 months (59.8% vs. 36.6%; $p = 0.021$) and 12 months of age (75.9% vs. 36.6%; AOR, 5.45; 95% CI, 2.22–13.4; $p < 0.001$), after adjusting for birthweight. There were no significant differences in the prevalence of anemia at these time-points when comparing Nn to Pn groups; however, at 6 weeks of age, sTfR was significantly higher in Pn infants (4.1 mg/L; 95% CI, 4.0–4.3) compared to Nn infants (3.5 mg/L; 95% CI, 3.2–3.8; $p = 0.001$).

In a prospective analysis conducted as part of the TOV study among 829 HIV-infected and HIV-uninfected children born to HIV-infected mothers, maternal WHO HIV stage 2 or greater was associated with increased risk of anemia in children up into the first year of life compared to maternal HIV stage 1 (RR, 1.31; 95% CI, 1.14–1.51; $p < 0.05$). Child HIV infection was also independently associated with increased risk of anemia during 24 months of follow-up (RR, 1.61; 95% CI, 1.40–1.85; $p < 0.05$). Children who had IDA (Hb < 8.5 g/dL with hypochromasia and microcytosis) had significantly increased risk of death in the first 24 months of life (HR, 1.99; 95% CI, 1.06–3.72; $p < 0.05$). Similar observations were not noted for severe anemia alone (Hb < 8.5 g/dL) (HR, 1.38; 95% CI, 0.96–3.61], $p = 0.07$) (Chatterjee et al., 2010). In an analysis in HIV-infected and HIV-uninfected infants as part of the ZVITAMBO project, maternal HIV infection was associated with increased total body iron (TBI) in infants at birth ($p < 0.001$) (Miller et al., 2003).

Post-ART Era: Associations between HIV/AIDS and Hematological Status Outcomes in the Context of ART and HAART

Of the 68 studies included, 6 investigated the associations of ART with iron status. One of these studies was categorized as an RCT, with the intervention being HAART (Widen et al., 2015). In an observational analysis in a prevention of mother-to-child transmission (PMTCT) trial in Pune, India, HIV-infected pregnant women taking ZDV (300 mg twice daily beginning at 36 weeks gestation, duration ≥ 2 weeks) had higher mean Hb values (11.5 vs. 11.3 g/dL; $p = 0.02$) and lower odds of anemia (Hb < 10.0 g/dL) (OR, 0.28; 95% CI, 0.14–0.57; $p < 0.01$) at delivery compared to women not taking ZDV (Sinha et al., 2007). However, women who took ZDV also had a significantly greater duration of iron–folic acid supplementation as standard prenatal care (48 vs. 24.3 days; $p < 0.01$). Maternal ZDV use was also associated with infant hematological status: Children born to women who took ZDV had significantly lower Hb concentrations at birth and at 4 weeks of age compared to infants of mothers who did not take ZDV: birth—ZDV, Hb = 16.5 g/dL (95% CI, 16.2–16.9) vs. no ZDV, Hb = 17.2 g/dL (95% CI, 16.9–17.5; $p = 0.02$); 4 weeks—ZDV, Hb = 12.1 g/dL (95% CI, 11.4–11.9) vs. no ZDV, Hb = 12.1 g/dL (95% CI, 1.19–12.3; $p = 0.03$). Maternal ZDV was also associated with lower mean corpuscular volume in infants at 4 weeks of age, and no infants had clinical anemia at any time-point.

In a nested cohort study that examined stored plasma from 138 initially HAART-naïve, HIV-infected patients who participated in the STACCATO HAART (stavudine [d4T]/didanosine [ddI] plus ritonavir-boosted saquinavir) interruption trial in Thailand, low baseline serum ferritin (<30.0 µg/L) was associated with a shorter time to meeting criteria for HAART interruption (CD4 T-cells ≥ 350 cells/µL) (Boom et al., 2007). HAART interruption was also associated with decline in SF (−8.8 ng/mL; IQR, −65.9–10.5; $p = 0.0005$) and MCV (−5.3; 95% CI, −9.9 to −2.7; $p = 0.0002$) during the interruption phase; however, 62% of patients with higher baseline SF had elevated concentrations (>200 ng/mL) during the interruption phase. Notably, in assessing whether ferritin was affected by inflammation, the authors found no significant differences between mean CRP levels in individuals with low and high baseline SF ($p = 0.15$).

In a cohort study conducted among 838 HIV-infected adults in Tanzania, Hb concentrations were assessed pre- and post-ART initiation (zidovudine/stavudine + lamivudine + efavirenz/nevirapine) (Johannessen et al., 2011). In the substudy on ART and anemia, 102 non-pregnant patients were anemic at ART initiation (Hb < 12 g/dL for women, < 13 g/dL for men) and had a follow-up Hb measurement 12 months post-ART initiation, having been given the following regimens: 62 patients (60.8%) stavudine + lamivudine + nevirapine; 17 patients (16.7%) stavudine + lamivudine + efavirenz; 16 patients (15.7%) zidouvine + lamivudine + nevirapine; and 7 patients (6.9%) zidovudine + lamivudine + efavirenz. Over one year, mean Hb concentrations increased by 2.5 g/dL ($p < 0.001$) in these 102 patients, with the greatest in change in Hb (+4.6 g/dL) being found in patients with severe anemia at ART initiation. In patients with moderate anemia at ART initiation, the change in Hb concentration was +3.0 g/dL; in patients with mild anemia at ART initiation, the change was +1.8g/dL. However, 38.2 % of these 102 patients were still anemic after one year. Taking ZDV initially was associated with increased odds of persistent anemia (defined as anemic after 12 months of ART) (OR, 2.91; 95% CI, 1.03–8.19; $p = 0.043$). Low mean cell volume (<76.0 fL) at ART initiation was also associated with increased odds of persistent anemia (OR, 2.91; 95% CI, 1.03–8.19; $p > 0.05$). The study also measured Hb after one year in 18 patients who did not initiate ART. Individuals who did not initiate ART had sixfold greater odds of persistent anemia after one year (OR, 5.99; 95% CI, 1.82–19.8; $p = 0.003$) compared to individuals who did initiate ART.

In prospective analyses among 10 children with advanced HIV disease (clinical class B or C and immunological class 3 according to the Centers for Disease Control and Prevention [CDC]), serum iron was assessed at enrollment and at three months and six months of HAART therapy, comprised of 400 mg/m² ritonavir every 12 hours in combination with stavudine and lamivudine (five children), zidovudine and lamivudine (three children), and stavudine and didanosine (two children). Difference in serum iron (µg/dL) between baseline and three months was significant, as well as between baseline and six months ($p < 0.05$) (graph shown but no numbers given) (Canani et al., 1999).

The BAN study conducted in Lilongwe, Malawi, randomized 2369 mothers and infants to one of the following 28-week interventions at delivery: (1) HAART ($n = 425$); (2) lipid-based nutrient supplement (LNS) (140 g/day) ($n = 334$); (3) HAART and LNS ($n = 424$); or (4) no HAART or LNS (control; $n = 334$) (Flax et al., 2015). HAART consisted of the following combination regimens: the first-line drug was a combination of lamivudine + zidovudine; the second-line drug was nelfinavir; and, last, lopinavir + ritonavir was used. Iron–folic acid (40 mg elemental iron and 0.25 mg folic acid given daily) was given to all mothers from the first visit during pregnancy through one week postpartum.

In analyses among 537 HIV-infected Malawian mothers (CD4 T-cells > 200 cells/µL) and their infants in the BAN study, maternal HAART alone, without LNS, was associated with increased risk of tissue iron depletion (sTfR > 8.3 mg/L) at 24 weeks postpartum (RR, 3.1; 95% CI [1.32–7.32], $p = 0.01$), compared to the control group. However, maternal HAART, without LNS, was not associated with increased risk of depleted iron stores as measured by ferritin (<15 ng/mL) at 24 weeks (RR, 0.99; 95% CI, 0.68–1.44; $p = 0.94$) and was not associated with risk of anemia (Hb < 120 g/L) at 24 weeks (RR, 1.14; 95% CI, 0.78–1.68; $p = 0.49$) compared to the control group. Women who received HAART and LNS did not have an increased risk of iron deficiency at 24 weeks postpartum compared to the control group (Widen et al., 2015). HAART was not associated with infant iron deficiency during 24 weeks of breastfeeding. In analyses among 690 lactating women in the BAN study, HAART (protease inhibitor-based triple therapy) was not associated with ferritin or Hb concentrations but was associated with greater sTfR concentrations (suggesting poorer iron status) and lower plasma folate concentrations (–12%; $p = 0.04$) (Flax et al., 2015).

DISCUSSION

Iron deficiency and anemia are common among HIV-infected individuals, and both low and high iron stores have been associated with increased risk of HIV disease progression and other adverse HIV-associated outcomes. Iron supplementation is the standard of care in the treatment of iron deficiency and anemia. However, several factors complicate the use of iron supplementation in HIV-infected individuals. Cell-based studies have found that iron promotes HIV growth and replication (Chang et al., 2015), and pathology-based studies have found associations between tissue iron and the prevalence of HIV-associated infections, including TB (Moyo et al., 1997; Gangaidzo et al., 2001; Lounis et al., 2001; McDermid et al., 2013). Studies have also observed decreased HIV replication and proliferation with iron chelators (Shatrov et al., 1997; Georgiou et al., 2000, 2002; Meyer, 2006; Debebe et al., 2007). Epidemiological studies have also observed that higher iron stores independently predict HIV-related mortality, and some studies have noted that prolonged iron supplementation may increase disease progression in individuals at an advanced stage of disease (Jacobus, 1996). However, HIV-infected individuals with anemia have poorer prognoses than HIV-infected individuals without anemia. Due to evidence suggesting a "double-edged sword"—the association between iron and advanced HIV/AIDS (Clark et al., 2001)—the use of iron supplementation for HIV-infected individuals warrants caution.

EVIDENCE FROM TRIALS ON IRON SUPPLEMENTATION

The safety and efficacy of iron supplementation for HIV-infected individuals has not been extensively studied through randomized trials. To date, only one randomized trial has been conducted with the explicit purpose of assessing the effects of iron supplementation without other micronutrients on health outcomes in HIV-infected populations. Among HIV-infected children with moderate anemia (7.0–9.9 g/dL Hb), iron supplementation was not associated with worsened HIV disease progression but was associated with increased risk of malaria (Esan et al., 2013); however, findings from a randomized study suggest that iron supplementation in patients at later stages of disease may worsen disease progression (Salmon-Ceron et al., 1995; Jacobus 1996). A recent analysis of a historical, randomized, low-dose iron supplementation trial conducted in 1994 found that low-dose (60 mg) iron supplementation provided twice weekly for four months did not increase viral load (Olsen et al., 2004). A randomized trial of iron supplementation in combination with other micronutrients (iron + micronutrients vs. micronutrients alone) in HIV-infected female drug users indicated that iron reduces anemia without increasing HIV RNA levels (Semba et al., 2007). To date, the majority of evidence regarding the association between outcomes in iron and hematological status with HIV/AIDS comes from observational studies. Findings from these studies consistently suggest that HIV is associated with worsened hematological outcomes, including anemia, although findings from observational studies regarding the association between iron and hematological status with HIV-related outcomes are less consistent.

EVIDENCE FROM OBSERVATIONAL STUDIES

Outcomes Related to HIV Disease Progression and HIV-Related Mortality

There is strong and consistent evidence that anemia is associated with increased risk of HIV disease progression and HIV-related mortality (Eley et al., 2002; Mugisha et al., 2013). Studies from the TOV study have consistently found that anemia in HIV-infected women is associated with increased risk of mortality and that the greater the severity of anemia, the greater the risk of mortality (O'Brien et al., 2005; Kupka et al., 2007; Chatterjee et al., 2010; Isanaka et al., 2012). Cohort studies have also found that anemia among HIV-infected children (Shet et al., 2015) and among adults (Minchella et al., 2015) is associated with disease progression, as measured by CD4 T-cell counts.

The association between elevated iron stores with HIV disease progression and HIV-related mortality is less clear, and no randomized trials have been conducted to assess this association. Observational cohort studies have found associations between elevated iron stores, as measured by SF, and both HIV-related and all-cause mortality (Gordeuk et al., 2006; McDermid et al., 2007; McDermid et al., 2009; Rawat et al., 2009). Elevated hepcidin has also been associated with HIV-related TB (Minchella et al., 2014) and mortality (Minchella et al., 2015) in cohort studies. Case-control studies have also found associations between higher serum hepcidin and patients with detectable viral load compared to lower hepcidin levels in patients with undetectable viral load (Malvoisin et al., 2014) and an inverse relationship between serum hepcidin and CD4 T-cell count (Wisaksana et al., 2013). A cohort analysis of ZVITAMBO found associations between SF above 45 μg/L and increased viral load, and between higher SF and mortality when controlling for AGP (Rawat et al., 2009). A cross-sectional analysis found inverse associations between ferritin levels and CD4 T-cell count (López-Calderón et al., 2015). However, in an analysis of the TOV study, high SF, as compared to low SF, was not associated with a greater risk of mortality (Kupka et al., 2007). Additionally, a study among 135 anemic patients (42 HIV-infected, 93 HIV-uninfected) found no difference in SF levels between HIV-infected and HIV-uninfected individuals (Camacho et al., 1992).

Outcomes Related to Iron and Hematological Status

There is strong and consistent evidence from observational epidemiological studies and laboratory studies that HIV is associated with increased risk of anemia. Case-control studies have consistently found that anemia is more prevalent among HIV-infected children than HIV-uninfected children (Totin et al., 2002; Miller et al., 2006). Evidence from cohort studies also provides support that HIV is associated with increased risk of anemia; however, findings also suggest that HIV is associated with elevated iron stores (Banjoko et al., 2012; Visser and Mostert, 2013), although the directionality of this association is unclear from observational studies.

Outcomes Related to Maternal, Infant, and Child Health

To date, no randomized trials have assessed the impact of maternal iron supplementation in HIV-infected mothers on infant iron and/or HIV status. Most evidence regarding the association between iron supplementation and HIV relating to maternal and child health comes from observational studies. Studies included in this review suggest that, although maternal anemia may lead to adverse HIV-related neonatal and infant outcomes, the long-term effects of maternal iron supplementation on child health are unclear. An analysis of the TOV study found that maternal anemia among HIV-infected mothers was associated with the risk of child HIV infection and an increased risk of child mortality compared to those without maternal anemia (O'Brien et al., 2005). One cohort study found that receipt of iron supplementation in the postpartum period did not increase the HIV RNA viral load in breast milk (Phiri et al., 2006). A cohort study that examined the association between maternal iron supplementation in mothers infected with HIV and infant outcomes found no adverse health outcomes with regard to HIV disease progression (Shet et al., 2015). However, the evidence for providing maternal iron supplementation is weak, and further research is needed to identify how iron supplementation in HIV-infected mothers may affect infant HIV status.

Post-ART Era

Certain ARVs are known to impact iron metabolism. ZDV is known to decrease Hb levels, impair iron metabolism, and increase the risk of anemia (Ezechi et al., 2013; Phe et al., 2013). Maternal ARVs have been shown to decrease infant Hb levels (Bae et al., 2008; Dryden-Peterson et al., 2011). A large-scale study assessing differences in incidence of severe anemia among HIV-uninfected infants born to HIV-infected mothers on various *in utero* and postnatal ARV regimes, all of which included ZDV, found that most cases of infant anemia were resolved with cessation of ZDV or with provision of multivitamin and iron supplementation (Dryden-Peterson et al., 2011). However, one study found that, although maternal initiation with ZDV increased the risk of anemia among newborns, ZDV unexpectedly decreased the risk of maternal anemia at the end of pregnancy (Pinnetti et al., 2011). There is consistent evidence that iron supplementation may be warranted in HIV-infected individuals taking HAART, which has generally been shown to improve hematological status and increase Hb levels (Masaisa et al., 2011). There is moderately strong and consistent evidence that HAART, combined with iron supplementation, improves HIV and hematological status more than

HAART alone (Shet et al., 2015). Further research is needed to assess the impact of combined iron supplementation and HAART together on HIV-related health outcomes, as well as the association between HAART and iron/hematological status.

RESEARCH GAPS

Findings from this review highlight the need for further research to elucidate the directionality of the association between HIV-related health outcomes and iron/hematological status. The majority of studies to date that assess this association are observational. The most recent Cochrane Systematic Review (Adetifa et al., 2009) concluded that there was weak evidence from observational studies and expert opinions that iron supplementation should be provided to HIV-infected children. Since then, one randomized trial in anemic HIV-infected children has been conducted (Esan et al., 2013). Iron supplementation was found to protect against the progression to AIDS in children and, therefore, may be recommended in children; however, further research is needed to assess whether this recommendation would apply to adults and pregnant women living with HIV, as well as to populations living in areas where other infections, such as TB, are endemic. No randomized trial has observed a relationship between iron supplementation and incidence of TB in an HIV-infected population. Further research is also needed to assess the proper dosage and timing of iron supplementation that would reduce anemia and not result in adverse HIV-related health outcomes.

IMPLICATIONS FOR CLINICAL CARE AND PUBLIC HEALTH PRACTICE

Iron and hematological abnormalities are prevalent in HIV-infected individuals and have been associated with increased risk of adverse health outcomes. Iron supplementation is the standard of care for iron deficiency and anemia. Based on evidence from observational studies, the safety and efficacy of therapeutic iron in individuals with HIV likely vary by population and location. The one randomized trial to date, which assessed the safety of iron supplementation in HIV-infected anemic children in a malaria-endemic region, found that iron reduced progression to AIDS yet increased the risk of malaria. Other randomized trials, including trials of iron and other micronutrients, have found beneficial effects of iron supplementation on hematological status in HIV-infected individuals, both on ART and ART-naïve patients. However, further research is urgently needed to assess the safety of therapeutic iron in adult populations, in pregnant women, and in populations where other infections are endemic. To date, randomized trials have demonstrated the benefit of iron supplementation in combination with ART on HIV disease progression and HIV-related health outcomes. Current evidence supports the use of iron supplementation at the single RDA level for HIV-infected and anemic individuals on ART.

REFERENCES

Adetifa, I. and U. Okomo. (2009). Iron supplementation for reducing morbidity and mortality in children with HIV. *Cochrane Database of Systematic Reviews* (1): CD006736).
Antelman, G., G. I. Masamanga, D. Spiegelman et al. (2000). Nutritional factors and infectious disease contribute to anemia among pregnant women with human immunodeficiency virus in Tanzania. *Journal of Nutrition* 130(8): 1950–7.
Armitage, A. E., A. R. Stacey, E. Giannoulatou et al. (2014). Distinct patterns of hepcidin and iron regulation during HIV-1, HBV, and HCV infections. *Proceedings of the National Academies of Science (USA)* 111(33): 12187–92.
Bae, W. H., C. Wester, L. M. Smeaton et al. (2008). Hematologic and hepatic toxicities associated with antenatal and postnatal exposure to maternal highly active antiretroviral therapy among infants. *AIDS* 22(13): 1633–40.
Banjoko, S. O., F. A. Oseni, R. A. Togun, O. Onayemi, B. O. Emma-Okon, and J. B. Fakunle. (2012). Iron status in HIV-1 infection: implications in disease pathology. *BMC Clinical Pathology* 12: 26.

Berlim, M. T. and A. M. Abeche. (2001). Evolutionary approach to medicine. *Southern Medical Journal* 94(1): 26–32.

Boelaert, J. R., G. A. Weinberg, and E. D. Weinberg. (1996). Altered iron metabolism in HIV infection: mechanisms, possible consequences, and proposals for management. *Infectious Agents and Disease* 5(1): 36–46.

Boom, J., E. Kösters, C. Duncombe et al. (2007). Ferritin levels during structured treatment interruption of highly active antiretroviral therapy. *HIV Medicine* 8(6): 388–95.

Camacho, J., F. Poveda, A. F. Zamorano, M. E. Valencia, J. J. Vazquez, and F.Arnalich. (1992). Serum erythropoietin levels in anaemic patients with advanced human immunodeficiency virus infection. *British Journal of Haematology* 82(3): 608–14.

Camaschella, C. (2017). New insights into iron deficiency and iron deficiency anemia. *Blood Reviews* 31(4): 225–33.

Canani, R. B., M. I. Spagnuolo, P. Cirillo, and A. Guarino. (1999). Ritonavir combination therapy restores intestinal function in children with advanced HIV disease. *Journal of Acquired Deficiency Syndrome* 21(4): 307–12.

Castaldo, A., L. Tarallo, E. Palomba et al. (1996). Iron deficiency and intestinal malabsorption in HIV disease. *Journal of Pediatric Gastroenterology and Nutrition* 22(4): 359–63.

Castella, A., T. S. Croxson, D. Mildvan, D. H. Witt, and R. Zalusky. (1985). The bone marrow in AIDS. A histologic, hematologic, and microbiologic study. *American Journal of Clinical Pathology* 84(4): 425–32.

Chang, H. C., M. Bayeva, B. Taiwo, F. J. Palella, Jr., T. J. Hope, and H. Ardehali. (2015). Short communication: high cellular iron levels are associated with increased HIV infection and replication. *AIDS Research and Human Retroviruses* 31(3): 305–12.

Chatterjee, A., R. J. Bosch, R. Kupka, D. J. Hunter, G. I. Msamanga, and W. W. Fawzi. (2010). Predictors and consequences of anaemia among antiretroviral-naive HIV-infected and HIV-uninfected children in Tanzania. *Public Health Nutrition* 13(2): 289–96.

Clark, T. D. and R. D. Semba. (2001). Iron supplementation during human immunodeficiency virus infection: a double-edged sword? *Medical Hypotheses* 57(4): 476–9.

Coyle, T. E. (1997). Hematologic complications of human immunodeficiency virus infection and the acquired immunodeficiency syndrome. *Medical Clinics of North America* 81(2): 449–70.

Dairo, M. D., T. O. Lawoyin, M. O. Onadeko, E. O. Asekun-Olarinmoye, and A. O. Adeniji. (2005). HIV as an additional risk factors for anaemia in pregnancy: evidence from primary care level in Ibadan, Southwestern Nigeria. *African Journal of Medicine and Medical Sciences* 34(3): 275–9.

de Monyé, C., D. S. Karcher, J. R. Boelaert, and V. R. Gordeuk. (1999). Bone marrow macrophage iron grade and survival of HIV-seropositive patients. *AIDS* 13(3): 375–80.

Debebe, Z., T. Ammosova, M. Jerebtsova et al. (2007). Iron chelators ICL670 and 311 inhibit HIV-1 transcription. *Virology* 367(2): 324–33.

Dikshit, B., A. Wanchu, R. K. Sachdeva, A. Sharma, and R. Das. (2009). Profile of hematological abnormalities of Indian HIV infected individuals. *BMC Blood Disorders* 9: 5.

Dryden-Peterson, S., R. L. Shapiro, M. D. Hughes et al. (2011). Increased risk of severe infant anemia after exposure to maternal HAART, Botswana. *Journal of Acquired Immune Deficiency Syndrome* 56(5): 428–36.

Eley, B. S., A. A. Sive, M. Shuttleworth, and G. D. Hussey. (2002). A prospective, cross-sectional study of anaemia and peripheral iron status in antiretroviral naïve, HIV-1 infected children in Cape Town, South Africa. *BMC Infectious Diseases* 2: 3.

Esan, M. O., M. B. van Hensbroek, E. Nkhoma et al. (2013). Iron supplementation in HIV-infected Malawian children with anemia: a double-blind, randomized, controlled trial. *Clinical Infectious Diseases* 57(11): 1626–34.

Ezechi, O. C., O. O. Kalejaiye, C. V. Gab-Okafor et al. (2013). The burden of anaemia and associated factors in HIV positive Nigerian women. *Archives of Gynecology and Obstetrics* 287(2): 239–44.

Fawzi, W. W., G. I. Msamanga, D. Spiegelman, E. J. Urassa, and D. J. Hunter. (1999). Rationale and design of the Tanzania Vitamin and HIV Infection Trial. *Controlled Clinical Trials* 20(1): 75–90.

Finkelstein, J. L., S. Mehta, C. P. Duggan et al. (2012). Predictors of anaemia and iron deficiency in HIV-infected pregnant women in Tanzania: a potential role for vitamin D and parasitic infections. *Public Health Nutrition* 15(5): 928–37.

Flax, V. L., L. S. Adair, L. H. Allen et al. (2015). Plasma micronutrient concentrations are altered by antiretroviral therapy and lipid-based nutrient supplements in lactating HIV-infected Malawian women. *Journal of Nutrition* 145(8): 1950–7.

Friis, H., E. Gomo, P. Kæstel et al. (2001). HIV and other predictors of serum folate, serum ferritin, and hemoglobin in pregnancy: a cross-sectional study in Zimbabwe. *American Journal of Clinical Nutrition* 73(6): 1066–73.

Friis, H., E. Gomo, N. Nyazema et al. (2003). Iron, haptoglobin phenotype, and HIV-1 viral load: a cross-sectional study among pregnant Zimbabwean women. *Journal of Acquired Immune Deficiency Syndrome* 33(1): 74–81.

Fuchs, D., R. Zangerle, E. Artner-Dworzak et al. (1993). Association between immune activation, changes of iron metabolism and anaemia in patients with HIV infection. *European Journal of Haematology* 50(2): 90–4.

Gangaidzo, I. T., V. M. Moyo, E. Mvundura et al. (2001). Association of pulmonary tuberculosis with increased dietary iron. *Journal of Infectious Diseases* 184(7): 936–9.

Georgiou, N. A., T. van der Bruggen, M. Oudshoorn, H. H. Nottet, J. J. Marx, and B. S. van Asbeck. (2000). Combining iron chelators with the nucleoside analog didanosine in anti-HIV therapy. *Transfusion Science* 23(3): 249–50.

Georgiou, N. A., T. van der Bruggen, M. Oudshoorn, R. C. Hider, J. J. Marx, and B. S. van Asbeck. (2002). Human immunodeficiency virus type 1 replication inhibition by the bidentate iron chelators CP502 and CP511 is caused by proliferation inhibition and the onset of apoptosis. *European Journal of Clinical Investigation* 32(Suppl. 1): 91–6.

Gomes, M. S., G. Dom, J. Pedrosa, J. R. Boelaert, and R. Appelberg. (1999). Effects of iron deprivation on *Mycobacterium avium* growth. *Tuberculosis and Lung Disease* 79(5): 321–8.

Gordeuk, V. R., J. R. Delanghe, M. R. Langlois, and J. R. Boelaert. (2001). Iron status and the outcome of HIV infection: an overview. *Journal of Clinical Virology* 20(3): 111–5.

Gordeuk, V. R., G. Onojobi, M. F. Schneider et al. (2006). The association of serum ferritin and transferrin receptor concentrations with mortality in women with human immunodeficiency virus infection. *Haematologica* 91(6): 739–43.

Gordeuk, V. R., V. M. Moyo, M. Nouraie et al. (2009). Circulating cytokines in pulmonary tuberculosis according to HIV status and dietary iron content. *International Journal of Tuberculosis and Lung Disease* 13(10): 1267–73.

Isanaka, S., D. Spiegelman, S. Aboud et al. (2012). Post-natal anaemia and iron deficiency in HIV-infected women and the health and survival of their children. *Maternal & Child Nutrition* 8(3): 287–98.

Jacobus, D. P. (1996). Randomization to iron supplementation of patients with advanced human immunodeficiency virus disease—an inadvertent but controlled study with results important for patient care. *Journal of Infectious Diseases* 173(4): 1044–5.

Johannessen, A., E. Naman, S. G. Gundersen, and J. N. Bruun. (2011). Antiretroviral treatment reverses HIV-associated anemia in rural Tanzania. *BMC Infectious Diseases* 11: 190.

Jonker, F. A. M. and M. B. van Hensbroek. (2014). Anaemia, iron deficiency and susceptibility to infections. *Journal of Infection* 69(Suppl. 1): S23–S27.

Kagu, M. B. K., M. I. Khalil, and S. G. Ahmed. (2007). Bone marrow macrophage iron stores in patients with HIV infection and AIDS-associated Kaposi's sarcoma. *African Journal of Medicine and Medicine Sciences* 36(2): 125–8.

Kerkhoff, A. D., R. Wood, F. G. Cobelens, A. Gupta-Wright, L. G. Bekker, and S. D. Lawn. (2014). Resolution of anaemia in a cohort of HIV-infected patients with a high prevalence and incidence of tuberculosis receiving antiretroviral therapy in South Africa. *BMC Infectious Diseases* 14: 3860.

Koka, P. S., B. D. Jamieson, D. G. Brooks, and J. A. Zack. (1999). Human immunodeficiency virus type 1-induced hematopoietic inhibition is independent of productive infection of progenitor cells in vivo. *Journal of Virology* 73(11): 9089–97.

Kosalaraksa, P., T. Bunupuradah, S. Vonthanak et al. (2012). Prevalence of anemia and underlying iron status in naïve antiretroviral therapy HIV-infected children with moderate immune suppression. *AIDS Research and Human Retroviruses* 28(12): 1679–86.

Kreuzer, K. A. and J. K. Rockstroh. (1997). Pathogenesis and pathophysiology of anemia in HIV infection. *Annals of Hematology* 75(5–6): 179–87.

Kruger, H. S., L. J. Balk, M. Viljoen, and T. M. Meyers. (2013). Positive association between dietary iron intake and iron status in HIV-infected children in Johannesburg, South Africa. *Nutrition Research* 33(1): 50–8.

Kupka, R. M., G. I. Msamanga, F. Mugusi, P. Petraro, D. J. Hunter, and W. W. Fawzi. (2007). Iron status is an important cause of anemia in HIV-infected Tanzanian women but is not related to accelerated HIV disease progression. *Journal of Nutrition* 137(10): 2317–23.

Lewis, D. K., C. J. M. Whitty, H. Epino, E. A. Letsky, J. M. Mukiibi, and N. R. van den Broek. (2007). Interpreting tests for iron deficiency among adults in a high HIV prevalence African setting: routine tests may lead to misdiagnosis. *Transactions of the Royal Society of Tropical Medicine and Hygiene* 101(6): 613–7.

López-Calderón, C., R. Palacios, and A. Cobo et al. (2015). Serum ferritin in HIV-positive patients is related to immune deficiency and inflammatory activity. *International Journal of STD & AIDS* 26(6): 393–7.

Lounis, N., C. Truffot-Pernot, J. Grosset et al. (2001). Iron and *Mycobacterium tuberculosis* infection. *Journal of Clinical Virology* 20(3): 123–6.

Makubi, A., J. Okuma, D. Spiegelman et al. (2015). Burden and determinants of severe anemia among HIV-infected adults: results from a large urban HIV program in Tanzania, East Africa. *Journal of the International Association of Providers of AIDS Care* 14(2): 148–55.

Malvoisin, E., D. Makhloufi, and J. M. Livrozet. (2014). Serum hepcidin levels in women infected with HIV-1 under antiviral therapy. *Journal of Medical Virology* 86(10): 1656–60.

Masaisa, F., J. B. Gahutu, J. Mukiibi, J. Delanghe, and J. Philippé. (2011). Anemia in human immunodeficiency virus-infected and uninfected women in Rwanda. *American Journal of Tropical Medicine and Hygiene* 84(3): 456–60.

McDermid, J. M., A. Jaye, M. F. Schim van der Loeff et al. (2007). Elevated iron status strongly predicts mortality in West African adults with HIV infection. *Journal of Acquired Deficiency Syndrome* 46(4): 498–507.

McDermid, J. M., M. F. van der Loeff, A. Jaye et al. (2009). Mortality in HIV infection is independently predicted by host iron status and SLC11A1 and HP genotypes, with new evidence of a gene-nutrient interaction. *American Journal of Clinical Nutrition* 90(1): 225–33.

McDermid, J. M., B. J. Hennig, M. van der Sande et al. (2013). Host iron redistribution as a risk factor for incident tuberculosis in HIV infection: an 11-year retrospective cohort study. *BMC Infectious Diseases* 13: 48.

Meda, N., L. Mandelbrot, M. Cartoux, B. et al. (1999). Anaemia during pregnancy in Burkina Faso, west Africa, 1995–96: prevalence and associated factors. DITRAME Study Group. *Bulletin of the World Health Organization* 77(11): 916–22.

Meidani, M., F. Rezaei, M. R. Maracy, M. Avijgan, and K. Tayeri. (2012). Prevalence, severity, and related factors of anemia in HIV/AIDS patients. *Journal of Research in Medical Sciences* 17(2): 138–42.

Meyer, D. (2006). Iron chelation as therapy for HIV and *Mycobacterium tuberculosis* co-infection under conditions of iron overload. *Current Pharmaceutical Design* 12(16): 1943–7.

Miller, M. F., R. J. Stoltzfus, N. V. Mbuya et al.; ZVITAMBO Study Group. (2003). Total body iron in HIV-positive and HIV-negative Zimbabwean newborns strongly predicts anemia throughout infancy and is predicted by maternal hemoglobin concentration. *Journal of Nutrition* 133(11): 3461–8.

Miller, M. F., J. H. Humphrey, P. J. Iliff et al.; ZVITAMBO Study Group. (2006). Neonatal erythropoiesis and subsequent anemia in HIV-positive and HIV-negative Zimbabwean babies during the first year of life: a longitudinal study. *BMC Infectious Diseases* 6: 1.

Minchella, P. A., A. E. Armitage, B. Darboe et al. (2014). Elevated hepcidin at HIV diagnosis is associated with incident tuberculosis in a retrospective cohort study. *International Journal of Tuberculosis and Lung Disease* 18(11): 1337–39.

Minchella, P. A., A. E. Armitage, B. Darboe et al. (2015). Elevated hepcidin is part of a complex relation that links mortality with iron homeostasis and anemia in men and women with HIV infection. *Journal of Nutrition* 145(6): 1194–1201.

Mlisana, K., S. C. Auld, A. Grobler et al. (2008). Anaemia in acute HIV-1 subtype C infection. *PLoS One* 3(2): e1626.

Moses, A. V., S. Williams, M. L. Heneveld et al. (1996). Human immunodeficiency virus infection of bone marrow endothelium reduces induction of stromal hematopoietic growth factors. *Blood* 87(3): 919–25.

Moyo, V. M., I. T. Gangaidzo, V. R. Gordeuk, C. F. Kiire, and A. P. Macphail. (1997). Tuberculosis and iron overload in Africa: a review. *Central African Journal of Medicine* 43(11): 334–9.

Mugisha, J. O., K. Baisley, G. Asiki, J. Seeley, and H. Kuper. (2013). Prevalence, types, risk factors and clinical correlates of anaemia in older people in a rural Ugandan population. *PLoS One* 8(10): e78394.

Murray, M. J., A. B. Murray, M. B. Murray, and C. J. Murray. (1978). The adverse effect of iron repletion on the course of certain infections. *British Medical Journal* 2(6145): 1113–5.

O'Brien, M. E., R. Kupka, G. I. Msamanga, E. Saathoff, D. J. Hunter, and W. W. Fawzi. (2005). Anemia is an independent predictor of mortality and immunologic progression of disease among women with HIV in Tanzania. *Journal of Acquired Immune Deficiency Syndrome* 40(2): 219–25.

Odhiambo, C., C. Zeh, F. Angira et al. (2016). Anaemia in HIV-infected pregnant women receiving triple antiretroviral combination therapy for prevention of mother-to-child transmission: a secondary analysis of the Kisumu breastfeeding study (KiBS). *Tropical Medicine & International Health* 21(3): 373–84.

Ogbe, P. J., O. A. Idoko, A. C. Ezimah, K. A. Digban, and B. O. Oguntayo. (2012). Evaluation of iron status in anemia of chronic disease among patients with HIV infection. *Clinical Laboratory Science* 25(1): 7–12.

Olsen, A., J. Nawiri, and H. Friis. (2000). The impact of iron supplementation on reinfection with intestinal helminths and *Schistosoma mansoni* in western Kenya. *Transactions of the Royal Society of Tropical Medicine and Hygiene* 94(5): 493–9.

Olsen, A., D. Mwaniki, H. Krarup, and H. Friis. (2004). Low-dose iron supplementation does not increase HIV-1 load. *Journal of Acquired Immune Deficiency Syndrome* 36(1): 637–8.

Omoregie, R., E. U. Omokaro, O. Palmer et al. (2009). Prevalence of anaemia among HIV-infected patients in Benin City, Nigeria. *Tanzania Journal of Health Research* 11(1): 1–4.

Pal, R., S. Hameed, and Z. Fatima. (2015). Iron deprivation affects drug susceptibilities of mycobacteria targeting membrane integrity. *Journal of Pathogens* 2015: 938523.

Parkes-Ratanshi, R., D. Katende, J. Levin et al. (2015). Development of severe anemia and changes in hemoglobin in a cohort of HIV-infected Ugandan adults receiving Zidovudine-, Stavudine-, and Tenofovir-containing antiretroviral regimens. *Journal of the International Association of Providers of AIDS Care* 14(5): 455-62.

Petraro, P., C. Duggan, W. Urassa et al. (2013). Determinants of anemia in postpartum HIV-negative women in Dar es Salaam, Tanzania. *European Journal of Clinical Nutrition* 67(7): 708–17.

Petraro, P., C. Duggan, D. Spiegelman et al. (2016). Determinants of anemia among human immunodeficiency virus-positive adults at care and treatment clinics in Dar es Salaam, Tanzania. *American Journal of Tropical Medicine and Hygiene* 94(2): 384–92.

Phe, T., S. Thai, C. Veng, S. Sok, L. Lynen, and J. van Griensven. (2013). Risk factors of treatment-limiting anemia after substitution of zidovudine for stavudine in HIV-infected adult patients on antiretroviral treatment. *PLoS One* 8(3): e60206.

Phiri, W., L. Kasonka, S. Collin et al. (2006). Factors influencing breast milk HIV RNA viral load among Zambian women. *AIDS Research and Human Retroviruses* 22(7): 607–14.

Pinnetti, C., S. Baroncelli, A. Molinari et al. (2011). Common occurrence of anaemia at the end of pregnancy following exposure to zidovudine-free regimens. *Journal of Infection* 63(2): 144–150.

Porter, M., M. A. Davies, M. K. Mapani et al. (2015). Outcomes of infants starting antiretroviral therapy in southern Africa, 2004–2012. *Journal of Acquired Deficiency Syndrome* 69(5): 593–601.

Rawat, R., J. H. Humphrey, R. Ntozini, K. Mutasa, P. Iliff, and R. J. Stoltzfus. (2009). Elevated iron stores are associated with HIV disease severity and mortality among postpartum women in Zimbabwe. *Public Health Nutrition* 12(9): 1321–9.

Redig, A. J. and N. Berliner. (2013). Pathogenesis and clinical implications of HIV-related anemia in 2013. *Hematology: American Society of Hematology Program* 2013: 377–81.

Riera, A., E. Gimferrer, J. Cadafalch, A. Remacha, and S. Martin. (1994). Prevalence of high serum and red cell ferritin levels in HIV-infected patients. *Haematologica* 79(2): 165–7.

Salmon-Ceron, D., A. Fontbonne, J. Saba et al. (1995). Lower survival in AIDS patients receiving dapsone compared with aerosolized pentamidine for secondary prophylaxis of *Pneumocystis carinii* pneumonia. Study Group. *Journal of Infectious Diseases* 172(3): 656–64.

Salomé, M. A. and H. Z. W. Grotto. (2004). Human immunodeficiency virus-related anemia of chronic disease: relationship to hematologic, immune, and iron metabolism parameters, and lack of association with serum interferon-γ levels. *AIDS Patient Care and STDs* 16(8): 361–5.

Sarcletti, M, G. Quirchmair, G. Weiss, D. Fuchs, and R. Zangerle. (2003). Increase of haemoglobin levels by anti-retroviral therapy is associated with a decrease in immune activation. *European Journal of Haematology* 70(1): 17–25.

Sebitloane, H. M. and D. Moodley. (2017). The impact of highly active antiretroviral therapy on obstetric conditions: a review. *European Journal of Obstetrics & Gynecology and Reproductive Biology* 210: 126–31.

Selvam, A., I. A. Buhimschi, J. D. Makin, R. C. Pattinson, R. Anderson, and B. W. Forsyth. (2015). Hyperferritinemia and markers of inflammation and oxidative stress in the cord blood of HIV-exposed, uninfected (HEU) infants. *HIV Medicine* 16(6): 375–80.

Semba, R. D., N. Shah, S. A. Strathdee, and D. Vlahov. (2002). High prevalence of iron deficiency and anemia among female injection drug users with and without HIV infection. *Journal of Acquired Immune Deficiency Syndrome* 29(2): 142–4.

Semba, R. D., E. P. Ricketts, S. Mehta et al. (2007). Effect of micronutrients and iron supplementation on hemoglobin, iron status, and plasma hepatitis C and HIV RNA levels in female injection drug users: a controlled clinical trial. *Journal of Acquired Immune Deficiency Syndrome* 45(3): 298–303.

Shatrov, V. A., J. R. Boelaert, S. Chouaib, W. Dröge, and V. Lehmann. (1997). Iron chelation decreases human immunodeficiency virus-1 Tat potentiated tumor necrosis factor-induced NF-kappa B activation in Jurkat cells. *European Cytokine Network* 8(1): 37–43.

Shen, Y., Z. Wang, H. Lu et al. (2013). Prevalence of anemia among adults with newly diagnosed HIV/AIDS in China. *PLoS One* 8(9): e73807.

Shet, A., S. Mehta, N. Rajagopalan et al. (2009). Anemia and growth failure among HIV-infected children in India: a retrospective analysis. *BMC Pediatrics* 9: 37.

Shet, A., K. Arumugam, N. Rajagopalan et al. (2012). The prevalence and etiology of anemia among HIV-infected children in India. *European Journal of Pediatrics* 171(3): 531–40.

Shet, A., P. K. Bhavani, N. Kumarasamy et al. (2015). Anemia, diet and therapeutic iron among children living with HIV: a prospective cohort study. *BMC Pediatrics* 15(1): 164.

Silva, E. B., M. T. N. da Silva, and M. M. S. Vilela. (1999). Evolução de parâmetros hematológicos em um grupo de crianças infectadas pelo vírus da imunodeficiência humana do tipo 1 HIV-1. [Evolution of hematological parameters in a group of children with human immunodeficiency virus infection – HIV-1.] *Jornal de Pediatria* 75(6): 442–8.

Silva, E. B., H. Z. Grotto, and M. M. S. Vilela. (2001). Aspectos clínicos e o hemograma em crianças expostas ao HIV-1: comparação entre pacientes infectados e soro-reversores. [Clinical aspects and complete blood counts in children exposed to HIV-1: Comparison between infected patients and seroreverters.] *Jornal de Pediatria* 77(6): 503–11.

Sinha, G., T. J. Choi, U. Nayak et al. (2007). Clinically significant anemia in HIV-infected pregnant women in India is not a major barrier to zidovudine use for prevention of maternal-to-child transmission. *Journal of Acquired Immune Deficiency Syndrome* 45(2): 210–17.

Sullivan, P. S., D. L. Hanson, S. Y. Chu, J. L. Jones, and J. W. Ward. (1998). Epidemiology of anemia in human immunodeficiency virus (HIV)-infected persons: results from the multistate adult and adolescent spectrum of HIV disease surveillance project. *Blood* 91(1): 301–8.

Sunder-Plassmann, G., S. I. Patruta, and W. H. Hörl. (1999). Pathobiology of the role of iron in infection. *American Journal of Kidney Diseases* 34(4, Suppl.): S25–S29.

Swetha, G. K., R. Hemalatha, U. V Prasad, V. Murali, K. Damayanti, and V. Bhaskar. (2015). Health & nutritional status of HIV infected children in Hyderabad, India. *Indian Journal of Medical Research* 141(1): 46–54.

Tohill, B. C., C. M. Heilig, R. S. Klein et al. (2007). Nutritional biomarkers associated with gynecological conditions among US women with or at risk of HIV infection. *American Journal of Clinical Nutrition* 85(5): 1327–34.

Totin, D., C. Ndugwa, F. Mmiro, R. T. Perry, J. B. Jackson, and R. D. Semba. (2002). Iron deficiency anemia is highly prevalent among human immunodeficiency virus-infected and uninfected infants in Uganda. *Journal of Nutrition* 132(3): 423–9.

Traoré, H. N. and D. Meyer. (2004). The effect of iron overload on in vitro HIV-1 infection. *Journal of Clinical Virology* 31(Suppl. 1): S92–8.

van Eijk, A. M., J. G. Ayisi, L. Slutsker et al. (2007). Effect of haematinic supplementation and malaria prevention on maternal anaemia and malaria in western Kenya. *Tropical Medicine and International Health* 12(3): 342–52.

Visser, A. and C. Mostert. (2013). Causes of hyperferritinaemia classified by HIV status in a tertiary-care setting in South Africa. *Epidemiology & Infection* 141(1): 207–11.

Weinberg, E. D. (1996). Iron withholding: a defense against viral infections. *Biometals* 9(4): 393–9.

WHO. (2012). *Guideline: Daily Iron and Folic Acid Supplementation in Pregnant Women.* Geneva: World Health Organization.

WHO. (2015). *The Global Prevalence of Anaemia in 2011.* Geneva: World Health Organization.

WHO. (2017). *Micronutrient Deficiencies: Iron Deficiency Anemia.* World Health Organization (http://www.who.int/nutrition/topics/ida/en/).

Widen, E. M., M. E. Bentley, C. S. Chasela et al. (2015). Antiretroviral treatment is associated with iron deficiency in HIV-infected Malawian women that is mitigated with supplementation, but is not associated with infant iron deficiency during 24 weeks of exclusive breastfeeding. *Journal of Acquired Immune Deficiency Syndrome* 69(3): 319–28.

Wisaksana, R., R. Sumantri, A. R. Indrati et al. (2011). Anemia and iron homeostasis in a cohort of HIV-infected patients in Indonesia. *BMC Infectious Diseases* 11: 213.

Wisaksana, R., Q de Mast, B. Alisjahbana et al. (2013). Inverse relationship of serum hepcidin levels with CD4 cell counts in HIV-infected patients selected from an Indonesian prospective cohort study. *PLoS One* 8(11): e79904.

4 Vitamin D and HIV

Elaine A. Yu and Saurabh Mehta

CONTENTS

INTRODUCTION

BACKGROUND

In 1981, rare opportunistic infections (Kaposi's sarcoma and *Pneumocystis carinii* pneumonia) were reported as clinical cases (Gottlieb et al., 1981) and later identified as acquired immunodeficiency syndrome (AIDS). Worldwide, 39 million deaths are cumulatively related to AIDS (UNAIDS, 2014), and 36.9 million individuals were living with HIV in 2014 (UNAIDS, 2015). Despite substantial progress, including increased global access to antiretroviral therapy (ART), the burden of disease from HIV disproportionately affects individuals in low- and middle-income countries (United Nations, 2015). The remaining major challenges in HIV prevention and treatments have heightened interest in the roles of treatment adjuncts, such as micronutrient supplementation. In certain resource-limited settings with higher prevalence of HIV, individuals often face the additional challenges of malnutrition (including vitamin D deficiency) and food insecurity (United Nations, 2015).

Suboptimal vitamin D status is considered by some as the most common medical condition globally (Holick, 2010); however, estimates of deficiency prevalence range widely (6 to 100%) among individuals living with HIV (Orkin et al., 2014). Aside from the established role of vitamin D in skeletal health, the immunomodulatory effects of vitamin D have more recently been recognized (Cantorna et al., 2004; Baeke et al., 2010; Cantorna, 2010; Hewison, 2012; Prietl et al., 2013). In the early 1980s, studies identified a nuclear receptor in immune cells (including lymphocytes and monocytes) (Bhalla et al., 1983; Provvedini et al., 1983), which binds specifically to the biologically active vitamin D metabolite. Furthermore, other key laboratory findings (Wang et al., 2004; Liu et al., 2006, 2007; Adams and Hewison, 2008) corroborated the dynamic interaction between vitamin D and the human host response against infectious diseases.

Separately, other studies have provided mechanisms of how certain ART pharmacokinetics could result in vitamin D deficiency (Dao et al., 2011; Yin and Stein, 2011). One non-nucleoside analog reverse transcriptase inhibitor (efavirenz [EFV]) induces cytochrome P450 enzymes (Vrouenraets et al., 2007), including CYP24 (Landriscina et al., 2008). CYP24A1 is a key enzyme in vitamin D metabolism that degrades the physiologically active vitamin D metabolite $1,25(OH)_2D$ to $24,25(OH)_2D$ (Jones et al., 2012). Over the past two decades, a number of published case reports have documented a link between vitamin D status and patients with HIV/AIDS on ART (Playford et al., 2001; Gyllensten et al., 2006; Kumar et al., 2012).

Preliminary evidence supports the complex associations between vitamin D and HIV (including host immunity and treatments); however, a number of research gaps remain. Therefore, our objective was to review current evidence of the bidirectional linkages between vitamin D and HIV/AIDS, including clinical health outcomes and ART treatments.

METHODS

We searched PubMed with "(HIV or AIDS) and vitamin D" as search terms and the restrictions of publication date (on or prior to June 30, 2015) and language (English; $n = 511$) (Figure 4.1). Inclusion screening criteria included (1) vitamin D (e.g., serum or plasma concentration, treatment regimen, exogenous administration in laboratory studies); (2) HIV infection and/or exposure status of study participants (or simian immunodeficiency virus [SIV] in animal studies); (3) outcomes related to morbidity and mortality; and (4) intervention studies, including randomized controlled trials (RCTs). A number of studies that satisfied the first three criteria were highlighted, although not comprehensively included, in this review. We included randomized controlled trials with study participants receiving treatment regimens other than vitamin D (such as ART) if individuals were living with HIV and vitamin D status was measured. Exclusion criteria included case reports, publications without primary data (such as literature reviews, editorials, letters), and studies that only reported outcomes directly related to skeletal health (and not vitamin D).

OVERVIEW

Broadly, this review addressed three themes: (1) the association between vitamin D and HIV, (2) vitamin D supplementation among individuals with HIV, and (3) linkages between ART and vitamin D among individuals living with HIV. The first theme highlights some *in vitro* and *ex vivo* laboratory studies (including animal models, human cell lines, and cultures) and observational human studies. The second theme focuses on 25 intervention studies with vitamin D supplementation. The third theme includes two RCTs that randomly assigned ART among individuals with HIV and assessed vitamin D. Finally, the last section of this chapter discusses some key limitations and research gaps.

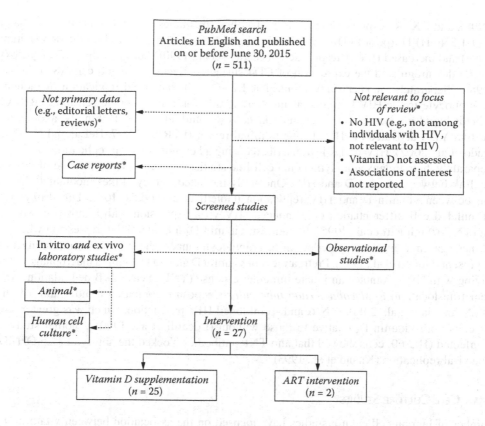

FIGURE 4.1 Study selection. Search terms: (("hiv"[MeSH Terms] OR "hiv"[All Fields]) OR ("acquired immunodeficiency syndrome"[MeSH Terms] OR ("acquired"[All Fields] AND "immunodeficiency"[All Fields] AND "syndrome"[All Fields]) OR "acquired immunodeficiency syndrome"[All Fields] OR "aids"[All Fields])) AND ("vitamin d"[MeSH Terms] OR "vitamin d"[All Fields] OR "ergocalciferols"[MeSH Terms] OR "ergocalciferols"[All Fields]) AND ("0001/01/01"[PDAT] : "2015/06/30"[PDAT]) AND English[lang].

ASSOCIATION BETWEEN VITAMIN D AND HIV

ANIMAL MODELS

Two primate studies found that simian immunodeficiency virus (SIV) infection was associated with decreased vitamin D serum concentrations (two weeks post-infection) (Kewenig et al., 1999), as well as vitamin D-binding protein during acute infection (Wiederin et al., 2010). HIV transgenic mice had reduced vitamin D receptor (VDR) expression in proximal tubular epithelial cells compared to control mice (FVB/N) (Salhan et al., 2012).

HUMAN CELL LINE STUDIES

Several *in vitro* studies with leukemia–lymphoma cell lines assessed the effects of vitamin D on indicators of HIV-1 transmission and disease severity, including U937 promonocytic (Pauza et al., 1993; Biswas et al., 1998) and HL-60 promyelocytic cell lines (Schlesinger et al., 1989; Kitano et al., 1990, 1993). In two studies, U937 cell clones with 1,25-dihydroxyvitamin D_3 pretreatment showed increased HIV-1 viral replication (Biswas et al., 1998; Pauza et al., 1993), proviral DNA (Biswas et al., 1998), and CXCR4 expression (Biswas et al., 1998). In studies with HL-60 cell lines, the presence of $1,25(OH)_2D_3$ (prior to HIV infection) delayed the induction of viral production (Kitano et al., 1993) and increased HIV virus production (Kitano et al., 1990). Additionally, 1,25-dihydroxyvitamin D_3 downregulated the expression of CD4 surface antigens in HL-60 cells (Schlesinger et al., 1989). Separately, another study found that $1,25(OH)_2D_3$ increased replication of monocyte- and lymphocyte-tropic HIV-1 strains (as much as 10,000-fold) in monocyte cell lines (BT4A3.5), peripheral blood monocytes, and mononuclear cells (Skolnik et al., 1991). Finally, another study found that VDR activated the HIV-1 long terminal repeat (LTR) in U937, HeLa, and Cos-1 cells (Nevado et al., 2007). HIV-1 LTR is transcribed during a key step for viral replication.

Separately, human leukemia–lymphoma cell line studies have considered the role of cytokines in the link between vitamin D and HIV. One study indicated that cytokines modulated the interaction between vitamin D and HIV replication (Goletti et al., 1995). $1\alpha,25$-Dihydroxyvitamin D_3-stimulated cell differentiation only induced HIV viral expression with tumor necrosis factor alpha (TNF-α) (Goletti et al., 1995). In contrast, vitamin D_3 inhibited HIV expression when other cytokines (gamma interferon, interleukin-6, granulocyte–macrophage colony-stimulating factor) were present (Goletti et al., 1995). Pretreatment of vitamin D among U1 human macrophages of people living with HIV promoted an innate immune response (TNF release, IκB degradation, NF-κB nuclear translocation) to *Mycobacterium tuberculosis* exposure compared to no vitamin D treatment (Anandaiah et al., 2013). IFN-α and -β inhibited HIV production, which was greater among U937 cells with vitamin D_3 relative to those without (Locardi et al., 1990). Another study with HIV-infected (HL-60) cells showed that anti-TNF antibodies blocked the ability of $1,25(OH)_2D_3$ to induce viral replication (Kitano et al., 1993).

HUMAN CELL CULTURE STUDIES

A number of human cell culture studies have focused on the association between vitamin D and HIV, including the role of vitamin D receptor (VDR). VDR polymorphisms (rs1544410_GG, rs1544410_AA) were associated with altered (1) response to vitamin D_3 in cell differentiation markers (CD14 inhibition, CD209 induction), and (2) HIV-1-LTR reporter gene activity with vitamin D_3 presence (Torres et al., 2010). This finding was supported by previous literature, including computational (Tastan et al., 2009) and cell line studies (Nevado et al., 2007). Other human cell culture studies more specifically focused on the bidirectional relationship between vitamin D and HIV and addressed the following questions: (1) How does vitamin D affect HIV (including disease progression and host response, as well as in the context of other comorbidities)? and (2) How does HIV infection affect vitamin D metabolism?

How Does Vitamin D Affect HIV?

A number of studies considered the effects of vitamin D (pretreatment or blood concentration) on HIV-related outcomes in leukocytes isolated from patients. Some studies involved cell cultures from patients with HIV infection, or no infection (to assess HIV exposure). HIV outcome indicators included (1) HIV disease progression and severity (HIV-1 infection, viral replication), (2) immunological and cellular responses to HIV (autophagy), and (3) other comorbidities (tuberculosis).

HIV Disease Progression and Severity

Studies that pretreated monocytes or macrophages with vitamin D_3 ($1,25(OH)_2D_3$, including its analog $1,25(OH)_2$-16-ene-23-yne-26,27-F_6-D_3) and subsequent HIV infection reported inconsistent findings. $1,25(OH)_2D$ pretreatment of freshly isolated blood monocytes reduced HIV-1 infection (Connor and Rigby, 1991) and inhibited HIV viral replication (Pauza et al., 1993) in two studies. In contrast, other studies reported that vitamin D_3 and analogs enhanced HIV infection 3.5-fold (Kizaki et al., 1993) and that there were no effects of 25-hydroxyvitamin D (25(OH)D) on HIV-1 production or CD4 expression (Connor and Rigby, 1991).

Immunological and Cellular Responses to HIV

Several human macrophage studies have established a potential autophagic mechanism involving $1,25(OH)_2D_3$ inhibition of HIV. Physiological concentrations of $1\alpha,25(OH)_2D_3$ induced autophagy (in a mechanism dependent on phosphatidyl 3-kinase, ATG-5, and Beclin-1), which has a dose-dependent inhibition of HIV-1 replication (Campbell and Spector, 2011). Subsequent studies delineated the role of an antimicrobial peptide (cathelicidin), which further corroborated the previous result. The activation of toll-like receptor (TLR) 8 was associated with increased expression of cathelicidin, vitamin D receptor (VDR), and cytochrome P450, family 27, subfamily B, polypeptide 1 (CYP27B1) (Campbell and Spector, 2012a). Physiological concentrations of 1,25-dihydroxycholecalciferol induced cathelicidin (LL37) production and autophagy in macrophages from patients with HIV–tuberculosis (TB) co-infections (Campbell and Spector, 2012b). Moreover, another study confirmed that the inhibition of HIV replication occurred via an autophagic pathway dependent on vitamin D and cathelicidin (Campbell and Spector, 2012a). Several studies found that vitamin D improved the function (motility, maturation, activation) of monocytes and macrophages. In monocytes from patients with AIDS, the exogenous administration of $1,25(OH)_2D_3$ improved migratory capacity, which was related to a chemoattractant (formyl peptide [FMLP]) and its receptor (Girasole et al., 1990). Separately, in monocytes from individuals with HIV infections (symptomatic and asymptomatic), $1,25(OH)_2D$ was associated with improved growth and maturation (Haug et al., 1996); a negative correlation was observed between response to $1,25(OH)_2D$ and CD4+ lymphocyte counts in the blood of patients with HIV. In another study involving peripheral blood monocytes/macrophages of patients with HIV, the addition of vitamin D-binding protein (Gc protein) macrophage-activating factor (MAF) resulted in monocyte/macrophage activation (Yamamoto et al., 1995).

Other Comorbidities

Three studies considered the role of vitamin D in *Mycobacterium* co-infections with HIV. Among macrophages with HIV–TB co-infection, physiological concentrations of $1\alpha,25$-dihydroxycholecalciferol $(1,25(OH)_2D_3)$ inhibited replication of HIV and TB via an autophagic mechanism dependent on cathelicidin and phagosomal maturation (Campbell and Spector, 2012c). Additionally, authors confirmed that the autophagic flux involves cAMP and phagosomal maturation (not only autophagy) (Campbell and Spector, 2012b). Separately, another study found that $1,25(OH)_2D$ supplementation resulted in decreased or no change in bacterial replication of *Mycobacterium avium* complex (MAC) in macrophages of individuals with HIV; however, $1,25(OH)_2D$ increased bacteria in cells of individuals without HIV (Haug et al., 1998a).

How Does HIV Infection Affect Vitamin D Metabolism?

Several studies considered the effects of HIV infection on vitamin D and key factors in vitamin D metabolism, including VDR. One study with monocytes (from human patients) showed that, in the presence of 25-hydroxyvitamin D_3, the p17 matrix protein of HIV-1 is able to induce 1α-hydroxylase activity and fructose 1,6-bisphosphatase gene expression (Besancon et al., 1997). Given the structural similarities between p17 and interferon-gamma (IFN-γ) and shared function in inducing 1α-hydroxylase, the authors posited that their findings suggest that p17 and IFN-γ facilitate selective conversion of 25-hydroxyvitamin D_3 to 1,25-dihydroxyvitamin D_3 (Besancon et al., 1997). Separately, in an epigenetic study considering the effects of HIV-induced methylation of vitamin D receptor on T cells, HIV-infected T cells showed increased VDR–cytosine–phosphate–guanine (CpG) dinucleotide methylation and DNA-(cytosine-5-)-methyltransferase-3-beta (Dnmt3b) expression, but reduced VDR expression (Chandel et al., 2013). The authors suggest that VDR methylation (by HIV) is one factor that mediates T-cell apoptosis through the reactive oxygen species (ROS) response.

OBSERVATIONAL STUDIES AMONG INDIVIDUALS LIVING WITH HIV

For this section, we included any studies that reported (1) cross-sectional or baseline data, regardless of the overall study design (such as randomized control trials and observational studies with longitudinal data); and (2) associations between vitamin D and health indicators among individuals living with HIV.

Vitamin D Status

Over 160 studies have assessed vitamin D status among individuals living with HIV. Most studies were conducted among individuals in North America (United States and Canada) or Europe (including Spain, Italy, France, Norway, Denmark, Belgium, Germany, Netherlands, United Kingdom, Austria, Switzerland, and Slovenia). Other studies included individuals residing in Africa (Zimbabwe, Uganda, Malawi, Tanzania, Guinea Bissau, and South Africa), Asia (Thailand, India, China, Cambodia, Nepal, Turkey, Israel, and Iran), South America (Brazil and Colombia), and Australia. Assessments of vitamin D status included radioimmunoassays (RIAs), chemiluminescence immunoassays (CLIAs), liquid chromatography/mass spectroscopy/tandem spectroscopy (LC/MS/TS), high-performance liquid chromatography (HPLC), enzyme-linked immunosorbent assays (ELISA), enzyme immunoassays (EIA), electrochemiluminescence immunoassays (ECLIA), competitive binding assays (CBAs), and automated immunoassays. Study population sizes ranged widely, from 16 to 2994 individuals (Jaeger et al., 1994; Allavena et al., 2012). Among *in vivo* studies reporting blood concentrations of vitamin D, a smaller proportion of studies were among infants, children, and adolescents (<18 years).

From available data of 25(OH)D concentrations in plasma or serum of study populations (or subpopulations), mean (8.1–61.8 ng/mL) and median (6–57 ng/mL) levels included wide ranges. $1,25(OH)_2D$ concentrations ranged considerably also, based on mean (22.3–56.0 pg/mL) and median (22–97 pg/mL) values. Although definitions of low vitamin D status (deficient, insufficient) varied across studies, common 25(OH)D cut points were between 10 and 30 ng/mL (or, equivalently, between 25 and 75 nmol/L).

Several studies found lower vitamin D status (or greater deficiency) among people with HIV compared to those with no infection (Teichmann et al., 2003; Madeddu et al., 2004; García Aparicio et al., 2006; Ross et al., 2011; Rutstein et al., 2011; Li Vecchi et al., 2012). In contrast, two studies observed that HIV infection was associated with higher vitamin D (or lower vitamin D deficiency) (Adeyemi et al., 2011; Ormesher et al., 2011; Friis et al., 2013; Lambert et al., 2014). Also, other studies reported no differences in vitamin D between subgroups stratified by HIV status (Stephensen et al., 2006; Friis et al., 2008; Sherwood et al., 2012; Hamill et al., 2013; Zhang et al., 2013).

Vitamin D and HIV Disease Progression

Studies that considered HIV disease progression included cohort (prospective, retrospective) and nested case-control and -cohort studies (Table 4.1; $n = 9$) (Barber et al., 2001; Nieto et al., 2004; Mehta et al., 2010a, 2013; Viard et al., 2011; Moodley et al., 2013; Havers et al., 2014a; Shepherd et al., 2014; Theodorou et al., 2014). Definitions of HIV disease progression varied, including WHO disease stages ≥3 or 4 (WHO, 2007); AIDS, according to the 1987 and 1993 Centers for Disease Control and Prevention (CDC) definitions (CDC, 1992); and other HIV-related outcomes (mortality, weight growth failure, ≥2 opportunistic infections, CD4 T-lymphocyte counts). The exposures of interest included suboptimal vitamin D status (lowest quantile, <10 and <32 ng/mL; $n = 6$) and genetic polymorphisms relating to vitamin D: CCR5 chemokine receptor wtΔ32, vitamin D receptor (VDR), *FokI* (C/T), *BsmI* (G/A), *DHCR7* (G/T), and *CYP2R1* (G/A) ($n = 3$).

Among three studies that considered the associations between genetic polymorphisms relating to vitamin D, all found increased risks or odds of HIV disease progression associated with particular genotypes (Barber et al., 2001; Nieto et al., 2004; Moodley et al., 2013). In a prospective cohort among patients living with HIV-1 in Spain (from an intravenous drug abuse risk group, Lleida AIDS

TABLE 4.1
Vitamin D and HIV Disease Progression among Individuals Living with HIV

ART Status at Baseline	Study Design	Location	Study Population	n	Age (yr)	Primary Exposures	Health Outcomes	Associations and Effect Estimates	Ref.
Heterogeneous	Prospective cohort	Spain	Patients with HIV (Caucasians with intravenous drug use)	185	Median 24 (IQR, 21–27)	VDR genetic polymorphisms	Progression to AIDS: CDC 1987 and 1993 criteria First decline of CD4 cells (<200/μL)	Progression to AIDS (CDC 1993 criteria): VDR-BB (vs. non-VDR-BB) ↑ ($p = 0.04$) Declining CD4 cells (<200/ μL): VDR-BB (vs. non-VDR-BB) ↑ ($p = <0.01$) *Sub-analyses* Progression to AIDS among patients on ART: VDR BB (vs. non-VDR-BB) ↑ (OR, 2.2; 95% CI, 0.98–5.00) Declining CD4 cells (<200/ μL among patients on ART: VDR-BB (vs. non-VDR-BB) ↑ (OR, 3.2; 95% CI, 1.4–7.0)	Barber et al. (2001)
Naïve	Nested case cohort (in RCT)	Brazil, Haiti, India, Malawi, Peru, South Africa, Thailand, United States, Zimbabwe	Adults with HIV	411	Median 35 (IQR, 30–41)	Low vitamin D (25(OH)D < 32 ng/mL)	HIV disease progression to WHO stage 3 or 4 or death (within 96 weeks of cART initiation) Virologic and immunologic failure	Virologic failure ↑ (AHR, 2.42; 95% CI, 1.33–4.41) Disease progression and death ↑ (AHR, 2.13; 95% CI, 1.09–4.18)	Havers et al. (2014a)
Naïve	Prospective cohort (in RCT)	Tanzania	Pregnant women with HIV	884	—	Low vitamin D (25(OH)D < 32 ng/mL; quintile)	HIV disease progression to greater than WHO stage 3 Mortality Hemoglobin	Greater than WHO stage 3 ↑ (RR, 1.25; 95% CI, 1.05–1.50) Death (highest vs. lowest vitamin D quintile) ↓ (RR, 0.58; 95% CI, 0.40–0.84) Severe anemia ↑ (RR, 1.46; 95% CI, 1.09–1.96)	Mehta et al. (2010a)

(continued)

TABLE 4.1 (continued)
Vitamin D and HIV Disease Progression among Individuals Living with HIV

ART Status at Baseline	Study Design	Location	Study Population	n	Age (yr)	Primary Exposures	Health Outcomes	Associations and Effect Estimates	Ref.
Naïve	Prospective cohort	Tanzania	Patients with TB (subgroup with HIV, n = 344)	677	HIV, 34.4 ± 8.6 No-HIV, 30.2 ± 9.2	Low vitamin D (25(OH)D < 30 ng/mL)	HIV disease progression to WHO stage 3 or 4 Mortality T-cell counts	HIV disease progression or death ↔ T-cell counts (CD_3, CD8) ↑	Mehta et al. (2013)
Naïve (<8 weeks prior to ART)	Prospective cohort	North America (multicenter)	Children with HIV	998	Median 2.3 (range, 0.1–18.0)	Genetic polymorphisms of Fok1 (C/T), Bsm1 (G/A), GC (A/C), DHCR7 (G/T), CYP2R1 (G/A)	Progression to HIV-related disease endpoint (≥2 opportunistic infection, weight growth failure) Mortality	HIV disease progression among children > 2 years: *DHCR7* G/G vs. T/T allele ↑ (HR, 5.0; $p = 0.035$) G/T vs. T/T ↑ (HR, 4.5; $p = 0.042$) G/G + G/T vs. T/T ↑ (HR, 4.8; $p = 0.036$) *Bsm1* A/G vs. G/G ↑ (HR, 2.2; $p = 0.014$) A/G + A/A vs. G/G ↑ (HR, 2.0; $p = 0.026$) HIV disease progression among children ≤ 2 years: *Bsm1* among Hispanics A/A vs. G/A + G/G ↑ (HR, 2.8; $p = 0.03$) A/A vs. G/G ↑ (HR, 2.8; $p = 0.046$) *Bsm1* among Caucasians A/A vs. G/G ↑ (HR, 6.6; $p = 0.025$) A/A vs. G/A + G/G ↑ (HR, 3.6; $p = 0.038$)	Moodley et al. (2013)

	Design	Country	Population	N	Age	Vitamin D measure	Outcome	Results	Reference
Heterogeneous	Prospective cohort	Spain	Patients with HIV (Caucasians with intravenous drug use)	185	Median 24 (IQR, 21–27)	VDR genetic polymorphisms: *FokI*	Progression to AIDS (CDC 1993 criteria) First decline of CD4 cells (<200/µL)	HIV disease progression (Ff vs. non-Ff) ↔ (RR, 1.38; 95% CI, 0.98–1.96) Decline in CD4 cell count (<200/µL) (Ff vs. non-Ff) ↑ (RR, 1.44; 95% CI, 1.02–2.03); ↑ (HR, 1.77; 95% CI, 1.1–2.8) Mean time to AIDS (Ff vs. non-Ff) ↑ (HR, 1.53; 95% CI, 1.00–2.33)	Nieto et al. (2004)
Heterogeneous	Nested case control (in prospective cohort)	Europe (33 countries), Argentina, Israel (multicenter; EuroSIDA)	Patients with and without HIV-1	250	>16	25(OH)D < 10 ng/mL	Cases: AIDS (1993 CDC criteria), death categorized by Coding of Causes of Death in HIV (CoDe), non-AIDS defining event Controls: 1:1 matching	Among those with 2-fold increase in latest 25(OH)D: Death ↓ (odds, 46.0%; 95% CI, 2.0–70.0%) Severe vitamin D deficiency (<10 ng/mL) (cases vs. controls): AIDS ↔; non-AIDS defining events ↔; death ↔	Shepherd et al. (2014)
Heterogeneous	Retrospective cohort	Belgium	Patients with HIV	2044	Median 43 (range, 20–85)	Low vitamin D (<30, <10 ng/mL)	HIV disease stage (CDC disease severity classification) CD4 count (<200/µL) ART	Vitamin D deficiency (<10ng/mL): CDC stage C ↑ (AOR, 2.21; 95% CI, 1.50–3.26) Low CD4 count (<200/µL) ↑ (AOR, 1.38; 95% CI, 1.03–1.85) EFV treatment ↑ (AOR, 2.18; 95% CI, 1.47–3.22)	Theodorou et al. (2014)

(continued)

TABLE 4.1 (continued)

Vitamin D and HIV Disease Progression among Individuals Living with HIV

ART Status at Baseline	Study Design	Location	Study Population	n	Age (yr)	Primary Exposures	Health Outcomes	Associations and Effect Estimates	Ref.
Heterogeneous	Prospective cohort	Europe (33 countries), Argentina, Israel (multicenter; EuroSIDA)	Patients with HIV-1	1985	Stratified by 25(OH)D tertiles: Lowest (<12 ng/mL): median 39.3 (IQR, 33.2–46.1) Middle (12–20 ng/mL): median 38.1 (IQR, 32.4–45.2) Highest (>20 ng/mL): median 38.0 (IQR, 33.4–44.2)	Low vitamin D (tertiles; ng/mL)	AIDS (1993 CDC criteria), non-AIDS events, all-cause mortality	AIDS: Middle vs. lowest ↔ (IRR, 0.53; 95% CI, 0.24–1.15) Highest vs. lowest ↔ (IRR, 0.61; 95% CI, 0.28–1.32) All-cause mortality: Middle vs. lowest ↔ (IRR, 0.67; 95% CI, 0.41–1.09) Highest vs. lowest ↓ (IRR, 0.60; 95% CI, 0.37–0.98)	Viard et al. (2011)

Note: AHR, adjusted hazard ratio; ART, antiretroviral therapy; cART, combination antiretroviral therapy; CDC, Centers for Disease Control and Prevention; CI, confidence interval; CoDe, Coding Causes of Death in HIV; Ff, *Fok*I polymorphism; HR, hazard ratio; IQR, interquartile range; IRR, incidence rate ratio; OR, odds ratio; RCT, randomized controlled trial; RR, relative risk; VDR, vitamin D receptor; WHO, World Health Organization.

Cohort), the VDR BB genotype was associated with increased odds of progression to AIDS as well as T cells < 200/µL (Barber et al., 2001). In another study among children (>2 years) with HIV in the United States and Puerto Rico, *DHCR7* alleles G/G vs. T/T (hazard ratio [HR], 5.0; $p = 0.035$); G/T vs. T/T (HR, 4.5; $p = 0.042$); and G/G + G/T vs. T/T (HR, 4.8; $p = 0.036$), as well as the *Bsm*I A allele, were associated with increased risk of progression to HIV-related endpoints (weight growth failure, ≥2 opportunistic infections, death) (Moodley et al., 2013). Heterozygous *Fok*I polymorphism (Ff) was associated with a shorter time to initial incidence of CD4 T-lymphocytes < 200/µL (risk ratio [RR], 1.44; 95% CI, 1.02–2.03) and AIDS ($p = 0.04$) (Nieto et al., 2004).

Six studies considered the association between low vitamin D concentration and HIV disease progression (Mehta et al., 2010a, 2013; Viard et al., 2011; Havers et al., 2014a; Shepherd et al., 2014; Theodorou et al., 2014). Three studies found that suboptimal vitamin D status was associated with HIV disease progression (including advanced clinical stages) or death (Mehta et al., 2010a; Havers et al., 2014a; Theodorou et al., 2014). In contrast, two studies showed no associations (Mehta et al., 2013; Shepherd et al., 2014), and one study reported protective effects between higher vitamin D and clinical progression as well as mortality (Viard et al., 2011).

Vitamin D, Other Health Indicators, and Comorbidities

Many studies assessed the links between vitamin D and a wide spectrum of clinical health indicators among patients living with HIV. The association between vitamin D and mortality has only been assessed by a few studies, which reported inconsistent findings (Mehta et al., 2010a; Sherwood et al., 2012; Sudfeld et al., 2012; Erlandson et al., 2014). Separately, other study findings indicated a negative correlation between vitamin D status and HIV duration (Eckard et al., 2013a) and no association with vertical HIV transmission (Mave et al., 2012). Other cross-sectional studies have also observed associations between vitamin D (25(OH)D and 1,25(OH)$_2$D) and other HIV-related indicators, including advanced disease stages (Theodorou et al., 2014) and clinical diagnoses such as oral thrush (Mehta et al., 2011; Sudfeld et al., 2013) and acute upper respiratory tract infection (Mehta et al., 2011). However, other studies also reported no associations between vitamin D and either HIV RNA (Chokephaibulkit et al., 2013; Poowuttikul et al., 2014) or viral load (Gedela et al., 2013).

Immunological Indicators

A number of studies showed that vitamin D (25(OH)D and 1,25(OH)$_2$D) was correlated with CD4 T-cell count (Haug et al., 1994; Teichmann et al., 2003; Mueller et al., 2010; Welz et al., 2010; Rutstein et al., 2011; Stein et al., 2011; Legeai et al., 2013; Poowuttikul et al., 2014), LL-37 (Honda et al., 2014), cytokine (TNF-α) (Haug et al., 1998b), erythrocyte sedimentation rate (Mehta et al., 2010b), virologic failure (Havers et al., 2014a), complete early virologic response (cEVR), and sustained virologic response (SVR) (Mandorfer et al., 2013) among individuals living with HIV. Serum neopterin (an indicator of cellular immune activation, including during HIV infection) (Murr et al., 2002) was observed to have a negative relationship with vitamin D (Haug et al., 1994). In contrast, a number of studies also reported no associations between vitamin D and T cells (van den Bout-van den Beukel 2008a; Mehta et al., 2010a; Stein et al., 2011), cytokines and inflammatory markers (including TNF-α and IFN-γ, IL-6) (van den Bout-van den Beukel, 2008b; Ross et al., 2011; Eckard et al., 2013a; Jarvis et al., 2014), TB-associated immune restoration disease (Price et al., 2012), and H1N1 vaccine response (Momplaisir et al., 2012) among people living with HIV.

Nutritional Status

Several studies confirmed the positive relationship between vitamin D intake (via consumption of natural food sources, fortified foods, or supplements) and vitamin D status of individuals living with HIV (Rodríguez et al., 2009; Crutchley et al., 2012; Etminani-Esfahani et al., 2012a). Daily calcium intake was also associated with vitamin D status among study participants with HIV (Etminani-Esfahani et al., 2012a). Blood concentrations of other micronutrients, including phosphate (Haug et al., 1998b), albumin (Frontini et al., 2012; Lambert et al., 2014), hemoglobin (Mehta et al., 2013), and vitamins A and E (Mehta et al., 2010b), were correlated with vitamin D status in studies. Other studies observed no associations between vitamin D and other nutritional indicators (Teichmann et al., 1997; Haug et al., 1998b; van den Bout-van den Beukel et al., 2008b; Nansera et al., 2011). Low 25(OH)D (<32 ng/mL) was associated with severe anemia (HR, 1.41; 95% CI, 1.05–1.89), and hypochromic microcytosis (HR, 2.38; 95% CI, 1.58–3.58) in a study among pregnant women living with HIV in Tanzania (Finkelstein et al., 2012a). In contrast, however, other studies showed no association between vitamin D status and anemia (Finkelstein et al., 2012b) or hemoglobin (Nansera et al., 2011).

In terms of anthropometric indicators, body weight and body mass index (BMI) were associated with vitamin D status among individuals living with HIV (Mueller et al., 2010; Dao et al., 2011; Mehta et al., 2011; Nansera et al., 2011; Rutstein et al., 2011; Crutchley et al., 2012; Eckard 2013a; Gangcuangco et al., 2013; Porter et al., 2013; Sudfeld et al., 2013; Havers et al., 2014a). Higher BMI was associated with low vitamin D status among individuals living with HIV (Dao et al., 2011; Rutstein 2011; Crutchley et al., 2012; Eckard et al., 2013a; Havers et al., 2014a). Among pregnant women with HIV, vitamin D was inversely associated with risk of low BMI (<18.5 kg/m^2) (Mehta et al., 2011). Another study found a positive association between vitamin D and BMI among adults in Uganda with TB and HIV (Nansera et al., 2011). Wasting (BMI < 18.5) was also associated with low vitamin D status among individuals with HIV (Mehta et al., 2011; Sudfeld et al., 2013).

Bone Health

Several studies confirmed the associations between vitamin D and skeletal health, as well as metabolic indicators among people living with HIV. Vitamin D was inversely associated with plasma parathyroid hormone (PTH) (Childs et al., 2010; Rosenvinge et al., 2010; Chokephaibulkit et al., 2013; Pinzone et al., 2013) and other markers for bone turnover (including alkaline phosphatase) (Kwan et al., 2012). Also, vitamin D status was associated with differences in bone mineral density and loss (Dolan et al., 2006; Yin et al., 2010; Shahar et al., 2013), including lumbar spine, femoral neck, and hip assessments. Yet, a number of studies also reported null associations between vitamin D and bone health indicators among individuals living with HIV, including osteoporosis (Hileman et al., 2014), osteopenia (Ramayo et al., 2005; Hileman et al., 2014), and other indicators (Yin et al., 2005; Chokephaibulkit et al., 2013; El-Maouche et al., 2013).

Diabetes Mellitus and Metabolic Syndrome

A study in Italy found vitamin D deficiency increased the risk of type-2 diabetes mellitus among patients with HIV (Szep et al., 2011). Similarly, other studies have confirmed low vitamin D associated with poor diabetes indicators, including insulin resistance (Eckard et al., 2013a; Moreno-Pérez et al., 2013) and insulin (Hammond et al., 2012) among individuals living with HIV. Further, studies showed links between vitamin D and random blood glucose (Rosenvinge et al., 2010), triglycerides (Portilla et al., 2014; Schwartz et al., 2014), beta cell function (Moreno-Pérez et al., 2013), and lipoatrophy among people living with HIV (Lerma et al., 2012). However, several studies found no association between vitamin D and metabolic syndrome (Szep et al., 2011) or other lipid measurements (van den Bout-van den Beukel et al., 2008b; Eckard et al., 2013a).

Other Noncommunicable Diseases

Among studies that considered cardiovascular health of individuals living with HIV, most indicated associations with vitamin D. Vitamin D was associated with hypertension (Dao et al., 2011), subclinical coronary artery disease (CAD) (Lai et al., 2012a, 2013a), coronary stenosis (Lai et al., 2012b), coronary artery calcification (Lai et al., 2013b), carotid intima–media thickness (cIMT) (Choi et al., 2011), flow-mediated dilatation (Shikuma et al., 2012), and plasminogen activator inhibitor-1 (Portilla et al., 2014). Separately, studies showed relationships between vitamin D and renal function, including glomerular filtration rate (Rosenvinge et al., 2010; Etminani-Esfahani et al., 2012a), urinary protein excretion (among individuals with diabetes, and injection drug users) (Estrella et al., 2012), and renal insufficiency (Dao et al., 2011), among study participants with HIV. However, a few studies found no relationships between vitamin D and cardiovascular health indicators (Eckard et al., 2013a; Portilla et al., 2014; Shikuma et al., 2012).

Sociodemographic and Additional Factors Associated with Vitamin D

A number of studies considered well-established influences of vitamin D status, including sociodemographics and factors affecting exposure to ultraviolet irradiation (which affects endogenous production of vitamin D), among people living with HIV. Generally, these factors were similar to studies that have assessed the influences of risk factors of vitamin D status among healthy individuals. Briefly, a few examples include *race or ethnicity* (Welz et al., 2010; Dao et al., 2011; Fox et al., 2011; Rutstein et al., 2011; Vescini et al., 2011; Viard et al., 2011; Crutchley et al., 2012; Frontini et al., 2012; Kim et al., 2012; Lerma et al., 2012; Price et al., 2012; Eckard et al., 2013b; Gangcuangco et al., 2013; Porter et al., 2013; Havers et al., 2014a; Lambert et al., 2014), *sex* (Etminani-Esfahani et al., 2012a; Pinzone et al., 2013; Theodorou et al., 2014), *age* (Rutstein et al., 2011; Vescini et al., 2011; Viard et al., 2011; Meyzer et al., 2013), *seasonality* (Welz et al., 2010; Fox et al., 2011; Rutstein et al., 2011; Viard et al., 2011; Gangcuangco et al., 2013; Gedela et al., 2013; Porter et al., 2013; Havers et al., 2014a,b; Jarvis et al., 2014; Lambert et al., 2014; Theodorou et al., 2014), *skin pigmentation* (van den Bout-van den Beukel et al., 2008a; Eckard et al., 2012; Meyzer et al., 2013), *sun (or ultraviolet light) exposure* (Dao et al., 2011; Etminani-Esfahani et al., 2012a), physical activity (Dao et al., 2011; Portilla et al., 2014), *smoking* (Legeai et al., 2013), and *geographic location and country of residence* (Viard et al., 2011; Havers et al., 2014b).

Other Clinical Signs and Symptoms

In a study among mother–child dyads in Tanzania, low maternal vitamin D status was associated with 50% higher risk of mother-to-child transmission (MTCT) of HIV through breastfeeding between birth and 6 weeks of age (Mehta et al., 2009); however, maternal vitamin D status was not associated with other pregnancy outcomes (low birthweight, preterm birth). Vitamin D was associated with serum anti-Müllerian hormone (AMH), which is associated with polycystic ovarian syndrome, in another study (Merhi et al., 2012).

Additionally, low vitamin D was associated with pulmonary TB (Martineau et al., 2011; Sudfeld et al., 2013) and hepatitis C virus (HCV) co-infections (Mueller et al., 2010; Etminani-Esfahani et al., 2012a) in individuals living with HIV. In a study of patients with HIV–HCV co-infection, higher vitamin D was associated with an ART (ritonavir) (Branch et al., 2013). Other studies have indicated associations between vitamin D and a spectrum of clinical diagnoses or symptoms, including cough (among children of mothers with low vitamin D status during pregnancy) (Finkelstein et al., 2012b), significant fibrosis (Milazzo et al., 2011; Terrier et al., 2011; Guzmán-Fulgencio et al., 2014), cirrhosis (Branch et al., 2014), bacterial vaginosis (French et al., 2011), and oral candidiasis (Sroussi et al., 2012). Other studies showed that vitamin D was not associated with other respiratory symptoms and diarrhea (among infants of mothers with suboptimal vitamin D concentrations) (Finkelstein et al., 2012b), fibrosis (El-Maouche et al., 2013), or TB-associated immune reconstitution inflammatory syndrome (Conesa-Botella et al., 2012a,b).

VITAMIN D SUPPLEMENTATION STUDIES AMONG INDIVIDUALS LIVING WITH HIV

Vitamin D supplementation studies among individuals living with HIV include randomized controlled trials ($n = 17$) and intervention studies ($n = 8$) (see Table 4.2). Most of the randomized controlled trials were double-blinded; however, a few trials were exceptions. In some intervention

TABLE 4.2
Vitamin D Supplementation among Individuals Living with (or Exposed to) HIV/AIDS in Intervention Studies[a]

ART Status at Baseline	Location	Study Population	n[b]	Age (yr)	Vitamin D Treatment Regimen						Referent Group	Assessed Outcomes	Associations and Effect Estimates	Ref.
					Vitamin D Form	Administration Method	Dose	Frequency	Duration	Other				
ART[e]	New York, NY	Youth with HIV	56 (29 intervention; 27 placebo)	Range, 6–16	D_3	Oral	100,000 IU	Every 2 months	12 months	Calcium (1 g/d)	Double placebo	Serum 25(OH)D concentration; serum and urine calcium; HIV (CD4 [count, %], viral load)	*Intervention vs. placebo* Serum 25(OH)D (mean; AUC) ↑ Δ in CD4 count ↔ Δ in CD4% ↔ Δ in viral load ↔	1
ART[f]	New York, NY	Youth with HIV	59 (30 intervention; 29 placebo)	Range, 6–16	D_3	Oral	100,000 IU	Every 2 months	24 months	Calcium (1 g/d)	Double placebo	TBBMC, TBBMD, SBMC, SBMD	*Intervention vs. placebo* Δ in TBBMC ↔ Δ in TBBMD ↔ Δ in SBMC ↔ Δ in SBMD ↔	2
ART	Denmark	Adult men with HIV-1	51 (17, Group 1; 19, Group 2; 15, Group 3)	Group 1 mean 49 (SD 11) Group 2 mean 48 (SD 7) Group 3 mean 45 (SD 7)	Group 1: D_3 Group 2: D_3, calcitriol	Injection (baseline) Oral	*Group 1* Baseline 100,000 IU D_3 Tablet 1: D_3 (1200 IU), calcium (1200 mg) Tablet 2: placebo	Daily	16 weeks	—	Baseline: saline Tablet 1: calcium (1200 mg) Tablet 2: placebo	Primary: T-cell subsets Secondary: PTH, ionized calcium, 25(OH)D, HIV-1 RNA, 1,25(OH)2D	*Overall between groups* Δ in % of T cell subsets ↔ Δ in 25(OH)D ↔ ($p < 0.01$)	3

See above.	See above.	See above.	See above.	See above.	See above.	See above.	See above.	See above.	See above.	See above.	See above.	CTx, PINP, PTH, ionized calcium, 25(OH)D, 1,25(OH)2D, T-cell subsets	Group 2 vs. 3 Δ in PINP ↓ (p < 0.01) Δ in CTx ↓ (p < 0.01) Group 1 vs. 3 Δ in PINP ↔ Δ in CTx ↔	4
ART (containing TDF)	—[c]	Patients with HIV	32 (24, Group 1; 8, Group 2)	Group 1 mean 46 (SE 2) Group 2 mean 48 (SE 4)	D_3	Oral	Loading dose (IU = 40 × 75 − 25(OH)D) × body weight); rounded up to next 25,000 IU Maintenance dose (50,000 IU)	Provided as 50,000 IU/week until full dose reached Monthly	1 year	Group 1: Deficient baseline 25(OH)D (<50 nmol/L) and/or calcium (<4 mmol/24 hr urinary excretion) Group 2: Sufficient baseline 25(OH)D and calcium	No treatment	Vitamin D, serum PTH, calcium, bone mineral density, PTH-rp, FGF-23, serum phosphate, renal phosphate loss	Overall Vitamin D, serum PTH, calcium balance, BMD ↑ PTH-rp, FGF-23, serum phosphate, renal phosphate ↔	5

(continued)

TABLE 4.2 (continued)
Vitamin D Supplementation among Individuals Living with (or Exposed to) HIV/AIDS in Intervention Studies[a]

ART Status at Baseline	Study Population	Location	n[b]	Age (yr)	Vitamin D Treatment Regimen						Referent Group	Assessed Outcomes	Associations and Effect Estimates	Ref.
					Vitamin D Form	Administration Method	Dose	Frequency	Duration	Other				
ART	Caucasian adults with HIV, current cART, and 25(OH)D < 30 ng/mL	Italy	153 (47 IM; 67 oral; 39 none)	Mean 45.0 (SD 10.6)	D_3	IM injection; oral	300,000 IU (IM) 25,000 IU (oral)	Every 10 months Every 30 days	10 months	—	No treatment	Serum 25(OH)D	Intervention groups vs. no intervention 25(OH)D ↑ 25(OH)D < 15 ng/mL (post supplementation) 4.2% (IM) vs. 8.9% (oral) vs. 56.4% (control) ($p < 0.001$)	6
Heterogeneous	Youth with HIV	Italy	48	Range, 8–26	D_3	Oral	100,000 IU	Every 3 months	12 months	—	Placebo	PTH, 25(OH)D, 1,25(OH)2D, CD4+ T cells, VDR	Intervention vs. placebo Vitamin D insufficiency (12 months) ↓ CD4+ T cells (3 months) ↔ Th17:Treg (3 months) ↓	7

Category	Location	Population	N	Age	Form	Route	Dose	Frequency	Duration			Measures	Results	Ref
Hetero-geneous	Pennsyl-vania	Youth with HIV	44	Range, 8–24	D_3	Oral	4000 IU 7000 IU	Daily	12 weeks	—	—	Serum 25(OH)D, whole blood lead	*Overall 25(OH)D ↑ Intervention group vs. control Whole blood lead ↔*	8
ART	United States and Puerto Rico (multisite)	Youth with HIV	203 (118 cART with TDF; 85 cART without TDF); groups randomized to intervention (n = 102) or placebo (n = 101)	Range, 18–25; range, 18–24	D_3	Oral	50,000 IU	Every 4 weeks	12 weeks	—	Placebo	Total and free 1,25(OH)2D, DBP, FGF-23	*Intervention vs. placebo Total and free 1,25(OH)2D ↑ Δ in FGF-23 (across 4 groups, stratified by TDF use) ↑ (p = 0.04)*	9
												Serum 25(OH)D, efavirenz	*Intervention vs. placebo 25(OH)D ↑ (no effect of EFV)*	10
												BAP, CTX	*Δ in 25(OH)D (% ≥ 20 ng/mL) Vitamin D group ↑ Placebo ↔ Δ in PTH Vitamin D (TDF) ↓ Vitamin D (no TDF) ↔ Placebo ↔*	

(continued)

TABLE 4.2 (continued)
Vitamin D Supplementation among Individuals Living with (or Exposed to) HIV/AIDS in Intervention Studies[a]

ART Status at Baseline	Location	Study Population	n[b]	Age (yr)	Vitamin D Form	Administration Method	Dose	Frequency	Duration	Other	Referent Group	Assessed Outcomes	Associations and Effect Estimates	Ref.
							Vitamin D Treatment Regimen							
Hetero-geneous	Toronto, Canada	Youth with HIV	53	Mean 10.3 (SD 3.9)	D$_3$	Oral (liquid drops)	5600 IU 11,200 IU	Weekly	6 months	—	No treatment (Group 1)	Viral load, CD4 (count, %), 25(OH)D, 1,25(OH)2D	*Δ in 25(OH)D* Group 1 ↔ Group 2 ↑ Group 3 ↑ *Group 3 vs. 2* Δ in 25(OH)D ↑ *Inter-group differences* CD4 (count, %), viral load ↔	11
ART	Ohio	Adults with HIV and low baseline vitamin D concentration (≤20 ng/mL)	45	Inter-vention mean 47 (SD 8) Placebo mean 40 (SD 10)	D$_3$	Oral	4000 IU	Daily	12 weeks	Randomized 2:1 (intervention: placebo)	Placebo	FMD and other metabolic indicators	*Intervention vs. placebo* Δ in 25(OH)D ↑ Δ in FMD ↔ Cholesterol (total, non-HDL), insulin resistance indicators ↓	12

	Location	Population	N	Age	Form	Route	Dose	Frequency	Duration	Placebo	Outcomes	Results	Ref
Hetero-geneous	Guinea-Bissau	Adults with TB (initiating anti-TB treatment)	281 (136 intervention; 145 placebo)	Intervention mean 37 (SD 13) Placebo mean 38 (SD 14)	D_3	Oral	100,000 IU	0, 5, 8 months	12 months	—	Primary: TB score (clinical severity score) Secondary: mortality at 12 months	*Sub-group analyses (among patients with HIV-1; n = 95); intervention vs. placebo:* Mortality ↔ (HR, 1.8; 95% CI, 0.8–4.1) TB score ↔	13
Naïve	Cape Town, South Africa	Healthy young adults	100 (2 ethnic groups: 50 Xhosa; 50 Cape Mixed)	Range, 18–24	D_3	Oral	50,000 IU	Weekly	6 weeks	Winter supplemen-tation	HIV-1 replication, leukocytes, macrocytic anemia (winter-associated)	HIV-1 replication ↓ Leukocytes ↑ Macrocytic anemia ↓	14
Hetero-geneous	Pennsyl-vania	Children and young adults with HIV	44	Range, 8–25	D_3	Oral	4000 IU 7000 IU	Daily	12 weeks	—	25(OH)D, 1,25(OH)2D, PTH	*Δ in 25(OH)D (0 vs. 12 weeks)* 4000 IU ↑ 7000 IU ↑ *Subgroup receiving EFV vs. other ART* Δ in 25(OH)D ↑ Δ in 1,25(OH)₂D ↔ Δ in PTH ↔ *Subgroup receiving TDF* Δ in 25(OH)D ↔ Δ in 1,25(OH)₂D ↔ Δ in PTH ↔	15

(continued)

TABLE 4.2 (continued)
Vitamin D Supplementation among Individuals Living with (or Exposed to) HIV/AIDS in Intervention Studies[a]

ART Status at Baseline	Location	Study Population	n[b]	Age (yr)	Vitamin D Form	Administration Method	Dose	Frequency	Duration	Other	Referent Group	Assessed Outcomes	Associations and Effect Estimates	Ref.
ART	Paris, France	Adults with HIV-1, on ART ≥ 3 years, and CD4+ T cells ≥ 350 cells/μL	53 (supplementation subgroup, n = 17)	Range, 40–55	—[c]	—[c]	100,000 IU	Every 14 days (1st phase); monthly (2nd phase)	3 months (1st phase); 9 months (2nd phase)	Supplementation among those severely deficient (25(OH)D₃ < 12 ng/mL) at baseline	—	Immune activation (activated memory CD8+ T cells), T and B cell subsets	Vitamin D supplementation T cell subsets ↔ B cell subsets ↔ Immune activation ↓	16
ART	California	Adults with HIV	122 (82 vitamin D insufficient; 40 sufficient)	Vitamin D insufficient median 49 (IQR, 41–55) Vitamin D sufficient median 49 (IQR, 43–56)	D₃	Oral	50,000 IU (1st phase); 2000 IU (2nd phase)	Twice weekly (1st phase); daily (2nd phase)	5 weeks (1st phase); 7 weeks (2nd phase)	Supplementation among those insufficient (<30 ng/mL) at baseline	Historical controls (no HIV)	Serum 25(OH)D	Supplementation group vs. historical controls 25(OH)D (≥30 ng/mL) ↔ (p = 0.32)	17

Group	Location	Population	N		Vitamin D	Route	Dose	Frequency	Duration	Calcium	Placebo	Outcomes	Results	Ref
Naïve	United States and Puerto Rico (multisite)	Adults with HIV	165 (79 vitamin D/ calcium; 86 placebo)	Intervention median 36 (IQR, 28–47) Control median 31 (IQR, 25–44)	D_3	Oral	4000 IU	Once daily	48 weeks	Calcium carbonate (500 mg twice daily)	Placebo (vitamin D and calcium)	Serum 25(OH)D, bone loss	*Placebo vs. vitamin D/ calcium at 48 wk* Total hip BMD loss ↑ Lumbar spine BMD loss ↑ *Δ in 25(OH)D$_3$* Vitamin D/ calcium group ↑ Placebo ↔	18
ART	Rome, Italy	Men with HIV-1 and osteoporosis or osteopenia	41 (20 with fractures; 21 without fractures)	—	D_3	Oral	800 IU	Daily	12 months (1st phase); 12 months (2nd phase)	1st phase: calcium (daily, oral, 1000 mg) 2nd phase fracture group: risedronate added (75 mg) 2nd phase no-fracture group: continued vitamin D/ calcium	—	Bone turnover markers	*Risedronate group* Δ in BMD ↑ *No-risedronate group* Δ in BMD ↔	19

(continued)

TABLE 4.2 (continued)
Vitamin D Supplementation among Individuals Living with (or Exposed to) HIV/AIDS in Intervention Studies[a]

ART Status at Baseline	Study Population	Location	n[b]	Age (yr)	Vitamin D Treatment Regimen						Referent Group	Assessed Outcomes	Associations and Effect Estimates	Ref.
					Vitamin D Form	Administration Method	Dose	Frequency	Duration	Other				
Heterogeneous	Children and young adults with HIV	Pennsylvania (8 centers)	58	Mean 20.7 (SD 3.7) Range, 5.0–24.9	D_3	Oral (capsules, drops)	7000 IU	Daily	12 months	—	Placebo	Serum 25(OH)D concentration, immunologic indicators	*Supplementation vs. placebo* Δ in 25(OH)D ↑ Δ in naïve T-helper cells ↑ Δ in T-helper cells (CD4%) ↑ Δ in RNA viral load ↓	20
ART	Children and adults with HIV	Botswana	60	Mean 19.5 (SD 11.8) Range, 5.0–50.9	D_3	Oral	4000 IU 7000 IU	Daily	12 weeks	—	—	Serum 25(OH)D concentration, HIV RNA viral load (VL), anthropometric and immunologic indicators	*Δ in 25(OH)D$_3$* Overall ↑ (*p* = 0.02) EFV or NVP vs. PI ↑ (*p* = 0.03) *7000 IU Group* HAZ↑ CD4%↑ VL↓	21
Heterogeneous	Adults with HIV and vitamin D deficiency	Netherlands	20	Mean 45.0 (SD 10.0)	D_3	Oral	2000 IU (0–14 wk); 1000 IU (14–48 wk)	Daily	48 weeks	—	—	Serum 25(OH)D, 1,25(OH)2D concentrations Indicators of bone (PTH, BMD) and metabolic health (insulin sensitivity, cholesterol, triglycerides)	*Δ in 25(OH)D* 24 weeks ↑ 48 weeks ↑ *Δ in 1,25(OH)2D* 24 weeks ↑ 48 weeks ↔ *Δ in PTH and insulin sensitivity* 24 weeks ↓ 48 weeks ↔	22

ART (containing EFV)	Tehran, Iran	Adults with HIV	121	(supplementation group: baseline vitamin D < 35 nmol/mL)	Mean 40.3 (SD 9.0)	—[c]	IM injection	300,000 IU	Once at baseline	3 months	—	Serum 25(OH)D concentration, Indicators of bone health	Post- vs. pre-supplementation: Δ in 25(OH)D ↑, Δ in PTH ↓, Δ in ALP, osteocalcin, CTx ↑	23
Heterogeneous	Switzerland	Patients with HIV and low vitamin D (<30 ng/mL)	77[b]	ART mean 43 (SD 9) No ART mean 43 (SD 9)	D₃	Oral	300,000 IU	Once	3 months	—	Serum 25(OH)D concentration, Indicators of bone health	Post- vs. pre-supplementation: Δ in 25(OH)D ↑, Δ in BSAP, PYR, DPD ↓	24

[a] 17 randomized controlled trials and 8 intervention studies (van den Bout-van den Beukel et al., 2008b; Bech et al., 2012; Etminani-Esfahani et al., 2012; Piso et al., 2013; Fabre-Mersserman et al., 2014; Pepe et al., 2014; Coussens et al., 2015; Lake et al., 2015).

[b] Sample size of individuals completing the RCT or intervention and included in analyses.

[c] Not specified.

[d] Only abstract available.

[e] Enrolled in treatment program.

[f] Exception of one patient not on ART.

Note: ALP, alkaline phosphatase; ART, antiretroviral therapy; BAP, bone alkaline phosphatase; BMD, bone mineral density; BSAP, bone-specific alkaline phosphatase; cART, combination antiretroviral therapy; CTx, type 1 collagen trimeric cross-linked C-telopeptide; DPD, desoxypyridinoline; EFV, efavirenz; FGF, fibroblast growth factor; FMD, flow-mediated brachial artery dilatation; HR, hazard ratio; IM, intramuscular; IQR, interquartile range; NVP, nevirapine; P1NP, procollagen type 1 N-terminal peptide; PI, protease inhibitor; PTH, parathyroid hormone; PTH-rp, PTH-related peptide; PYR, pyridinoline; SBMC, spine bone mineral content; SBMD, spine bone mineral density; SD, standard deviation; TBBMC, total-body bone mineral content; TBBMD, total-body bone mineral density; TRP, tubular reabsorption of phosphate; VDR, vitamin D receptor; VL, viral load.

References: [1]Arpadi et al. (2009); [2]Arpadi et al (2012); [3]Bang et al. (2012); [4]Bang et al. (2013); [5]Bech et al. (2012); [6]Falasca et al. (2014); [7]Giacomet et al. (2013); [8]Groleau et al. (2013); [9]Havens et al. (2014); [10]Havens et al. (2012a,b); [11]Kakalia et al. (2011); [12]Longenecker et al. (2012); [13]Wejse et al. (2009); [14]Coussens et al. (2015); [15]Dougherty et al. (2014); [16]Fabre-Mersserman et al. (2014); [17]Lake et al. (2015); [18]Overton et al. (2015); [19]Pepe et al. (2014); [20]Stallings et al. (2015); [21]Steenhoff et al. (2015); [22]van den Bout-van den Beukel et al. (2008b); [23]Etminani-Esfahani et al. (2012b); [24]Piso et al. (2013).

studies, vitamin D supplementation was determined by the vitamin D concentration of individual study participants at baseline. Vitamin D supplementation varied considerably in terms of dosage (including 1200 and 300,000 IU), form (D_3, cholecalciferol; D_2, ergocalciferol), frequency (daily, weekly, monthly, bimonthly, every three months, once at baseline), and administration (singly vs. jointly with other micronutrients, such as calcium by capsule, drop, or intramuscular injection). The study duration (or follow-up) ranged widely from 12 weeks to 2 years. A number of outcomes were assessed, including vitamin D (25(OH)D) status, T-lymphocyte subsets (CD4+, CD8+), HIV viral load, and other related health outcomes, including parathyroid hormone (PTH), total body bone mineral content (TBBMC), bone mineral density (BMD), calcium, phosphate, and fibroblast growth factor 23 (FGF-23), among study participants with HIV. Most referent groups received placebo, although a few studies included comparisons that received either no or lower dosage supplementation.

Study populations differed considerably across intervention studies, with samples sizes ranging from 20 to 281 individuals. Other characteristics included geographic location of residence (including the United States, Puerto Rico, Denmark, Italy, Canada, and Guinea-Bissau), age, and ART received during and prior to study participation. Among individuals living with HIV, several studies confirmed improved vitamin D status (increased 25(OH)D or 1,25(OH)$_2$D concentrations) after vitamin D supplementation (van den Bout-van den Beukel et al., 2008b; Etminani-Esfahani et al., 2012b; Piso et al., 2013).

OUTCOMES RELEVANT TO VITAMIN D AND BONE HEALTH

In terms of bone health indicators, a study found reduced collagen type 1 trimeric cross-linked peptide and procollagen type 1 N-terminal peptide among adult men living with HIV-1, who were randomized to receive vitamin D (calcitriol, 0.5–1.0 µg; cholecalciferol, 1200 IU), compared to the placebo group (Bang et al., 2013). From a study among patients (n = 24) with HIV and ART treatment containing tenofovir (TDF), vitamin D supplementation (dosage according to body weight) was associated with decreased serum PTH and improved calcium balance and bone mineral density (Bech et al., 2012). FGF-23 increased among patients with HIV receiving vitamin D and TDF relative to those receiving placebo or no TDF (Havens et al., 2014). In another study among patients with HIV, bone biomarkers (collagen telopeptidase, osteocalcin) increased with vitamin D supplementation (Etminani-Esfahani et al., 2012b). Other studies observed no effects of vitamin D supplementation on bone health indicators among people with HIV, including total body and spine bone mineral content and density (Arpadi et al., 2012), as well as PTH-related peptide, FGF-23, serum phosphate, or renal phosphate loss (Bech et al., 2012).

IMMUNOLOGICAL INDICATORS

High-dosage vitamin D_3 supplementation (50,000 IU per week for six weeks) was associated with reduced HIV-1 replication (p24) during the winter (Coussens et al., 2015). Oral cholecalciferol supplements (100,000 IU received every two months) with calcium (1 g/day) did not affect HIV viral load among youth (6 to 16 years old) compared to the placebo group (Arpadi et al., 2009). Pharmacological (100,000 IU) and physiological (4000 or 7000 IU) dosages of vitamin D were associated with increased CD4:CD8 ratio (Fabre-Mersseman et al., 2014) and CD4% (Stallings et al., 2015; Steenhoff et al., 2015). Separately, a study among individuals (8 to 26 years old) with HIV observed a decreased Th17:Treg ratio among those receiving vitamin D supplementation (100,000 IU) compared to the placebo group at three months (Giacomet et al., 2013). However, several studies reported no changes of T-cell subsets between adults and children who were randomized to receive vitamin D supplementation compared to referent groups (Arpadi et al., 2009; Kakalia et al., 2011; Bang et al., 2012; Giacomet et al., 2013).

OTHER OUTCOMES

From a study in Guinea-Bissau among patients with TB who were ≥15 years old, a subgroup analysis among individuals with HIV indicated no effects of vitamin D supplementation on mortality (HR, 1.8; 95% CI, 0.8–4.1) among those randomly assigned to receive vitamin D_3 (100,000 IU) compared to placebo (Wejse et al., 2009). Vitamin D supplementation (4000 IU daily oral cholecalciferol) and placebo treatment regimens for individuals living with HIV showed no effect with respect to changes in diabetic indicators, including insulin, glucose, homeostatic model assessment of insulin resistance (HOMA-IR), blood pressure (systolic, diastolic), cholesterol (total, non-HDL), and triglycerides (Longenecker et al., 2012). Flow-mediated brachial artery dilatation (FMD) was not affected by vitamin D supplementation in a study among 45 individuals with HIV and low baseline serum 25(OH)D (≤20 ng/mL). A study among children and adolescents in the United States living with HIV confirmed the safety of vitamin D supplementation in terms of blood lead (Groleau et al., 2013).

ART AND VITAMIN D AMONG INDIVIDUALS LIVING WITH HIV

BIOLOGICAL EVIDENCE FROM *IN VITRO* AND *EX VIVO* STUDIES

Results from three human cell studies suggest bidirectional interactions between ART and vitamin D. HIV-1 protease inhibitors (ritonavir, indinavir, nelfinavir) were observed to reduce hepatic production of 25(OH)D and macrophage synthesis of $1,25(OH)_2D$ in dose-dependent, reversible relationships (Cozzolino et al., 2003). Separately, $1,25(OH)_2D_3$ was protective against mitochondrial DNA depletion of human skeletal muscle myoblasts and myotubes following nucleoside reverse transcriptase inhibitor (didanosine and stavudine) pretreatment (Campbell et al., 2013). In human airway epithelium-derived Calu-3 cell monolayers, $1\alpha,25(OH)_2D_3$ pretreatment increased differentiation (based on greater cilia and mucus secretion) and P-glycoprotein expression compared to untreated controls (Patel et al., 2002). Additionally, cellular transport of ART (ritonavir and sasquinavir) was higher among untreated cells compared to those treated at three hours post-treatment (Patel et al., 2002). Moreover, several studies have found links between ART and CYP24A1, which is a key 25-hydroxylase enzyme involved with converting the active vitamin D metabolite $1,25(OH)_2D_3$ to an inactive metabolite form ($24,25(OH)_2D_3$, or calcitroic acid). Another study confirmed that ritonavir pretreatment reduced CYP24A1 expression and was associated with increased intracellular $1,25(OH)_2D_3$ (Ikezoe et al., 2006). Efavirenz, phenobarbital, and calcitriol affected the expression and activity of certain 25-hydroxylases in dermal fibroblasts and prostate cancer LNCaP cells (Ellfolk et al., 2009). In human renal carcinoma cells, efavirenz and nevirapine upregulated VDR, calbindin 28k, and *CYP24A1* genes (Landriscina et al., 2008).

OBSERVATIONAL STUDIES AMONG INDIVIDUALS LIVING WITH HIV

A number of observational studies provided evidence of the association between vitamin D and antiretroviral therapy among individuals living with HIV (Ramayo et al., 2005; Paul et al., 2010; Conrado et al., 2011; Allavena et al., 2012; Cervero et al., 2013; Mastala et al., 2013; Portilla et al., 2014). Some studies confirmed links between vitamin D and specific HIV drug therapies, including efavirenz (EFV) (Brown and McComsey, 2010; Welz et al., 2010; Dao et al., 2011; Fox et al., 2011; Allavena et al., 2012; Cervero et al., 2012; Wiboonchutikul et al., 2012; Meyzer et al., 2013; Schwartz et al., 2014; Theodorou et al., 2014), ritonavir (RTV) (Dao et al., 2011), zidovudine (ZDV) (Fox et al., 2011; Gangcuangco et al., 2013), and tenofovir (TDF) (Mueller et al., 2010; Klassen et al., 2012; Havens et al., 2013). Three studies reported suboptimal vitamin D among individuals living with HIV and receiving non-nucleoside reverse transcriptase inhibitors (NNRTIs), compared to protease inhibitors (PIs) (Conesa-Botella et al., 2010; Wasserman and Rubin, 2010). Additionally, studies indicate associations between low vitamin D and longer ART duration (Theodorou et al.,

2014), as well as cumulative ART use (Eckard et al., 2013a) in people with HIV. In contrast, studies also show null associations between vitamin D and ART (Masiá et al., 2012; Sherwood et al., 2012; Foissac et al., 2013), including EFV (Chokephaibulkit et al., 2013). One study found no differences in vitamin D among patients receiving TDF or EFV relative to other ART (Poowuttikul et al., 2014).

RANDOMIZED CONTROLLED TRIALS OF ART WITH ASSESSMENT OF VITAMIN D

Two RCTs assessed the effects of different ART on vitamin D or related indicators among individuals living with HIV (see Table 4.3) (Gupta et al., 2013; Wohl et al., 2014). In a multicountry, double-blinded Phase III trial, 690 adults living with HIV were randomly assigned to receive either rilpivirine (RPV, 25 mg) or efavirenz (EFV, 600 mg) with TDF and emtricitabine (FTC) once daily (Wohl et al., 2014). Among study participants with vitamin D deficiency or insufficiency at baseline, a greater proportion of individuals receiving EFV (8%) had severe vitamin D deficiency at 48 weeks compared to RPV (2%; $p = 0.0079$) (Wohl et al., 2014). In another study, no differences in 25(OH)D concentration, flow-mediated dilatation, or PTH were observed among 30 patients with HIV who received either: (1) TDF, FTC, and EFV, or (2) TDF, FTC, and raltegravir (Gupta et al., 2013). However, study participants in the group receiving raltegravir had decreased total cholesterol, C-reactive protein, serum alkaline phosphatase, sCD14 concentrations, and renal function, as well as increased sCD163 concentrations (Gupta et al., 2013).

CONCLUSION

In summary, *ex vivo* studies involving cell cultures from patients have characterized biological pathways between physiological concentrations of $1,25(OH)_2D_3$ and the inhibition of HIV-1 viral replication (via cathelicidin and autophagy) (Campbell and Spector, 2012a–c). Similarly, studies with human leukemia–lymphoma cell lines corroborated a role of vitamin D in HIV replication (Kitano et al., 1990; Skolnik et al., 1991; Pauza et al., 1993; Biswas et al., 1998). VDR, including specific genetic polymorphisms and methylation (Chandel et al., 2013), has been associated with indicators of HIV, such as LTR activation (Nevado et al., 2007; Torres et al., 2010). Cross-sectional studies found associations between vitamin D status and HIV infection (based on viral load, disease stage, clinical signs and symptoms). Observational studies showed increased HIV disease progression among individuals with certain VDR genotypes and low vitamin D status. However, results were not consistent across all epidemiological studies, and null findings were also reported. Among RCTs with vitamin D as treatment regimens, most reported positive associations between supplementation and improved vitamin D status, as well as bone-health outcomes among individuals with HIV. Available RCTs observed protective or no effects of vitamin D supplementation on other outcomes, including immunological indicators.

From this review, a number of key research gaps remain. The majority of studies were observational or cross-sectional, although longitudinal data are necessary for an improved understanding of vitamin D and HIV transmission, disease progression, clinical relevance, and etiology. Additionally, although a number of studies have assessed vitamin D status among individuals living with HIV, many included study participants in Europe or North America instead of sub-Saharan Africa and other regions with the highest burden of disease from HIV. Comparisons between RCTs are difficult due to the heterogeneity of study designs, especially substantial differences in vitamin D treatment dosage, frequency, and duration. Despite the potential clinical relevance, only two RCTs with ART as the treatment regimens have considered interactions between ART and vitamin D. Finally, a number of studies assessed the effects of vitamin D on HIV transmission and disease progression; however, there are limited longitudinal studies regarding the influence of HIV infection on vitamin D metabolism.

TABLE 4.3

Effects of ART on Vitamin D Status among Individuals Living with HIV/AIDS in Randomized Controlled Trials

ART Status at Baseline	Location	Study Population	n	Age	Treatment Regimen				Health Outcomes	Associations and Effect Estimates	Ref.
					ART	Dose	Frequency	Duration			
ART (tenofovir, emtricitabine, efavirenz)	Indiana	Patients with HIV	30	≥18 years	Group 1: tenofovir, emtricitabine, efavirenz; Group 2: tenofovir, emtricitabine, raltegravir	Group 1: not specified; Group 2: TDF/FTC (not specified); raltegravir (400 mg)	Twice daily	24 wk	FMD, 25(OH)D, PTH, total cholesterol, hs-CRP, serum ALP, sCD14 levels, renal function, sCD163	Group 2 vs. Group 1 FMD, 25(OH)D, PTH ↔ Total cholesterol, hs-CRP, serum ALP, sCD14 levels, renal function ↓ sCD163 ↑	Gupta et al. (2013)
Naïve	Multisite (21 countries)	Adults with HIV	690 (rilpivirine, 346; efavirenz, 344)	≥18 years	Group 1: rilpivirine (with tenofovir, emtricitabine, efavirenz)	25 mg	Once daily	48 wk	25(OH)D	Δ in 25(OH)D EFV ↓ ($p < 0.0001$) RPV ↔ ($p = 0.57$) Development of severe 25(OH)D deficiency, among those insufficient or deficient at baseline, week 48: RFV (2%) vs. EFV (8%; $p = 0.0079$)	Wohl et al. (2014)

Note: ALP, alkaline phosphatase; EFV, efavirenz; FMD, flow-mediated dilatation; FTC, TDF + 3TC (lamivudine); hs-CRP, high-sensitivity C-reactive protein; PTH, parathyroid hormone; RPV, rilpivirine; TDF/FTC, emtricitabine/tenofovir disoproxil fumarate.

Currently, there are no international policies or nutritional recommendations regarding vitamin D status or supplementation among individuals living with HIV. The growing preliminary evidence of the association between vitamin D and HIV infection emphasizes the need for further research in order to improve our understanding of etiology and clinical implications.

REFERENCES

Adams, J. S. and M. Hewison. (2008). Unexpected actions of vitamin D: new perspectives on the regulation of innate and adaptive immunity. *Nature Clinical Practice Endocrinology & Metabolism* 4(2): 80–90.

Adeyemi, O. M., D. Agniel, A. L. French et al. (2011). Vitamin D deficiency in HIV-infected and HIV-uninfected women in the United States. *Journal of Acquired Immune Deficiency* 57(3): 197–204.

Allavena, C., C. Delpierre, L. Cusin et al. (2012). High frequency of vitamin D deficiency in HIV-infected patients: effects of HIV-related factors and antiretroviral drugs. *Journal of Antimicrobial Chemotherapy* 67(9): 2222–30.

Anandaiah, A., S. Sinha, M. Bole et al. (2013). Vitamin D rescues impaired *Mycobacterium tuberculosis*-mediated tumor necrosis factor release in macrophages of HIV-seropositive individuals through an enhanced Toll-like receptor signaling pathway *in vitro*. *Infection and Immunity* 81(1): 2–10.

Arpadi, S. M., D. McMahon, E. J. Abrams et al. (2009). Effect of bimonthly supplementation with oral cholecalciferol on serum 25-hydroxyvitamin D concentrations in HIV-infected children and adolescents. *Pediatrics* 123(1): e121–6.

Arpadi, S. M., D. J. McMahon, E. J. Abrams et al. (2012). Effect of supplementation with cholecalciferol and calcium on 2-y bone mass accrual in HIV-infected children and adolescents: a randomized clinical trial. *American Journal of Clinical Nutrition* 95(3): 678–85.

Baeke, F., T. Takiishi, H. Korf, C. Gysemans, and C. Mathieu. (2010). Vitamin D: modulator of the immune system. *Current Opinion in Pharmacology* 10(4): 482–96.

Bang, U. C., L. Kolte, M. Hitz et al. (2012). Correlation of increases in 1,25-dihydroxyvitamin D during vitamin D therapy with activation of CD4+ T lymphocytes in HIV-1-infected males. *HIV Clinical Trials* 13(3): 162–70.

Bang, U. C., L. Kolte, M. Hitz et al. (2013). The effect of cholecalciferol and calcitriol on biochemical bone markers in HIV type 1-infected males: results of a clinical trial. *AIDS Research and Human Retroviruses* 29(4): 658–64.

Barber, Y., C. Rubio, E. Fernández, M. Rubio, and J. Fibla. (2001). Host genetic background at CCR5 chemokine receptor and vitamin D receptor loci and human immunodeficiency virus (HIV) type 1 disease progression among HIV-seropositive injection drug users. *Journal of Infectious Diseases* 184(10): 1279–88.

Bech, A., Van Bentum, D. Telting, J. Gisolf, C. Richter, and H. De Boer. (2012). Treatment of calcium and vitamin D deficiency in HIV-positive men on tenofovir-containing antiretroviral therapy. *HIV Clinical Trials* 13(6): 350–6.

Besançon, F., J. Just, M. F. Bourgeade et al. (1997). HIV-1 p17 and IFN-gamma both induce fructose 1,6-bisphosphatase. *Journal of Interferon & Cytokine Research* 17(8): 461–7.

Bhalla, A. K., E. Amento, T. L. Clemons, M. F. Holick, and S. M. Krane. (1983). Specific high-affinity receptors for 1,25-dihydroxyvitamin D_3 in human peripheral blood mononuclear cells: presence in monocytes and induction in T lymphocytes following activation. *Journal of Clinical Endocrinology & Metabolism* 57(6): 1308–10.

Biswas, P., M. Mengozzi, B. Mantelli et al. (1998). 1,25-Dihydroxyvitamin D_3 upregulates functional CXCR4 human immunodeficiency virus type 1 coreceptors in U937 minus clones: NF-kappaB-independent enhancement of viral replication. *Journal of Virology* 72(10): 8380–3.

Branch, A. D., M. Kang, K. Hollabaugh, C. M. Wyatt, R. T. Chung, and M. J. Giesby. (2013). In HIV/hepatitis C virus co-infected patients, higher 25-hydroxyvitamin D concentrations were not related to hepatitis C virus treatment responses but were associated with ritonavir use. *American Journal of Clinical Nutrition* 98(2): 423–9.

Branch, A. D., B. Barin, A. Rahman, Stock, and T. D. Schiano. (2014). Vitamin D status of human immunodeficiency virus-positive patients with advanced liver disease enrolled in the solid organ transplantation in HIV: multi-site study. *Liver Transplantation* 20(2): 156–64.

Brown, T. T. and G. A. McComsey. (2010). Association between initiation of antiretroviral therapy with efavirenz and decreases in 25-hydroxyvitamin D. *Antiviral Therapy* 15(3): 425–9.

Campbell, G. R. and S. A. Spector. (2011). Hormonally active vitamin D_3 (1alpha,25-dihydroxycholecalciferol) triggers autophagy in human macrophages that inhibits HIV-1 infection. *Journal of Biological Chemistry* 286(21): 18890–902.

Campbell, G. R. and S. A. Spector. (2012a). Toll-like receptor 8 ligands activate a vitamin D mediated autophagic response that inhibits human immunodeficiency virus type 1. *PLoS Pathogens* 8(11): e1003017.

Campbell, G. R. and S.A. Spector. (2012b). Vitamin D inhibits human immunodeficiency virus type 1 and *Mycobacterium tuberculosis* infection in macrophages through the induction of autophagy. *PLoS Pathogens* 8(5): e1002689.

Campbell, G. R. and S. A. Spector. (2012c). Autophagy induction by vitamin D inhibits both *Mycobacterium tuberculosis* and human immunodeficiency virus type 1). *Autophagy* 8(10): 1523–5.

Campbell, G. R., Z. T. Pallack, and S. A. Spector. (2013). Vitamin D attenuates nucleoside reverse transcriptase inhibitor induced human skeletal muscle mitochondria DNA depletion. *AIDS* 27(9): 1397–401.

Cantorna, M. T. (2010). Mechanisms underlying the effect of vitamin D on the immune system. *Proceedings of the Nutrition Society* 69(3): 286–9.

Cantorna, M. T., Y. Zhu, M. Froicu, and A. Wittke. (2004). Vitamin D status, 1,25-dihydroxyvitamin D_3, and the immune system. *American Journal of Clinical Nutrition* 80(6, Suppl.): 1717S–20S.

CDC. (1992). 1993 revised classification system for HIV infection and expanded surveillance case definition for AIDS among adolescents and adults. *Morbidity and Mortality Weekly Report (MMWR) Recommendations and Reports* 41(RR-17): 1–19.

Cervero, M., J. L. Agud, C. García-Lacalle et al. (2012). Prevalence of vitamin D deficiency and its related risk factor in a Spanish cohort of adult HIV-infected patients: effects of antiretroviral therapy. *AIDS Research and Human Retroviruses* 28(9): 963–71.

Cervero, M., J. L. Agud, R. Torres et al. (2013). Higher vitamin D levels in HIV-infected out-patients on treatment with boosted protease inhibitor monotherapy. *HIV Medicine* 14(9): 556–62.

Chandel, N., M. Husain, H. Goel et al. (2013). VDR hypermethylation and HIV-induced T cell loss. *Journal of Leukocyte Biology* 93(4): 623–31.

Childs, K. E., S. L. Fishman, C. Constable et al. (2010). Short communication: inadequate vitamin D exacerbates parathyroid hormone elevations in tenofovir users. *AIDS Research and Human Retroviruses* 26(8): 855–9.

Choi, A. I., J. C. Lo, K. Mulligan et al. (2011). Association of vitamin D insufficiency with carotid intima–media thickness in HIV-infected persons. *Clinical Infectious Disease* 52(7): 941–4.

Chokephaibulkit, K., R. Saksawad, T. Bunupuradah et al. (2013). Prevalence of vitamin D deficiency among perinatally HIV-infected Thai adolescents receiving antiretroviral therapy. *Pediatric Infectious Disease Journal* 32(11): 1237–9.

Conesa-Botella, A., E. Florence, L. Lynen, R. Colebunders, J. Menten, and R. Moreno-Reyes. (2010). Decrease of vitamin D concentration in patients with HIV infection on a non-nucleoside reverse transcriptase inhibitor-containing regimen. *AIDS Research and Therapy* 7(1): 40.

Conesa-Botella, A., O. Goovaerts, M. Massinga-Loembé et al.; TB IRIS Study Group. (2012a). Low prevalence of vitamin D deficiency in Ugandan HIV-infected patients with and without tuberculosis. *International Journal of Tuberculosis and Lung Disease* 16(11): 1517–21.

Conesa-Botella, A., G. Meintjes, A. K. Coussens et al. (2012b). Corticosteroid therapy, vitamin D status, and inflammatory cytokine profile in the HIV-tuberculosis immune reconstitution inflammatory syndrome. *Clinical Infectious Diseases* 55(7): 1004–11.

Connor, R. I. and W. F. Rigby. (1991). 1 alpha,25-dihydroxyvitamin D_3 inhibits productive infection of human monocytes by HIV-1. *Biochemical and Biophysical Research Communications* 176(2): 852–9.

Conrado, T., D. de B. Miranda-Filho, R. A. Ximenes et al. (2011). Vitamin D deficiency in HIV-infected women on antiretroviral therapy living in the tropics. *Journal of the International Association of Physicians in AIDS Care* 10(4): 239–45.

Coussens, A. K., C. E. Naude, R. Goliath, G. Chaplin, R. J. Wilkinson, and N. G. Jablonski. (2015). High-dose vitamin D_3 reduces deficiency caused by low UVB exposure and limits HIV-1 replication in urban Southern Africans. *Proceedings of the National Academy of Sciences* 112(26): 8052–7.

Cozzolino, M., M. Vidal, M. V. Arcidiacono, Tebas, K. E. Yarasheski, and A. S. Dusso. (2003). HIV-protease inhibitors impair vitamin D bioactivation to 1,25-dihydroxyvitamin D. *AIDS* 17(4): 513–20.

Crutchley, R. D., J. Gathe, Jr., C. Mayberry, A. Trieu, S. Abughosh, and K. W. Garey. (2012). Risk factors for vitamin D deficiency in HIV-infected patients in the south central United States. *AIDS Research and Human Retroviruses* 28(5): 454–9.

Dao, C. N., Patel, E. T. Overton et al.; Study to Understand the Natural History of HIV and AIDS in the Era of Effective Therapy (SUN) Investigators. (2011). Low vitamin D among HIV-infected adults: prevalence of and risk factors for low vitamin D levels in a cohort of HIV-infected adults and comparison to prevalence among adults in the US general population. *Clinical Infectious Diseases* 52(3): 396–405.

Dolan, S. E., J. R. Kanter, and S. Grinspoon. (2006). Longitudinal analysis of bone density in human immunodeficiency virus-infected women. *Journal of Clinical Endocrinology & Metabolism* 91(8): 2938–45.

Dougherty, K. A., J. I. Schall, B. S. Zemel et al. (2014). Safety and efficacy of high-dose daily vitamin D_3 supplementation in children and young adults infected with human immunodeficiency virus. *Journal of the Pediatric Infectious Diseases Society* 3(4): 294–303.

Eckard, A. R., S. E. Judd, T. R. Ziegler et al. (2012). Risk factors for vitamin D deficiency and relationship with cardiac biomarkers, inflammation and immune restoration in HIV-infected youth. *Antiviral Therapy* 17(6): 1069–78.

Eckard, A. R., V. Tangpricha, S. Seydafkan et al. (2013a). The relationship between vitamin D status and HIV-related complications in HIV-infected children and young adults. *Pediatric Infectious Disease Journal* 32(11): 1224–9.

Eckard, A. R., T. Leong, A. Avery et al. (2013b). Short communication: high prevalence of vitamin D deficiency in HIV-infected and HIV-uninfected pregnant women. *AIDS Research and Human Retroviruses* 29(9): 1224–8.

El-Maouche, D., S. H. Mehta, C. G. Sutcliffe et al. (2013). Vitamin D deficiency and its relation to bone mineral density and liver fibrosis in HIV–HCV coinfection. *Antiviral Therapy* 18(2): 237–42.

Ellfolk, M., M. Norlin, K. Gyllensten, and K. Wikvall. (2009). Regulation of human vitamin D(3) 25-hydroxylases in dermal fibroblasts and prostate cancer LNCaP cells. *Molecular Pharmacology* 75(6): 1392–9.

Erlandson, K. M., I. Gudza, S. Fiorillo et al. (2014). Relationship of vitamin D insufficiency to AIDS-associated Kaposi's sarcoma outcomes: retrospective analysis of a prospective clinical trial in Zimbabwe. *International Journal of Infectious Diseases* 24: 6–10.

Estrella, M. M., G. D. Kirk, S. H. Mehta et al. (2012). Vitamin D deficiency and persistent proteinuria among HIV-infected and uninfected injection drug users. *AIDS* 26(3): 295–302.

Etminani-Esfahani, M., H. Khalili, N. Soleimani, A. Abdollahi, Z. Khazaelpour, and K. Gholami. (2012a). Serum vitamin D concentration and potential risk factors for its deficiency in HIV positive individuals. *Current HIV Research* 10(2): 165–70.

Etminani-Esfahani, M., H. Khalili, S. Jafari, A. Abdollahi, and S. Dashti-Khavidaki. (2012b). Effects of vitamin D supplementation on the bone specific biomarkers in HIV infected individuals under treatment with efavirenz. *BMC Research Notes* 5: 204.

Fabre-Mersseman, V., R. Tubiana, L. Papagno et al. (2014). Vitamin D supplementation is associated with reduced immune activation levels in HIV-1-infected patients on suppressive antiretroviral therapy. *AIDS* 28(18): 2677–82.

Falasca, K., C. Ucciferri, M. Di Nicola, F. Vignale, J. Di Blase, and J. Vecchiet. (2014). Different strategies of 25OH vitamin D supplementation in HIV+ subjects. *International Journal of STD & AIDS* 25(11): 785–92.

Finkelstein, J. L., S. Mehta, C. Duggan et al. (2012a). Predictors of anaemia and iron deficiency in HIV-infected pregnant women in Tanzania: a potential role for vitamin D and parasitic infections. *Public Health Nutrition* 15(5): 928–37.

Finkelstein, J. L., S. Mehta, C. Duggan et al. (2012b). Maternal vitamin D status and child morbidity, anemia, and growth in human immunodeficiency virus-exposed children in Tanzania. *Pediatric Infectious Disease Journal* 31(2): 171–5.

Foissac, F., J. M. Tréluyer, J. C. Souberbielle, H. Rostane, S. Urien, and J. Viard. (2013). Vitamin D_3 supplementation scheme in HIV-infected patients based upon pharmacokinetic modelling of 25-hydroxycholecalciferol. *British Journal of Clinical Pharmacology* 75(5): 1312–20.

Fox, J., B. Peters, M. Prakash, J. Arribas, A. Hill, and C. Moecklinghoff. (2011). Improvement in vitamin D deficiency following antiretroviral regime change: results from the MONET trial. *AIDS Research and Human Retroviruses* 27(1): 29–34.

French, A. L., O. M. Adeyemi, D. M. Agniel et al. (2011). The association of HIV status with bacterial vaginosis and vitamin D in the United States. *Journal of Women's Health* 20(10): 1497–503.

Friis, H., N. Range, M. L. Pedersen et al. (2008). Hypovitaminosis D is common among pulmonary tuberculosis patients in Tanzania but is not explained by the acute phase response. *Journal of Nutrition* 138(12): 2474–80.

Friis, H., N. Range, J. Changalucha et al. (2013). Vitamin D status among pulmonary TB patients and non-TB controls: a cross-sectional study from Mwanza, Tanzania. *PLoS One* 8(12): e81142.

Frontini, M., J. Nnadi, S. Bairu, T. Khan, J. Chotalia, and R. A. Clark. (2012). Risk factors for suboptimal vitamin D levels among adults with HIV attending an inner-city clinic of New Orleans, Louisiana. *Journal of the Louisiana State Medical Society* 164(1): 10–2.

Gangcuangco, L. M., D. C. Chow, C. Y. Liang et al. (2013). Predictors of 25-hydroxyvitamin D levels in HIV-infected patients in Hawai'i. *Hawai'i Journal of Medicine & Public Health* 72(6): 197–201.

García Aparicio, A. M., S. Muñoz Fernández, J. González et al. (2006). Abnormalities in the bone mineral metabolism in HIV-infected patients. *Clinical Rheumatology* 25(4): 537–9.

Gedela, K., S. G. Edwards, Benn, and A. D. Grant. (2013). Prevalence of vitamin D deficiency in HIV-positive, antiretroviral treatment-naive patients in a single centre study. *International Journal of STD & AIDS* 25(7): 488–92.

Giacomet, V., A. Vigano, V. Manfredini et al. (2013). Cholecalciferol supplementation in HIV-infected youth with vitamin D insufficiency: effects on vitamin D status and T-cell phenotype: a randomized controlled trial. *HIV Clinical Trials* 14(2): 51–60.

Girasole, G., J. M. Wang, M. Pedrazzoni et al. (1990). Augmentation of monocyte chemotaxis by 1 alpha,25-dihydroxyvitamin D_3. Stimulation of defective migration of AIDS patients. *Journal of Immunology* 145(8): 2459–64.

Goletti, D., A. L. Kinter, Biswas, S. M. Bende, G. Poli, and A. S. Fauci. (1995). Effect of cellular differentiation on cytokine-induced expression of human immunodeficiency virus in chronically infected promonocytic cells: dissociation of cellular differentiation and viral expression. *Journal of Virology* 69(4): 2540–6.

Gottlieb, M. S., R. Schroff, H. M. Schanker. (1981). *Pneumocystis carinii* pneumonia and mucosal candidiasis in previously healthy homosexual men: evidence of a new acquired cellular immunodeficiency. *New England Journal of Medicine* 305(24): 1425–31.

Groleau, V., R. A. Herold, J. I. Schall et al. (2013). Blood lead concentration is not altered by high-dose vitamin D supplementation in children and young adults with HIV. *Journal of Pediatric Gastroenterology and Nutrition* 56(3): 316–9.

Gupta, S. K., D. Mi, S. M. Moe, M. Dubé, and Z. Liu. (2013). Effects of switching from efavirenz to raltegravir on endothelial function, bone mineral metabolism, inflammation, and renal function: a randomized, controlled trial. *Journal of Acquired Immune Deficiency Syndromes* 64(3): 279–83.

Guzmán-Fulgencio, M., M. García-Alvarez, J. Berenguer et al. (2014). Vitamin D deficiency is associated with severity of liver disease in HIV/HCV coinfected patients. *Journal of Infection* 68(2): 176–84.

Gyllensten, K., F. Josephson, K. Lidman, and M. Sääf. (2006). Severe vitamin D deficiency diagnosed after introduction of antiretroviral therapy including efavirenz in a patient living at latitude 59 degrees N. *AIDS* 20(14): 1906–7.

Hamill, M. M., K. A. Ward, J. M. Pettifor, S. A. Norris, and A. Prentice. (2013). Bone mass, body composition and vitamin D status of ARV-naïve, urban, black South African women with HIV infection, stratified by CD(4) count. *Osteoporosis International* 24(11): 2855–61.

Hammond, E., E. McKinnon, P. Glendenning, R. Williams, S. Mallai, and E. Phillips. (2012). Association between 25-OH vitamin D and insulin is independent of lipoatrophy in HIV. *Clinical Endocrinology* 76(2): 201–6.

Haug, C., F. Müller, Aukrust, and S. S. Frøland. (1994). Subnormal serum concentration of 1,25-vitamin D in human immunodeficiency virus infection: correlation with degree of immune deficiency and survival. *Journal of Infectious Diseases* 169(4): 889–93.

Haug, C. J., F. Müller, H. Rollag, Aukrust, M. Degré, and S. S. Førland. (1996). The effect of 1,25-vitamin D_3 on maturation of monocytes from HIV-infected patients varies with degree of immunodeficiency. *Acta Pathologica, Microbiologica, et Immunologica Scandinavica (APMIS)* 104(7–8): 539–48.

Haug, C. J., F. Müller, Aukrust, and S. S. Frøland. (1998a). Different effect of 1,25-dihydroxyvitamin D_3 on replication of *Mycobacterium avium* in monocyte-derived macrophages from human immunodeficiency virus-infected subjects and healthy controls. *Immunology Letters* 63(2): 107–12.

Haug, C. J., Aukrust, E. Haug, L. Mørkrid, F. Müller, and S. S. Frøland. (1998b). Severe deficiency of 1,25-dihydroxyvitamin D_3 in human immunodeficiency virus infection: association with immunological hyperactivity and only minor changes in calcium homeostasis. *Journal of Clinical Endocrinology & Metabolism* 83(11): 3832–8.

Havens, L., K. Mulligan, R. Hazra et al.; Adolescent Medicine Trials Network (ATN) for HIV/AIDS Interventions 063 Study Team. (2012a). Serum 25-hydroxyvitamin D response to vitamin D_3 supplementation 50,000 IU monthly in youth with HIV-1 infection. *Journal of Clinical Endocrinology & Metabolism* 97(11): 4004–13.

Havens, L., C. B. Stephensen, R. Hazra et al.; Adolescent Medicine Trials Network (ATN) for HIV/AIDS Interventions 063 Study Team. (2012b). Vitamin D_3 decreases parathyroid hormone in HIV-infected youth being treated with tenofovir: a randomized, placebo-controlled trial. *Clinical Infectious Diseases* 54(7): 1013–25.

Havens, L., J. J. Kiser, C. B. Stephensen et al.; Adolescent Medicine Trials Network (ATN) for HIV/AIDS Interventions 063 Study Team. (2013). Association of higher plasma vitamin D binding protein and lower free calcitriol levels with tenofovir disoproxil fumarate use and plasma and intracellular tenofovir pharmacokinetics: cause of a functional vitamin D deficiency? *Antimicrobial Agents and Chemotherapy* 57(11): 5619–28.

Havens, L., R. Hazra, C. B. Stephensen et al.; Adolescent Medicine Trials Network (ATN) for HIV/AIDS Interventions 063 Study Team. (2014). Vitamin D_3 supplementation increases fibroblast growth factor-23 in HIV-infected youth treated with tenofovir disoproxil fumarate. *Antiviral Therapy* 19(6): 613–8.

Havers, F., L. Smeaton, N. Gupte et al.; ACTG PEARLS; NWCS 319 Study Teams. (2014a). 25-hydroxyvitamin D insufficiency and deficiency is associated with HIV disease progression and virological failure post-antiretroviral therapy initiation in diverse multinational settings. *Journal of Infectious Diseases* 210(2): 244–53.

Havers, F. P., B. Detrick, S. W. Cardosa et al.; ACTG A5175 PEARLS and NWCS319 Study Teams. (2014b). Change in vitamin D levels occurs early after antiretroviral therapy initiation and depends on treatment regimen in resource-limited settings. *PLoS One* 9(4): e95164.

Hewison, M. (2012). Vitamin D and immune function: an overview. *Proceedings of the Nutrition Society* 71(1): 50–61.

Hileman, C. O., D. E. Labbato, N. J. Storer, V. Tangpricha, and G. A. McComsey. (2014). Is bone loss linked to chronic inflammation in antiretroviral-naive HIV-infected adults? A 48-week matched cohort study. *AIDS* 28(12): 1759–67.

Holick, M. F., Ed. (2010). *Vitamin D: Physiology, Molecular Biology, and Clinical Applications.* New York: Humana Press.

Honda, J. R., E. Connick, S. MaWhinney, E. D. Chan, and S. C. Flores. (2014). Plasma LL-37 correlates with vitamin D and is reduced in HIV-1 infected individuals not receiving antiretroviral therapy. *Journal of Medical Microbiology* 63: 997–1003.

Ikezoe, T., K. Bandobashi, Y. Yang et al. (2006). HIV-1 protease inhibitor ritonavir potentiates the effect of 1,25-dihydroxyvitamin D_3 to induce growth arrest and differentiation of human myeloid leukemia cells via down-regulation of CYP24). *Leukemia Research* 30(8): 1005–11.

Jaeger, P., S. Otto, R. F. Speck et al. (1994). Altered parathyroid gland function in severely immunocompromised patients infected with human immunodeficiency virus. *Journal of Clinical Endocrinology & Metabolism* 79(6): 1701–5.

Jarvis, J. N., T. Bicanic, A. Loyse et al. (2014). Very low levels of 25OH vitamin D are not associated with immunologic changes or clinical outcome in South African patients with HIV-associated cryptococcal meningitis. *Clinical Infectious Diseases* 59(4): 493–500.

Jones, G., D. E. Prosser, and M. Kaufmann. (2012). 25-Hydroxyvitamin D-24-hydroxylase (CYP24A1): its important role in the degradation of vitamin D. *Archives of Biochemistry and Biophysics* 523(1): 9–18.

Kakalia, S., E. B. Sochett, D. Stephens, E. Assor, S. E. Read, and A. Bitnun. (2011). Vitamin D supplementation and CD4 count in children infected with human immunodeficiency virus. *Journal of Pediatrics* 159(6): 951–7.

Kewenig, S., T. Schneider, K. Hohloch et al. (1999). Rapid mucosal CD4(+) T-cell depletion and enteropathy in simian immunodeficiency virus-infected rhesus macaques. *Gastroenterology* 116(5): 1115–23.

Kim, J. H., V. Gandhi, G. Psevdos, Jr., F. Espinoza, J. Park, and V. Sharp. (2012). Evaluation of vitamin D levels among HIV-infected patients in New York City. *AIDS Research and Human Retroviruses* 28(3): 235–41.

Kitano, K., G. C. Baldwin, M. A. Raines, and D. W. Golde. (1990). Differentiating agents facilitate infection of myeloid leukemia cell lines by monocytotropic HIV-1 strains. *Blood* 76(10): 1980–8.

Kitano, K., C. I. Rivas, G. C. Baldwin, J. C. Vera, and D. W. Golde. (1993). Tumor necrosis factor-dependent production of human immunodeficiency virus 1 in chronically infected HL-60 cells. *Blood* 82(9): 2742–8.

Kizaki, M., Y. Ikeda, K. J. Simon, M. Nanjo, and H. Koeffler. (1993). Effect of 1,25-dihydroxyvitamin D_3 and its analogs on human immunodeficiency virus infection in monocytes/macrophages. *Leukemia* 7(10): 1525–30.

Klassen, K., A. R. Martineau, R. J. Wilkinson, G. Cooke, A. Courtney, and M. Hickson. (2012). The effect of tenofovir on vitamin D metabolism in HIV-infected adults is dependent on sex and ethnicity. *PLoS One* 7(9): e44845.

Kumar, N., M. Bower, and M. Nelson. (2012). Severe vitamin D deficiency in a patient treated for hepatitis B with tenofovir. *International Journal of STD & AIDS* 23(1): 59–60.

Kwan, C. K., B. Eckhardt, J. Baghdadi, and J. A. Aberg. (2012). Hyperparathyroidism and complications associated with vitamin D deficiency in HIV-infected adults in New York City, New York. *AIDS Research and Human Retroviruses* 28(9): 1025–32.

Lai, H., B. Detrick, E. K. Fishman et al. (2012a). Vitamin D deficiency is associated with the development of subclinical coronary artery disease in African Americans with HIV infection: a preliminary study. *Journal of Investigative Medicine* 60(5): 801–7.

Lai, H., G. Gerstenblith, E. K. Fishman et al. (2012b). Vitamin D deficiency is associated with silent coronary artery disease in cardiovascularly asymptomatic African Americans with HIV infection. *Clinical Infectious Diseases* 54(12): 1747–55.

Lai, H., E. K. Fishman, G. Gerstenblith et al. (2013a). Vitamin D deficiency is associated with development of subclinical coronary artery disease in HIV-infected African American cocaine users with low Framingham-defined cardiovascular risk. *Vascular Health and Risk Management* 9: 729–37.

Lai, S., E. K. Fishman, G. Gerstenblith et al. (2013b). Vitamin D deficiency is associated with coronary artery calcification in cardiovascularly asymptomatic African Americans with HIV infection. *Vascular Health and Risk Management* 9: 493–500.

Lake, J. E., R. M. Hoffman, C. H. Tseng, H. M. Wilhalme, J. S. Adams, and J. S. Currier. (2015). Success of standard dose vitamin D supplementation in treated human immunodeficiency virus infection. *Open Forum Infectious Diseases* 2(2): ofv068.

Lambert, A. A., M. B. Drummond, S. H. Mehta et al. (2014). Risk factors for vitamin D deficiency among HIV-infected and uninfected injection drug users. *PLoS One* 9(4): e95802.

Landriscina, M., S. A. Altamura, L. Roca et al. (2008). Reverse transcriptase inhibitors induce cell differentiation and enhance the immunogenic phenotype in human renal clear-cell carcinoma. *International Journal of Cancer* 122(12): 2842–50.

Legeai, C., C. Vigouroux, J.-C. Souberbielle et al.; ANRS–COPANA Cohort Study Group. (2013). Associations between 25-hydroxyvitamin D and immunologic, metabolic, inflammatory markers in treatment-naive HIV-infected persons: the ANRS CO9 «COPANA» cohort study. *PLoS One* 8(9): e74868.

Lerma, E., M. Ema Molas, M. Montero et al. (2012). Prevalence and factors associated with vitamin D deficiency and hyperparathyroidism in HIV-infected patients treated in Barcelona. *ISRN AIDS* 2012: 485307.

Li Vecchi, V., M. Soresi, L. Giannitrapani et al. (2012). Dairy calcium intake and lifestyle risk factors for bone loss in HIV-infected and uninfected Mediterranean subjects. *BMC Infectious Diseases* 12: 192.

Liu, T., S. Stenger, H. Li et al. (2006). Toll-like receptor triggering of a vitamin D-mediated human antimicrobial response. *Science* 311(5768): 1770–3.

Liu, T., S. Stenger, D. H. Tang, and R. L. Modlin. (2007). Cutting edge: vitamin D-mediated human antimicrobial activity against *Mycobacterium tuberculosis* is dependent on the induction of cathelicidin. *Journal of Immunology* 179(4): 2060–3.

Locardi, C., C. Petrini, and G. Boccoli. (1990). Increased human immunodeficiency virus (HIV) expression in chronically infected U937 cells upon *in vitro* differentiation by hydroxyvitamin D_3: roles of interferon and tumor necrosis factor in regulation of HIV production. *Journal of Virology* 64(12): 5874–82.

Longenecker, C. T., C. O. Hileman, T. L. Carman et al. (2012). Vitamin D supplementation and endothelial function in vitamin D deficient HIV-infected patients: a randomized placebo-controlled trial. *Antiviral Therapy* 17(4): 613–21.

Madeddu, G., A. Spanu, P. Solinas et al. (2004). Bone mass loss and vitamin D metabolism impairment in HIV patients receiving highly active antiretroviral therapy. *Quarterly Journal of Nuclear Medicine and Molecular Imaging* 48(1): 39–48.

Mandorfer, M., T. Reiberger, B. A. Payer et al.; HIV & Liver Study Group. (2013). Low vitamin D levels are associated with impaired virologic response to PEGIFN + RBV therapy in HIV-hepatitis C virus coinfected patients. *AIDS* 27(2): 227–32.

Martineau, A. R., S. Nhamoyebonde, T. Oni et al. (2011). Reciprocal seasonal variation in vitamin D status and tuberculosis notifications in Cape Town, South Africa. *Proceedings of the National Academy of Sciences* 108(47): 19013–7.

Masiá, M., S. Padilla, C. Robledano, N. López, J. M. Ramos, and F. Guiterrez. (2012). Early changes in parathyroid hormone concentrations in HIV-infected patients initiating antiretroviral therapy with tenofovir. *AIDS Research and Human Retroviruses* 28(3): 242–6.

Mastala, Y., Nyangulu, R. V. Banda, B. Mhemedi, S. A. White, and T. J. Allain. (2013). Vitamin D deficiency in medical patients at a central hospital in Malawi: a comparison with TB patients from a previous study. *PLoS One* 8(3): e59017.

Mave, V., D. Shere, N. Gupte et al.; WEN India and Byramjee–Jeejeebhoy Medical College Clinical Trials Unit Study Team. (2012). Vitamin D deficiency is common among HIV-infected breastfeeding mothers in Pune, India, but is not associated with mother-to-child HIV transmission. *HIV Clinical Trials* 13(5): 278–83.

Mehta, S., D. J. Hunter, F. M. Mugusi et al. (2009). Perinatal outcomes, including mother-to-child transmission of HIV, and child mortality and their association with maternal vitamin D status in Tanzania. *Journal of Infectious Diseases* 200(7): 1022–30.

Mehta, S., E. Giovannucci, F. M. Mugusi et al. (2010a). Vitamin D status of HIV-infected women and its association with HIV disease progression, anemia, and mortality. *PLoS One* 5(1): e8770.

Mehta, S., D. Spiegelman, S. Aboud et al. (2010b). Lipid-soluble vitamins A, D, and E in HIV-infected pregnant women in Tanzania. *European Journal of Clinical Nutrition* 64(8): 808–17.

Mehta, S., F. M. Mugusi, D. Spiegelman et al. (2011). Vitamin D status and its association with morbidity including wasting and opportunistic illnesses in HIV-infected women in Tanzania. *AIDS Patient Care and STDs* 25(10): 579–85.

Mehta, S., F. M. Mugusi, R. J. Bosch et al. (2013). Vitamin D status and TB treatment outcomes in adult patients in Tanzania: a cohort study. *BMJ Open* 3(11): e003703.

Merhi, Z. O., D. B. Seifer, J. Weedon et al. (2012). Circulating vitamin D correlates with serum antimüllerian hormone levels in late-reproductive-aged women: Women's Interagency HIV Study. *Fertility and Sterility* 98(1): 228–34.

Meyzer, C., P. Frange, H. Chappuy et al. (2013). Vitamin D deficiency and insufficiency in HIV-infected children and young adults. *Pediatric Infectious Disease Journal* 32(11): 1240–4.

Milazzo, L., C. Mazzali, G. Bestetti et al. (2011). Liver-related factors associated with low vitamin D levels in HIV and HIV/HCV coinfected patients and comparison to general population. *Current HIV Research* 9(3): 186–93.

Momplaisir, F., I. Frank, W. Meyer III, D. Kim, R. Kappes, and P. Tebas. (2012). Vitamin D levels, natural H1N1 infection and response to H1N1 vaccine among HIV-infected individuals. *Journal of AIDS & Clinical Research* 3(4): 152.

Moodley, A., M. Qin, K. K. Singh, and S. A. Spector. (2013). Vitamin D-related host genetic variants alter HIV disease progression in children. *Pediatric Infectious Disease Journal* 32(11): 1230–6.

Moreno-Pérez, O., J. Portilla, C. Escoín et al. (2013). Impact of vitamin D insufficiency on insulin homeostasis and beta cell function in nondiabetic male HIV-infected patients. *HIV Medicine* 14(9): 540–8.

Mueller, N. J., C. A. Fux, B. Ledergerber et al.; Swiss HIV Cohort Study. (2010). High prevalence of severe vitamin D deficiency in combined antiretroviral therapy-naive and successfully treated Swiss HIV patients. *AIDS* 24(8): 1127–34.

Murr, C., B. Widner, B. Wirleitner, and D. Fuchs. (2002). Neopterin as a marker for immune system activation. *Current Drug Metabolism* 3(2): 175–87.

Nansera, D., F. M. Graziano, D. J. Friedman, M. K. Bobbs, A. N. Jones, and K. E. Hansen. (2011). Vitamin D and calcium levels in Ugandan adults with human immunodeficiency virus and tuberculosis. *International Journal of Tuberculosis and Lung Disease* 15(11): 1522–7.

Nevado, J., S. Tenbaum, A. I. Castillo, A. Sánchez-Pacheco, and A. Aranda. (2007). Activation of the human immunodeficiency virus type I long terminal repeat by 1 alpha,25-dihydroxyvitamin D₃). *Journal of Molecular Endocrinology* 38(6): 587–601.

Nieto, G., Y. Barber, M. C. Rubio, M. Rubio, and J. Fibla. (2004). Association between AIDS disease progression rates and the Fok-I polymorphism of the VDR gene in a cohort of HIV-1 seropositive patients. *Journal of Steroid Biochemistry and Molecular Biology* 89–90(1–5): 199–207.

Orkin, C., D. A. Wohl, A. Williams, and H. Deckx. (2014). Vitamin D deficiency in HIV: a shadow on long-term management? *AIDS Reviews* 16(2): 59–74.

Ormesher, B., S. Dhaliwal, E. Nylen et al. (2011). Vitamin D deficiency is less common among HIV-infected African-American men than in a matched cohort. *AIDS* 25(9): 1237–9.

Overton, E. T., E. S. Chan, T. T. Brown et al. (2015). Vitamin D and calcium attenuate bone loss with antiretroviral therapy initiation: a randomized trial. *Annals of Internal Medicine* 162(12): 815–24.

Patel, J., D. Pal, V. Vangal, M. Gandhi, and A. L. Mitra. (2002). Transport of HIV-protease inhibitors across 1 alpha,25di-hydroxy vitamin D₃-treated Calu-3 cell monolayers: modulation of P-glycoprotein activity. *Pharmaceutical Research* 19(11): 1696–703.

Paul, T. V., H. S. Asha, N. Thomas et al. (2010). Hypovitaminosis D and bone mineral density in human immunodeficiency virus-infected men from India, with or without antiretroviral therapy. *Endocrine Practice* 16(4): 547–53.

Pauza, C. D., R. Kornbluth, Emau, D. D. Richman, and L. J. Deftos. (1993). Vitamin D_3 compounds regulate human immunodeficiency virus type 1 replication in U937 monoblastoid cells and in monocyte-derived macrophages. *Journal of Leukocyte Biology* 53(2): 157–64.

Pepe, J., A. M. Isidori, M. Falciano et al. (2014). Effect of risedronate in osteoporotic HIV males, according to gonadal status: a pilot study. *Endocrine* 47(2): 456–62.

Pinzone, M. R., M. Di Rosa, B. M. Celesia et al. (2013). LPS and HIV gp120 modulate monocyte/macrophage CYP27B1 and CYP24A1 expression leading to vitamin D consumption and hypovitaminosis D in HIV-infected individuals. *European Review for Medical and Pharmacological Sciences* 17(14): 1938–50.

Piso, R. J., M. Rothen, J. Rothen, M. Stahl, and C. Fux. (2013). Per oral substitution with 300000 IU vitamin D (Cholecalciferol) reduces bone turnover markers in HIV-infected patients. *BMC Infectious Diseases* 13: 577.

Playford, E. G., A. S. Bansal, D. F. M. Locke, M. Whitby, and G. Hogan. (2001). Hypercalcaemia and elevated 1,25(OH)(2)D(3) levels associated with disseminated *Mycobacterium avium* infection in AIDS. *Journal of Infection* 42(2): 157–8.

Poowuttikul, P., R. Thomas, B. Hart, and E. Secord. (2014). Vitamin D insufficiency/deficiency in HIV-infected inner city youth. *Journal of the International Association of Providers of AIDS Care* 13(5): 438–42.

Porter, T. R., X. Li, C. B. Stephensen et al.; Adolescent Medicine Trials Network for HIV/AIDS Interventions (ATN) 063 Study Team. (2013). Genetic associations with 25-hydroxyvitamin D deficiency in HIV-1-infected youth: fine-mapping for the GC/DBP gene that encodes the vitamin D-binding protein. *Frontiers in Genetics* 4: 234.

Portilla, J., O. Moreno-Pérez, C. Sema-Candel et al. (2014). Vitamin D insufficiency and subclinical athero-sclerosis in non-diabetic males living with HIV. *Journal of the International AIDS Society* 17: 18945.

Price, P., L. J. Haddow, J. Affandi et al. (2012). Short communication: plasma levels of vitamin D in HIV patients initiating antiretroviral therapy do not predict immune restoration disease associated with *Mycobacterium tuberculosis*. *AIDS Research and Human Retroviruses* 28(10): 1216–9.

Prietl, B., G. Treiber, T. R. Pieber, and K. Amrein. (2013). Vitamin D and immune function. *Nutrients* 5(7): 2502–21.

Provvedini, D. M., C. D. Tsoukas, L. J. Deftos, and S. C. Manolagas. (1983). 1,25-dihydroxyvitamin D_3 receptors in human leukocytes. *Science* 221(4616): 1181–3.

Ramayo, E., M. González-Moreno, J. Macías et al. (2005). Relationship between osteopenia, free testosterone, and vitamin D metabolite levels in HIV-infected patients with and without highly active antiretroviral therapy. *AIDS Research and Human Retroviruses* 21(11): 915–21.

Rodríguez, M., B. Daniels, S. Gunawardene, and G. K. Robbins. (2009). High frequency of vitamin D deficiency in ambulatory HIV-positive patients. *AIDS Research and Human Retroviruses* 25(1): 9–14.

Rosenvinge, M. M., K. Gedela, A. J. Copas et al. (2010). Tenofovir-linked hyperparathyroidism is independently associated with the presence of vitamin D deficiency. *Journal of Acquired Immune Deficiency Syndromes* 54(5): 496–9.

Ross, A. C., S. Judd, M. Kumari et al. (2011). Vitamin D is linked to carotid intima–media thickness and immune reconstitution in HIV-positive individuals. *Antiviral Therapy* 16(4): 555–63.

Rutstein, R., A. Downes, B. Zemel, J. Schall, and V. Stallings. (2011). Vitamin D status in children and young adults with perinatally acquired HIV infection. *Clinical Nutrition* 30(5): 624–8.

Salhan, D., M. Husain, A. Subrati et al. (2012). HIV-induced kidney cell injury: role of ROS-induced down-regulated vitamin D receptor. *American Journal of Physiology: Renal Physiology* 303(4): F503–14.

Schlesinger, M., Z. Bar-Shavit, R. Hadar, and R. Rabinowitz. (1989). Modulation of the expression of CD4 on HL-60 cells by exposure to 1,25-dihydroxyvitamin D_3). *Immunology Letters* 22(4): 307–11.

Schwartz, J. B., K. L. Moore, M. Yin et al. (2014). Relationship of vitamin D, HIV, HIV treatment, and lipid levels in the Women's Interagency HIV Study of HIV-infected and uninfected women in the United States. *Journal of the International Association of Providers of AIDS Care* 13(3): 250–9.

Shahar, E., E. Segal, G. S. Rozen et al. (2013). Vitamin D status in young HIV infected women of various ethnic origins: incidence of vitamin D deficiency and possible impact on bone density. *Clinical Nutrition* 32(1): 83–7.

Shepherd, L., J.-C. Souberbielle, J.-P. Bastard et al. (2014). Prognostic value of vitamin D level for all-cause mortality, and association with inflammatory markers, in HIV-infected persons. *Journal of Infectious Diseases* 210 (2): 234–43.

Sherwood, J. E., O. C. Mesner, A. C. Weintrob et al. (2012). Vitamin D deficiency and its association with low bone mineral density, HIV-related factors, hospitalization, and death in a predominantly black HIV-infected cohort. *Clinical Infectious Diseases* 55(12): 1727–36.

Shikuma, C. M., T. Seto, C. Y. Liang et al. (2012). Vitamin D levels and markers of arterial dysfunction in HIV. *AIDS Research and Human Retroviruses* 28(8): 793–7.

Skolnik, R., B. Jahn, M. Z. Wang, T. R. Rota, M. S. Hirsch, and S. M. Krane. (1991). Enhancement of human immunodeficiency virus 1 replication in monocytes by 1,25-dihydroxycholecalciferol. *Proceedings of the National Academy of Sciences* 88(15): 6632–6.

Sroussi, H. Y., J. Burke-Miller, A. L. French et al. (2012). Association among vitamin D, oral candidiasis, and calprotectinemia in HIV. *Journal of Dental Research* 91(7): 666–70.

Stallings, V. A., J. I. Schall, M. L. Hediger et al. (2015). High-dose vitamin D₃ supplementation in children and young adults with HIV: a randomized, placebo-controlled trial. *Pediatric Infectious Disease Journal* 34(2): e32–40.

Steenhoff, A. P., J. I. Schall, J. Samuel et al. (2015). Vitamin D(3)supplementation in Batswana children and adults with HIV: a pilot double blind randomized controlled trial. *PLoS One* 10(2): e0117123.

Stein, E. M., M. T. Yin, D. J. McMahon et al. (2011). Vitamin D deficiency in HIV-infected postmenopausal Hispanic and African-American women. *Osteoporosis International* 22(2): 477–87.

Stephensen, C .B., G. S. Marquis, L. A. Kruzich, S. D. Douglas, G. M. Aldrovandi, and C. M. Wilson. (2006). Vitamin D status in adolescents and young adults with HIV infection. *American Journal of Clinical Nutrition* 83(5): 1135–41.

Sudfeld, C. R., M. Wang, S. Aboud, E. L. Giovannucci, F. M. Mugusi, and W. W. Fawzi. (2012). Vitamin D and HIV progression among Tanzanian adults initiating antiretroviral therapy. *PLoS One* 7(6): e40036.

Sudfeld, C. R., E. L. Giovannucci, S. Isanaka et al. (2013). Vitamin D status and incidence of pulmonary tuberculosis, opportunistic infections, and wasting among HIV-infected Tanzanian adults initiating antiretroviral therapy. *Journal of Infectious Diseases* 207(3): 378–85.

Szep, Z., G. Guaraldi, S. S. Shah et al. (2011). Vitamin D deficiency is associated with type 2 diabetes mellitus in HIV infection. *AIDS* 25(4): 525–9.

Tastan, O., Y. Qi, J. G. Carbonell, and J. Klein-Seetharaman. (2009). Prediction of interactions between HIV-1 and human proteins by information integration. *Pacific Symposium on Biocomputing* 2009: 516–27.

Teichmann, J., E. Stephan, U. Lange, T. Discher, H. Stracke, K. Federlin. (1997). Elevated serum-calcium and parathormone-levels in HIV afflicted female heroin addicts. *European Journal of Medical Research* 2(8): 343–6.

Teichmann, J., E. Stephan, U. Lange et al. (2003). Osteopenia in HIV-infected women prior to highly active antiretroviral therapy. *Journal of Infection* 46(4): 221–7.

Terrier, B., F. Carrat, G. Geri et al. (2011). Low 25-OH vitamin D serum levels correlate with severe fibrosis in HIV–HCV co-infected patients with chronic hepatitis. *Journal of Hepatology* 55(4): 756–61.

Theodorou, M., T. Sersté, M. Van Gossum, and S. Dewit. (2014). Factors associated with vitamin D deficiency in a population of 2044 HIV-infected patients. *Clinical Nutrition* 33(2): 274–9.

Torres, C., M. Sánchez de la Torre, C. García-Moruja et al. (2010). Immunophenotype of vitamin D receptor polymorphism associated to risk of HIV-1 infection and rate of disease progression. *Current HIV Research* 8(6): 487–92.

UNAIDS. (2014). *Fact Sheet 2014*. Geneva: Joint United Nations Programme on HIV/AIDS (http://www.unaids.org/sites/default/files/en/media/unaids/contentassets/documents/factsheet/2014/20140716_FactSheet_en.pdf).

UNAIDS. (2015). *Fact Sheet 2015*. Geneva: Joint United Nations Programme on HIV/AIDS (http://www.unaids.org/en/resources/campaigns/HowAIDSchangedeverything/factsheet).

United Nations. (2015). *The Millenium Development Goals Report 2015*. New York: United Nations.

van den Bout-van den Beukel, C. J., L. Fievez, M. Michels et al.. (2008a). Vitamin D deficiency among HIV type 1-infected individuals in the Netherlands: effects of antiretroviral therapy. *AIDS Research and Human Retroviruses* 24(11): 1375–82.

van den Bout-van den Beukel, C. J., M. van den Bos, W. J. Oyen et al. (2008b). The effect of cholecalciferol supplementation on vitamin D levels and insulin sensitivity is dose related in vitamin D-deficient HIV-1-infected patients. *HIV Medicine* 9(9): 771–9.

Vescini, F., A. Cozzi-Lepri, M. Borderi et al.; Icona Foundation Study Group. (2011). Prevalence of hypovitaminosis D and factors associated with vitamin D deficiency and morbidity among HIV-infected patients enrolled in a large Italian cohort. *Journal of Acquired Immune Deficiency Syndromes* 58(2): 163–72.

Viard, J. P., J. C. Souderbielle, O. Kirk et al.; EuroSIDA Study Group. (2011). Vitamin D and clinical disease progression in HIV infection: results from the EuroSIDA study. *AIDS* 25(10): 1305–15.

Vrouenraets, S. M., F. W. Wit, J. van Tongeren, and J. M. Lange. (2007). Efavirenz: a review. *Expert Opinion on Pharmacotherapy* 8(6): 851–71.

Wang, T. T., F. Nestel, V. Bourdeau et al. (2004). Cutting edge: 1,25-dihydroxyvitamin D$_3$ is a direct inducer of antimicrobial peptide gene expression. *Journal of Immunology.* 173(5): 2909–12.

Wasserman, P. and D. S. Rubin. (2010). Highly prevalent vitamin D deficiency and insufficiency in an urban cohort of HIV-infected men under care. *AIDS Patient Care and STDS* 24(4): 223–7.

Wejse, C., V. F. Gomes, P. Rabna et al. (2009). Vitamin D as supplementary treatment for tuberculosis: a double-blind, randomized, placebo-controlled trial. *American Journal of Respiratory and Critcal Care Medicine* 179(9): 843–50.

Welz, T., K. Childs, F. Ibrahim et al. (2010). Efavirenz is associated with severe vitamin D deficiency and increased alkaline phosphatase. *AIDS* 24(12): 1923–8.

WHO. (2007). *WHO Case Definitions of HIV for Surveillance and Revised Clinical Staging and Immunological Classification of HIV-Related Disease in Adults and Children.* Geneva: World Health Organization.

Wiboonchutikul, S., S. Sungkanuparph, S. Kiertiburanakul et al. (2012). Vitamin D insufficiency and deficiency among HIV-1-infected patients in a tropical setting. *Journal of the International Association of Physicians in AIDS Care* 11(5): 305–10.

Wiederin, J. L., R. M. Donahoe, J. R. Anderson et al. (2010). Plasma proteomic analysis of simian immunodeficiency virus infection of rhesus macaques. *Journal of Proteome Research* 9(9): 4721–31.

Wohl, D. A., C. Orkin, M. Doroana et al. (2014). Change in vitamin D levels and risk of severe vitamin D deficiency over 48 weeks among HIV-1-infected, treatment-naive adults receiving rilpivirine or efavirenz in a Phase III trial (ECHO). *Antiviral Therapy* 2014). 19(2): 191–200.

Yamamoto, N., V. R. Naraparaju, and S. M. Srinivasula. (1995). Structural modification of serum vitamin D$_3$-binding protein and immunosuppression in AIDS patients. *AIDS Research and Human Retroviruses* 11(11): 1373–8.

Yin, M. and E. Stein. (2011). The effect of antiretrovirals on vitamin D. *Clinical Infectious Diseases* 52(3): 406–8.

Yin, M., J. Dobkin, K. Brudney et al. (2005). Bone mass and mineral metabolism in HIV+ postmenopausal women. *Osteoporosis International* 16(11): 1345–52.

Yin, M. T., D. Lu, S. Cremers et al. (2010). Short-term bone loss in HIV-infected premenopausal women. *Journal of Acquired Immune Deficiency Syndromes* 53(2): 202–8.

Zhang, L., Y. Su, E. Hsieh et al. (2013). Bone turnover and bone mineral density in HIV-1 infected Chinese taking highly active antiretroviral therapy—a prospective observational study. *BMC Musculoskeletal Disorders* 14(1): 224.

5 Antioxidants and HIV/ AIDS: Zinc, Selenium, and Vitamins C and E

Amanda L. Wilkinson, Samantha L. Huey, and Saurabh Mehta

CONTENTS

INTRODUCTION

The worldwide prevalence of HIV/AIDS was estimated to be 35 million in 2012 (UNAIDS, 2013). Although provision of antiretroviral therapy (ART) is essential to stop viral progression, complementary approaches to improving the overall health and quality of life among people living with HIV are important secondary objectives. Poor antioxidant status and deficiencies in other micronutrients are common among people living with HIV (Semba and Tang, 1999). HIV contributes to oxidative stress, thus increasing antioxidant demand, and an impaired antioxidant defense system promotes disease progression (Baruchel and Wainberg, 1992; Pace and Leaf, 1995). Reduced dietary intake and poor absorption of antioxidant micronutrients, secondary to HIV infection, further contribute to negative antioxidant balance and susceptibility to oxidative damage. For these reasons, antioxidant micronutrients have been examined in the context of HIV through observational investigations and clinical trials. Antioxidants are produced endogenously to neutralize reactive oxygen species and prevent excessive oxidative damage. Therefore, exogenous administration of antioxidants may have therapeutic benefits, especially among individuals experiencing persistent oxidative stress. Antioxidant supplementation trials among people living with HIV have been heterogeneous in design and have yielded somewhat conflicting results. This is a review of supplementation trials of antioxidant micronutrients vitamin C, vitamin E, zinc, and selenium, delivered alone or in combination. The populations of interest were adults and children living with HIV infection. Both ART-naïve and populations receiving ART were included. Observational studies related to the nutrients of interest are also briefly summarized.

METHODS

We conducted a literature search in PubMed to identify published studies through June 30, 2015; the search details are shown in Figure 5.1. Previous reviews on the topic were also searched for relevant articles that may have been missed. Inclusion criteria were human studies published in English that included individuals with known HIV infection receiving oral supplementation of antioxidant micronutrients. Because few randomized trials have examined the effects of antioxidants in the context of HIV, pilot studies and trials without control arms were included. Trials that delivered multiple micronutrients were included if the effects of the antioxidants of interest could be isolated (i.e., if trials included a comparison of groups receiving or not receiving one or more antioxidants as part of a multiple micronutrient supplement). The main outcomes of interest were mortality, CD4 cell count, viral load, HIV transmission, and pregnancy outcomes. Other clinical morbidities and assessments, such as hematological indicators and anthropometric measures, were also included.

RESULTS

The articles in this review were published between 1988 and 2015 (see Figure 5.1). Study populations included HIV-infected adults and children with varied ART regimens. In this section, articles are stratified into four groups based on the study population: (1) pregnant women living with HIV,

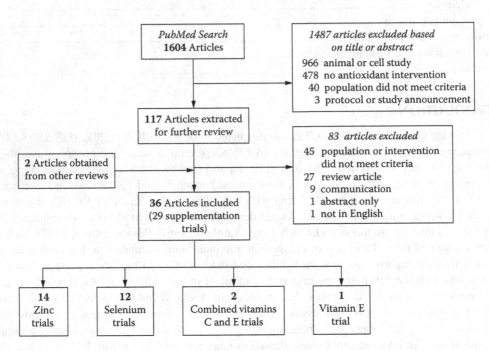

FIGURE 5.1 Study selection. Search terms: (HIV Infections[MeSH] OR HIV[MeSH] OR hiv[tw] OR hiv-1*[tw] OR hiv-2*[tw] OR hiv1[tw] OR hiv2[tw] OR hiv infect*[tw] OR human immunodeficiency virus[tw] OR human immunedeficiency virus[tw] OR human immuno-deficiency virus[tw] OR human immune deficiency virus[tw] OR ((human immun*) AND (deficiency virus[tw])) OR acquired immunodeficiency syndrome[tw] OR acquired immunedeficiency syndrome[tw] OR acquired immunodeficiency syndrome[tw] OR acquired immune-deficiency syndrome[tw] OR ((acquired immun*) AND (deficiency syndrome[tw])) OR "sexually transmitted diseases, viral"[MESH:NoExp]) AND ((("ascorbic acid"[MeSH Terms] OR "ascorbic acid deficiency"[MeSH Terms] OR ("ascorbic"[tw] AND "acid"[tw]) OR "vitamin c"[tw] OR ascorbate[tw]) OR ("vitamin e"[MeSH Terms] OR "vitamin e deficiency"[MeSH Terms] OR "vitamin e"[tw] OR "tocopherols"[MeSH Terms] OR "tocopherol*"[tw]) OR ("zinc"[MeSH Terms] OR "zinc"[tw]) OR ("selenium"[MeSH Terms] OR "selenium"[tw])).

(2) adults living with HIV and receiving ART, (3) adults living with HIV and receiving heterogeneous or unspecified ART, and (4) children living with HIV. Antioxidant supplementation trials among people living with HIV have been predominantly conducted in North America ($n = 9$) and sub-Saharan Africa ($n = 8$), with trials also conducted in Europe ($n = 6$), Asia ($n = 4$), and South America ($n = 2$).

EVIDENCE FROM SUPPLEMENTATION TRIALS

Fourteen trials have examined the effects of zinc supplementation among adults and children living with HIV (Table 5.1), and 12 trials have evaluated selenium (Table 5.2). Studies of zinc supplementation have been predominantly placebo-controlled, double-blind randomized controlled trials (RCTs), whereas much of the evidence regarding selenium supplementation comes from non-randomized trials. Two trials investigated the effects of combined vitamin C and E supplementation in people living with HIV, and one trial examined the effects of vitamin E delivered alone (Table 5.3).

Zinc

Pregnant Women

A study in Tanzania randomized 400 ART-naïve pregnant women with HIV to receive either 25 mg zinc sulfate or a placebo supplement beginning prenatally (12 to 27 weeks gestation) and continuing through six weeks postpartum (Fawzi et al., 2005; Villamor et al., 2006). All study participants were prescribed an antenatal supplement containing ferrous sulfate and folate and a multiple micronutrient supplement containing B vitamins, vitamin C, and vitamin E. Zinc supplementation had no effect on viral load (assessed in a subset of 100 participants), gestational weight gain, or mother-to-child transmission (MTCT) (Villamor et al., 2006). T-lymphocyte subsets and birth outcomes were also similar between treatment groups (Fawzi et al., 2005). Women receiving zinc were more likely to become wasted during the observation period, defined as a mid-upper arm circumference (MUAC) < 22 cm, and had lower MUAC during the second trimester of pregnancy (Villamor et al., 2006). In both treatment groups, hemoglobin concentration increased from baseline to six weeks postpartum; however, the change in hemoglobin was significantly lower among women supplemented with zinc ($p = 0.03$) (Fawzi et al., 2005).

Antiretroviral Therapy

Among adults in Italy with stage 3 and 4 HIV ($n = 57$), daily zinc supplementation of 200 mg for 30 days was associated with increased CD4 cell counts, increased thymulin levels, and reduced opportunistic infections compared with placebo (Mocchegiani et al., 1995). Zinc was also associated with patient weight gain or stabilization. All study participants also received zidovudine.

Heterogeneous or Unspecified ART

An RCT in the United States included 231 adults with HIV and low plasma zinc (<0.75 mg/L) (Baum et al., 2010). Study participants were assigned to either daily elemental zinc (12 mg for women and 15 mg for men) or placebo for 18 months. Zinc supplementation was associated with reduced immunological failure (defined as reaching a CD4 cell count < 200 cells/mm^3) and a lower rate of diarrhea. Mortality did not differ between treatment groups (Baum et al., 2010). Two studies examined the effects of zinc supplementation among people with HIV and CD4 cell count < 200 cells/mm^3 (Green et al., 2005; Asdamongkol et al., 2013). Among 66 adults in Singapore, daily zinc supplementation (220 mg zinc sulfate for 28 days) had no effect on T-lymphocyte subsets, thymic T-cell generation, or immune response to tuberculosis (Green et al., 2005). A randomized trial in Thailand observed that six months of daily zinc supplementation (15 mg chelated zinc) increased CD4 cell count among patients with low baseline plasma zinc (Asdamongkol et al., 2013).

TABLE 5.1
Trials of Zinc Supplementation in Adults and Children with HIV Infection

Reference	Location	Sample	Design	Results
Zazzo et al. (1989)	France	5 adults with AIDS-related complex	Trial without control group; 45 mg zinc gluconate every 8 hours for 15 days, and 15 mg every 8 hours for the following 8 days	Increased lymphocyte activation and improved phagocytic function
Isa et al. (1992)	Italy	11 adult drug users with AIDS	Trial without control group; 1 mg elemental zinc per kg as zinc sulfate daily for 10 weeks	Slight increase in CD4 cell count; Progressive weight gain
Reich and Church (1994)	United States	13 HIV-infected children	Trial without control group; 200 mg zinc sulfate (45.5 mg elemental zinc) daily for 1 month	No effect on CD4 cell count
Mocchegiani et al. (1995)	Italy	57 adults on AZT monotherapy	Randomized trial with partial blinding; 200 mg zinc sulfate daily for 30 days vs. zinc-untreated	Increased CD4 cell count and decreased infectious morbidity; Body weight gain or stabilization and increased active thymulin levels
Fawzi et al. (2005); Villamor et al. (2006)	Tanzania	400 pregnant women	Randomized controlled trial; 25 zinc as zinc sulfate daily from enrollment (between 12 and 27 weeks gestation) until 6 weeks postpartum vs. placebo	No effects on viral load, T-lymphocyte subsets, MTCT of HIV, or birth outcomes; Increased risk of wasting (RR = 2.7; 95% CI, 1.1–6.4; $p = 0.03$); Lower mid-upper arm circumference during the second trimester (mean difference = 4 mm; $p = 0.02$)
Bobat et al. (2005)	South Africa	96 HIV-infected children	Randomized controlled trial; 10 mg elemental zinc as zinc sulfate daily for 6 months vs. placebo	No effects on viral load, CD4 cell count, or hemoglobin concentration; Fewer occurrences of watery diarrhea ($p = 0.001$)
Green et al. (2005)	Singapore	66 adults	Randomized controlled trial; 50 mg elemental zinc as zinc sulfate daily for 28 days vs. placebo	No effects on CD4/8 cell levels, T-lymphocyte subsets, TREC, or viral load

Reference	Country	Population	Intervention	Findings
Deloria-Knoll et al. (2006)	United States	60 adult injection drug users	Randomized controlled trial; 6 × 50 mg zinc tablets delivered over 6 days vs. placebo	No effect on antibody response to vaccine
Range et al. (2006)	Tanzania	106 adults with tuberculosis	Randomized controlled trial; 45 mg elementary zinc as zinc gluconate for 2 months vs. placebo	No effect on viral load or CD4 cell count
Cárcamo et al. (2006)	Peru	159 adults with diarrhea ≥7 days	Randomized controlled trial; 100 mg elemental zinc as zinc sulfate daily for 14 days vs. placebo	No effect on duration of diarrhea
Baum et al. (2010)	United States	231 adults with low plasma zinc	Randomized controlled trial; 12 mg elemental zinc for women and 15 mg for men daily for 18 months vs. placebo	Reduced immunological failure (defined as CD4 count < 200 cells/mm^3 (RR = 0.24; 95% CI, 0.1–0.56; p < 0.002) Reduced diarrhea (OR = 0.4, 95% CI, 0.183–0.981; p = 0.02) No effect on mortality
Srinivasan et al. (2012)	Uganda	55 HIV-infected children with severe pneumonia	Randomized controlled trial; 20 mg zinc as zinc gluconate for children ≥ 12 months and 10 mg for those < 12 months daily for 7 days vs. placebo	Decreased risk of pneumonia fatality (RR = 0.1, 95% CI, 0.0–1.0)
Asdamongkol et al. (2013)	Thailand	31 adults	Pilot study with randomized controlled trial phase; 15 mg chelated zinc daily for 6 months vs. placebo	Increased CD4 cell count among those with low plasma zinc (p = 0.04)
Lodha et al. (2014)	India	52 HIV-infected children initiating HAART	Randomized controlled trial; 20 mg elemental zinc as zinc sulfate daily for 24 weeks vs. placebo	No effects on CD4%, viral load, anthropometric indicators, or infectious morbidity

Note: AZT, azidothymidine; CI, confidence interval; HAART, highly active antiretroviral therapy; MTCT, mother-to-child transmission; OR, odds ratio; RR, risk ratio; TREC, T-cell receptor excision circle.

TABLE 5.2
Trials of Selenium Supplementation in Adults and Children with HIV Infection

Reference	Location	Sample	Design	Results
Zazzo et al. (1988)	France	10 adults with AIDS and cardiomyopathy	Trial without control group; 800 µg sodium selenite daily for 15 days and 400 µg daily for 8 days	Normalization of left ventricular function among participants with low plasma selenium
Olmstead et al. (1989)	United States	50 adults with AIDS or AIDS-related complex	Trial without control group; 400 µg selenium as selenium yeast daily for 70 days	Increased whole blood selenium
Delmas-Beauvieux et al. (1996); Constans et al. (1996, 1998)	France	37 adults (participant number varied among articles)	Randomized trial; 250 µg l-selenomethionine (100 µg selenium) daily for 1 year vs. placebo	Increased glutathione peroxidase activity between 3 and 6 months ($p < 0.04$)
				Improved glutathione status after 12 months ($p < 0.001$)
				No effect on CD4 cell counts
				Improved oxidative stress markers
				Prevention of endothelial damage (indicated by stable thrombomodulin and von Willebrand factor)
Look et al. (1998)	Germany	24 adults	Randomized controlled trial; 500 mg selenium daily plus 600 mg N-acetylcysteine t.i.d. for either 24 or 12 weeks	Increased CD4/CD8 after 6 and 12 weeks of treatment ($p = 0.02$ and $p = 0.04$, respectively)
				No effects on glutathione peroxidase activity or plasma glutathione concentration
Burbano et al. (2002)	United States	186 adults	Randomized controlled trial; 200 µg selenium daily for 2 years vs. placebo	Reduced risk of hospitalization (RR = 0.38; $p = 0.002$)
Shor-Posner et al. (2003)	United States	115 adults with past or current drug use	Randomized controlled trial; 200 µg selenium daily for 1 year vs. placebo	No effects on depression or distress
				Reduced state and trait anxiety ($p = 0.05$ and $p = 0.02$, respectively) and increased vigor ($p = 0.004$)
Hurwitz et al. (2007)	United States	262 adults	Randomized controlled trial; 200 µg selenium as high selenium yeast daily for 9 months vs. placebo	Greater CD4 cell count increase and smaller viral load increase ($p < 0.02$, for both) in selenium responders

Study	Country	Sample	Intervention	Results
Durosinmi et al. (2008)	Nigeria	32 adults	Randomized controlled trial; 200 μg selenium daily plus multivitamin containing vitamins A, C, D, and B-complex with 300 mg aspirin 4 to 6 times daily for 6 months vs. without aspirin	Increased weight in both groups; Trend toward increased CD4 in both groups
Kupka et al. (2008, 2009); Sudfeld et al. (2014)	Tanzania	913 pregnant women	Randomized controlled trial; 200 μg selenium as selenomethionine daily from enrollment (12–27 weeks gestation) to 6 months postpartum (vs. placebo)	No significant effects on low birth weight (RR = 0.71; 95% CI, 0.49–1.05; $p = 0.09$), fetal death (RR = 1.58; 95% CI, 0.95–2.63; $p = 0.08$), or maternal mortality (RR = 1.02; 95% CI, 0.51–2.04; $p = 0.96$); Reduced child mortality after 6 weeks (RR = 0.43; 95% CI, 0.19–0.99; $p = 0.048$); No effect on maternal hemoglobin concentration; Reduced maternal diarrheal morbidity (RR = 0.60; 95% CI, 0.42–0.84; $p = 0.003$); Increased risk of detectable HIV-1 RNA in breast milk among women not receiving HAART (RR = 1.37; 95% CI, 1.03–1.82; $p = 0.03$)
Mansouri et al. (2011)	Iran	52 adults	Controlled trial; 200 μg selenium daily for 6 months vs. placebo	No effect on CD4 cell counts
Baum et al. (2013)	Botswana	439 adults	Randomized controlled trial; 200 μg selenium daily for 24 months vs. placebo	No effect on CD4 cell count, viral load, or disease progression
Kamwesiga et al. (2011)	Rwanda	300 adults	Randomized controlled trial; 200 μg selenium daily for 24 months vs. placebo	Reduced rate of CD4 cell count decline (43.8% reduction) (95% CI, 7.8–79.8); No effect on viral suppression

Note: CI, confidence interval; HAART, highly active antiretroviral therapy; RR, risk ratio; t.i.d., three times a day.

TABLE 5.3

Trials of Vitamin C and/or E Supplementation in Adults and Children with HIV Infection

Reference	Location	Sample	Design	Results
Allard et al. (1998)	Canada	49 adults	Randomized controlled trial of vitamins C and E; 800 IU α-tocopherol acetate plus 1000 mg vitamin C daily for 3 months vs. placebo	Reduced biomarkers of lipid peroxidation (breath pentane, $p < 0.025$; plasma lipid peroxides, $p < 0.01$; malondialdehyde, $p < 0.0005$) Trend toward reduced viral load
McComsey et al. (2003)	United States	10 adults	Trial without control group; 800 IU vitamin E, 1000 mg vitamin C, and 1200 mg N-acetylcysteine daily for 24 weeks	No significant changes in anthropometry; trend toward decreased waist-to-hip ratio (from 0.94 ± 0.06 at baseline to 0.92 ± 0.05 at endline; $p = 0.05$) Increased fasting glucose (from 84 ± 11 to 110 ± 21 mg/dL; $p = 0.017$) and HOMA-IR (from 2.75 ± 2.69 to 7.20 ± 5.77; $p = 0.03$)
de Souza et al. (2005)	Brazil	29 adults	Controlled trial; 800 mg α-tocopherol daily for 180 days vs. placebo	Greater increase in viable lymphocytes (2.49-fold increase vs. 1.95-fold increase in placebo group; $p = 0.047$) Greater reduction of lymphocytes in apoptosis ($p = 0.03$) No differences in HIV RNA or CD4 cell count between groups

Note: HOMA-IR, homeostatic model assessment of insulin resistance.

Among 106 adults with sputum-positive pulmonary tuberculosis (TB) and HIV co-infection in Tanzania, daily supplementation with 45 mg elemental zinc had no effect on viral load or CD4 cell count after two months (Range et al., 2006). In Peru, 159 adults with HIV who had experienced diarrhea for ≥7 days were randomly assigned to receive either 100 mg zinc or placebo daily for two weeks (Cárcamo et al., 2006). Loss to follow-up was high (>30%) but similar between treatment groups. Zinc supplementation had no effect on diarrhea duration. A trial in the United States randomized 60 adult intravenous drug users to receive either zinc (six tablets of 50-mg zinc gluconate delivered over six days) or placebo before being immunized with a pneumococcal conjugate vaccine. Zinc had no effect on antibody response to the vaccine (Deloria-Knoll et al., 2006).

ART-Naïve

Two small trials without control groups observed the benefits of zinc supplementation among adults with AIDS (Zazzo et al., 1989) and AIDS-related complex (Isa et al., 1992). In France, five adults supplemented with zinc daily for 30 days showed signs of immune recovery, including stimulation of lymphocytes and peripheral mononuclear cell chemiluminescence (Zazzo et al. 1989). Among 11 adult drug users with AIDS in Italy, zinc supplementation for 10 weeks was associated with increased CD4 cell count and weight gain (Isa et al., 1992).

Children

Trials in the United States, South Africa, Uganda, and India have investigated the effects of zinc supplementation among children with HIV infection (Reich and Church, 1994; Bobat et al., 2005; Srinivasan et al., 2012; Lodha et al., 2014). A study in the United States provided 45.5 mg elemental zinc to 13 children with HIV, daily for one month. In this non-controlled trial, zinc supplementation had no association with changes in CD4 cell count (Reich and Church, 1994). In South Africa, 96 children between the ages of 6 and 60 months were assigned to either daily zinc supplementation (10 mg of elemental zinc as zinc sulfate) or placebo. Zinc supplementation for six months had no effects on viral load, CD4 cell count, or hemoglobin concentration; however, children receiving zinc had significantly fewer occurrences of diagnosed watery diarrhea (Bobat et al., 2005).

A study in Uganda recruited HIV-infected and HIV-uninfected children (ages 6 to 59 months) with severe pneumonia. Study participants were assigned daily zinc as zinc gluconate (doses were 20 mg for children ≥ 12 months and 10 mg for children < 12 months) or placebo for seven days. All children also received antibiotics for pneumonia. Zinc supplementation had no effect on primary study outcomes (time until normalization of respiration rate, temperature, and oxygen saturation) but was associated with decreased risk of fatality (Srinivasan et al., 2012). It should be noted that death was a secondary outcome in this study. One study assessed the effects of daily zinc supplementation for 24 weeks among 52 children ages > 6 months that were newly initiating highly active ART (HAART). Children who received zinc (20 mg elemental zinc as zinc sulfate) and placebo had similar CD4%, viral load, anthropometric indicators, and morbidities (Lodha et al., 2014).

Selenium

Pregnant Women

In Tanzania, pregnant women with HIV were recruited between 12 and 27 weeks gestation ($n = 913$) and randomized to receive either 200 μg selenium (as selenomethionine) daily or a placebo supplement (Kupka et al., 2008, 2009). Treatment was initiated at enrollment and continued until six months postpartum. Study participants were also receiving daily antenatal supplements and multiple micronutrient supplements containing B-vitamin complex, vitamin C, and vitamin E. A small proportion of study participants ($n = 31$) were prescribed HAART during follow-up. Selenium supplementation was associated with a 40% reduced risk of diarrhea (Kupka et al., 2009). Treatment groups had similar average hemoglobin concentration and non-diarrhea morbidities (Kupka et al., 2009). Overall, selenium had no effect on maternal CD4 cell count, viral load, mortality risk, or birth outcomes (birthweight, small-for-gestational age, premature birth, and neonatal mortality) (Kupka et al. (2008). Although not statistically significant, selenium supplementation was associated with lower risk of low birthweight (risk ratio [RR], 0.71; 95% CI, 0.49–1.05; $p = 0.09$) and increased risk of fetal death (RR, 1.58; 95% CI, 0.95–2.63; $p = 0.08$) (Kupka et al., 2008). A reduced risk of child mortality after six weeks postpartum was observed in the treatment group (Kupka et al., 2008). In the same trial, the effect of selenium supplementation on HIV shedding in breast milk was also examined (Sudfeld et al., 2014). Selenium supplementation was marginally associated with an increased risk of having detectable HIV-1 RNA among the total cohort (RR, 1.32; 95% CI, 1.00–1.76; $p = 0.05$); the association was statistically significant in a subgroup analysis of women not receiving HAART (RR, 1.37; 95% CI, 1.03–1.82; $p = 0.03$) (Sudfeld et al., 2014).

Heterogeneous or Unspecified ART

A study in the United States investigated the effect of selenium supplementation (200 µg/day) on 186 men and women with HIV admitted to a hospital. Participants in the selenium group had significantly reduced risk of hospital admission over the two-year study duration (Burbano et al., 2002). Another selenium trial in the United States randomized 262 adults with HIV into supplementation (200 µg of high-selenium yeast daily) and placebo groups (Hurwitz et al., 2007). Treatment duration was 18 months, and increased selenium concentration as a result of supplementation was protective against HIV progression. Specifically, selenium responders (those with a >26.1 µg/L improvement in serum selenium) had less viral load increase and increased improvement in CD4 cell count compared to non-responders and to participants in the placebo group (Hurwitz et al., 2007).

In a substudy that included 115 adults with HIV that were identified as past or current drug users, the effects of selenium supplementation (200 µg/day) on psychological measures were examined (Shor-Posner et al., 2003). Participants supplemented with selenium for 12 months reported less anxiety and increased vigor, according to the Spielberger State–Trait Anxiety Inventory (STAI)–Form Y questionnaire, compared to participants in the placebo group. However, both groups receiving treatment or placebo were experiencing similar depression and distress based on the Beck Depression Inventory (BDI) and the Profile of Mood States (POMS) measures (Shor-Posner et al., 2003).

In France, adults with HIV and CD4 cell counts < 400 cells/mm^3 were assigned to receive selenium ($n = 15$), placebo ($n = 22$), or β-carotene (Constans et al., 1998). Participants in the selenium group received 250 µg selenomethionine (100 µg selenium) daily for one year. Pilot data indicated that selenium had no effect on CD4 cell counts but was associated with an improvement in measures of oxidative stress (Constans et al., 1996). Participants receiving selenium showed increased glutathione peroxidase activity—the main enzyme involved in scavenging reactive oxygen species and maintaining oxidative balance—and glutathione status, but supplementation had no effect on super-oxidase dismutase activity ($n = 14$ and $n = 18$ for the intervention and placebo groups, respectively) (Delmas-Beauvieux et al., 1996). In another article, it was reported that selenium supplementation had a protective effect against endothelial damage (Constans et al., 1998). Non-supplemented participants showed evidence of endothelial damage (increased thrombomodulin and von Willebrand factor), whereas endothelial damage indicators in the selenium group remained relatively stable over the year of supplementation (Constans et al., 1998).

ART Naïve

A trial in Botswana randomized ART-naïve adults to receive multivitamins with or without selenium, selenium alone ($n = 220$), or placebo ($n = 219$) (Baum et al., 2013). Selenium supplementation of 200 µg/day for 24 months had no effect on CD4 cell count, viral load, or disease progression (Baum et al., 2013). In Rwanda, 300 ART-naïve adults with HIV and CD4 cell counts between 400 and 650 cells/mm^3 were randomized to receive either 200 µg selenium daily for 24 months or placebo (Kamwesiga et al., 2011). Participants in the intervention group had a 43.8% reduction in CD4 cell count decline compared to the placebo group (95% CI, 7.8–79.8), but no other effects were observed (Kamwesiga et al., 2011).

A pilot trial of antioxidant supplementation with 500 μg/day sodium selenite and 1800 mg/day N-acetylcysteine (NAC) was performed among adults with HIV using a partial cross-over design (Look et al., 1998). NAC/selenium supplementation was significantly associated with an increased CD4/8 ratio at 6 and 12 weeks of treatment and was marginally associated with increased CD4% at 6 weeks ($p = 0.08$). No effects of NAC/selenium on glutathione peroxidase activity or plasma glutathione concentrations were observed (Look et al., 1998).

Two trials without control groups observed health improvements among people living with AIDS following selenium supplementation (Zazzo et al., 1988; Olmsted et al., 1989). In a small study in France, 10 adults with AIDS and cardiomyopathy were supplemented with daily selenium for 23 days (Zazzo et al., 1988). Participants received 800 μg sodium selenite daily for the first 15 days and 400 μg sodium selenite for the remaining eight days. Of the eight participants with low baseline selenium status, six showed improvement in left ventricular function after 21 days (Zazzo et al., 1988). In the United States, 19 adults with AIDS or AIDS-related complex received 400 μg selenium as selenium yeast for up to 70 days (Olmsted et al., 1989). Average whole blood selenium concentration increased following 70 days of supplementation (baseline mean ± SD, 0.142 + 0.040; endline, 0.280 + 0.08 μg/mL) (Olmsted et al., 1989).

In Iran, a trial with a 2×2 factorial design examined the effects of selenium supplementation and treatment with levamisole (an antihelminthic) on CD4 cell counts among adults with HIV and baseline CD4 < 350 cells/mm^3 who were not taking antiretroviral drugs (Mansouri et al., 2011). Daily supplementation with 200 μg selenium for six months had no effect on CD4 cell counts ($n = 17$ and $n = 35$ for the selenium and placebo groups, respectively) (Mansouri et al., 2011).

Other Outcomes

The Breastfeeding, Antiretroviral, and Nutrition (BAN) study was a trial conducted in Malawi among lactating women with HIV and included three treatment arms: (1) lipid-based nutrient supplements (LNS) containing sodium selenite, (2) ART, and (3) LNS and ART, as well as a control (Chasela et al., 2010). In a substudy, selenium was measured in maternal plasma and breast milk at two time points, either at 2 and 24 weeks ($n = 358$) or at 6 and 24 weeks ($n = 168$) postpartum. Changes in plasma and breast milk selenium concentrations were similar between treatment groups (Flax et al., 2014).

Vitamins C and E

Heterogeneous or Unspecified ART

In Canada, 49 adults with HIV on heterogeneous ART were randomized to receive either a combination vitamin C and E supplement, consisting of 800 IU α-tocopherol acetate plus 1000 mg vitamin C daily for three months, or placebo (Allard et al., 1998). Supplementation with vitamins C and E significantly decreased biomarkers of lipid peroxidation (breath pentane, $p < 0.025$; plasma lipid peroxides, $p < 0.01$; malondialdehyde, $p < 0.0005$). Mean viral load increased in the placebo group (increase of 0.50 ± 0.40 log$_{10}$ copies/mL) and decreased in the vitamins C and E group (decrease of 0.45 ± 0.39 log$_{10}$ copies/mL) following three months of supplementation (95% CI, -0.21 to -2.14; $p = 0.1$). In Brazil, 29 adults with HIV were assigned to receive either 800 mg α-tocopherol daily for 180 days or placebo; all patients were ART naïve prior to study entry and thereafter received heterogeneous ART (de Souza et al., 2005). Plasma levels of HIV-1 RNA decreased significantly ($p = 0.0001$) after 120 days of treatment. CD4+ counts increased significantly ($p = 0.0002$) for both the vitamin C-supplemented and control groups; however, no difference between the groups was observed (de Souza et al., 2005).

Antiretroviral Therapy

In the United States, 10 adults with HIV and either lipoatrophy or sustained hyperlactatemia participated in a non-controlled pilot trial of antioxidant supplementation (vitamins C and E plus NAC) (McComsey et al. (2003). All participants were receiving nucleoside reverse transcriptase inhibitor

(NRTI)-containing ART for at least one year. Supplementation was not significantly associated with any changes in anthropometric measures, although there was a trend toward decreased waist-to-hip ratio (from 0.94 ± 0.06 at baseline to 0.92 ± 0.05 at endline; $p = 0.05$). Average fasting glucose and homeostatic model assessment of insulin resistance (HOMA-IR) increased from baseline to 24 weeks (fasting glucose: 84 ± 11 to 110 ± 21 mg/dL, $p = 0.017$; HOMA: 2.75 ± 2.69 to 7.20 ± 5.77, $p = 0.03$).

DISCUSSION

This review examined the evidence regarding antioxidant supplementation in adults and children living with HIV. Overall, there is insufficient evidence to support blanket supplementation with antioxidant micronutrients in this population. Clinical trials of antioxidant micronutrients, alone or in combination, among people with HIV infection have yielded mostly null results, with a few studies observing mild benefits of supplementation with zinc (Zazzo et al., 1989; Isa et al., 1992; Bobat et al., 2005; Mocchegiani et al., 1995; Baum et al., 2010; Srinivasan et al., 2012; Asdamongkol et al., 2013) and selenium (Olmsted et al., 1989; Costans et al., 1996, 1998; Look et al., 1998; Zazzo et al., 1988; Kamwesiga et al., 2001; Burbano et al., 2002; Shor-Posner et al., 2003; Hurwitz et al., 2007; Kupka et al., 2009). It is likely that the effectiveness of antioxidant supplementation depends upon individual micronutrient status. Results from a selenium supplementation study suggest that HIV-infected people with deficiencies would benefit from supplementation to the point of becoming replete (Hurwitz et al., 2007). Furthermore, there is no evidence of adverse effects from supplementation with vitamins C and E, zinc, or selenium among people with HIV.

Despite a reasonable biological plausibility argument, results from antioxidant supplementation trials have been mostly disappointing. Laboratory evidence suggests that chronic oxidative stress not only impedes immune function by compromising T- and B-cell growth and function but also increases HIV replication (Hosein, 1997; Srinivas and Dias, 2008). It has been hypothesized by several authors that supplementation with antioxidant micronutrients could combat oxidative damage and slow the progression of HIV, among other benefits (Baruchel and Wainberg, 1992; Pace and Leaf, 1995; Tang et al., 2000; Jaruga et al., 2002; Srinivas and Dias, 2008; Kaio et al., 2013). One study found that among HIV-infected patients supplementation with vitamins A, C, and E resulted in decreased levels of modified DNA bases and partially restored antioxidant enzymes (superoxide dismutase and catalase) (Jaruga et al., 2002). However, antioxidant supplementation in human trials for the mitigation of HIV symptoms has shown little effect. Possible explanations for this lack of effect include that the efficacy of antioxidant supplementation may depend on the baseline serum levels of other micronutrients and that co-infections or other factors may mask the outcomes being studied. Additionally, many of these interventions were administered alongside other micronutrients, which may have impacted the effect of the micronutrient in question—for example, vitamins C and E were administered in the same micronutrient dose in several studies, sometimes also along with zinc (Allard et al., 1998; Fawzi et al., 2005; Villamor et al., 2006). Finally, it is possible that the micronutrient doses administered in previous studies were not optimal or were too low to effect outcomes among individuals with increased antioxidant demands due to chronic HIV infection (Stephenson et al., 2006).

An important limitation of this research is the relative absence of consistent functional outcomes to evaluate the potential effects of antioxidant supplementation. For example, potential functional indexes for zinc repletion include wound healing, taste acuity, and visual adaptation to the dark; however, these outcomes are not an exclusive result of zinc status (WHO and FAO, 2004). A recent review (King et al., 2016) identified plasma zinc concentration and serum zinc concentration as biomarkers of dietary zinc status and height for age (or stunting) as a functional indicator of zinc deficiency in populations, which will be useful in future zinc intervention studies involving children with HIV. Serum biomarkers for vitamins C and E include plasma ascorbate for vitamin C, and plasma α-tocopherol as well as α-tocopherol transport protein and γ-tocopherol for vitamin E, as assessed in one study of adolescents and young adults living with HIV (Stephensen et al., 2006). However, there are no widely recommended biomarkers for the accurate assessment of vitamins C or E. Finally, the outcomes measured varied across studies and included anthropometry, immune function, and survival.

FUTURE DIRECTIONS AND CONCLUSIONS

Although this review found no overall beneficial effect of vitamin C, vitamin E, selenium, and zinc supplementation on HIV/AIDS outcomes, correcting micronutrient deficiencies can improve health and quality of life. The lack of effect during micronutrient intervention trials may be due to several factors, which could be addressed in future research. In environments of food insecurity, particularly in low-income countries, an intervention utilizing micronutrient supplements alone may not have a large enough benefit for those who are energy or protein malnourished. There are also limitations with assessing impact, given the lack of reliable biomarkers or functional outcomes associated with the nutrients discussed in this chapter.

REFERENCES

Allard, J. P., E. Aghdassi, J. Chau et al. (1998). Effects of vitamin E and C supplementation on oxidative stress and viral load in HIV-infected subjects. *AIDS* 12(13): 1653–9.

Asdamongkol, N., P. Phanachet, and S. Sungkanuparph. (2013). Low plasma zinc levels and immunological responses to zinc supplementation in HIV-infected patients with immunological discordance after antiretroviral therapy. *Japanese Journal of Infectious Diseases* 66(6): 469–74.

Baruchel, S. and M. A. Wainberg. (1992). The role of oxidative stress in disease progression in individuals infected by the human immunodeficiency virus. *Journal of Leukocyte Biology* 52(1): 111–4.

Baum, M. K., S. Lai, S. Sales, J. B. Page, and A. Campa. (2010). Randomized, controlled clinical trial of zinc supplementation to prevent immunological failure in HIV-infected adults. *Clinical Infectious Diseases* 50(12):1653–60.

Baum, M. K., A. Campa, S. Lai et al. (2013). Effect of micronutrient supplementation on disease progression in asymptomatic, antiretroviral-naive, HIV-infected adults in Botswana: a randomized clinical trial. *JAMA* 310(20): 2154–63.

Bobat, R., H. Coovadia, C. Stephen et al. (2005). Safety and efficacy of zinc supplementation for children with HIV-1 infection in South Africa: a randomised double-blind placebo-controlled trial. *The Lancet* 366(9500): 1862–7.

Burbano, X., M. J. Miquez-Burban, K. McCollister et al. (2002). Impact of a selenium chemoprevention clinical trial on hospital admissions of HIV-infected participants. *HIV Clinical Trials* 3(6): 483–91.

Cárcamo, C., T. Hooton, N. S. Weiss et al. (2006). Randomized controlled trial of zinc supplementation for persistent diarrhea in adults with HIV-1 infection. *Journal of Acquired Immune Deficiency Syndromes* 43(2): 197–201.

Chasela, C. S., M. G. Hudgens, D. J. Jamieson et al.; BAN Study Group. (2010). Maternal or infant antiretroviral drugs to reduce HIV-1 transmission. *New England Journal of Medicine* 362: 2271–81.

Constans, J., M. C. Delmas-Beauvieux, C. Sergeant et al. (1996). One-year antioxidant supplementation with β-carotene or selenium for patients infected with human immunodeficiency virus: a pilot study. *Clinical Infectious Diseases* 23(3): 654–6.

Constans, J., M. Seigneur, A. Blann et al. (1998). Effect of the antioxidants selenium and beta-carotene on HIV-related endothelium dysfunction. *Thrombosis and Haemostatis* 80(6): 1015–7.

de Souza, J. O., A. Treitinger, G. L. Baggio et al. (2005). alpha-Tocopherol as an antiretroviral therapy supplement for HIV-1-infected patients for increased lymphocyte viability. *Clinical Chemistry and Laboratory Medicine* 43(4): 376–82.

Delmas-Beauvieux, M.-C., E. Peuchant, A. Couchouron et al. (1996). The enzymatic antioxidant system in blood and glutathione status in human immunodeficiency virus (HIV)-infected patients: effects of supplementation with selenium or beta-carotene. *American Journal of Clinical Nutrition* 64(1): 101–7.

Deloria-Knoll, M., M. Steinhoff, R. D. Semba, K. Nelson, D. Vlahov, and C. L. Meinert. (2006). Effect of zinc and vitamin A supplementation on antibody responses to a pneumococcal conjugate vaccine in HIV-positive injection drug users: a randomized trial. *Vaccine* 24(10): 1670–9.

Durosinmi, M. A., H. Armistead, N. O. Akinola et al. (2008). Selenium and aspirin in people living with HIV and AIDS in Nigeria. *Niger Postgraduate Medical Journal* 15(4): 215–8.

Fawzi, W. W., E. Villamor, G. I. Msamanga et al. (2005). Trial of zinc supplements in relation to pregnancy outcomes, hematologic indicators, and T cell counts among HIV-1-infected women in Tanzania. *American Journal of Clinical Nutrition* 81(1): 161–7.

Flax, V. L., M. E. Bentley, G. F. Combs, Jr. et al. (2014). Plasma and breast-milk selenium in HIV-infected Malawian mothers are positively associated with infant selenium status but are not associated with maternal supplementation: results of the Breastfeeding, Antiretrovirals, and Nutrition study. *American Journal of Clinical Nutrition* 99(4): 950–6.

Green, J. A., S. R. Lewin, F.Wightman, M. Lee, T. S. Ravindran, and N. I. Paton. (2005). A randomised controlled trial of oral zinc on the immune response to tuberculosis in HIV-infected patients. *International Journal of Tuberculosis and Lung Disease* 9(12): 1378–84.

Hosein. S. (1997). HIV and antioxidants. *Treatment Update* (7): 7.

Hurwitz, B. E., J. R. Klaus, M. M. Llabre et al. (2007). Suppression of human immunodeficiency virus type 1 viral load with selenium supplementation: a randomized controlled trial. *Archives of Internal Medicine* 167(2): 148–154.

Isa, L., A. Lucchini, S. Lodi, and M. Giachetti. (1992). Blood zinc status and zinc treatment in human immunodeficiency virus-infected patients. *International Journal of Clinical and Laboratory Research* 22(1): 45–7.

Jaruga, P., B. Jaruga, D. Gackowski et al. (2002). Supplementation with antioxidant vitamins prevents HIV-infected patients. *Free Radical Biology & Medicine* 32(5): 414–20.

Kaio D. J., P. H. Rondó, J. M. Souza, A. V. Firmino, L. A. Luzia, and A. A. Segurado. (2013). Vitamin A and beta-carotene concentrations in adults with HIV/AIDS on highly active antiretroviral therapy. *Journal of Nutritonal Science and Vitaminology* 59(6): 496–502.

Kamwesiga, J., V. Mutabazi, J. Kayumba et al. (2011). Effect of selenium supplementation on CD4 T-cell recovery, viral suppression, morbidity and quality of life of HIV-infected patients in Rwanda: study protocol for a randomized controlled trial. *Trials* 12:192.

King J. C., K. H. Brown, R. S. Gibson et al. (2016). Biomarkers of nutrition for development (BOND)—zinc review. *Journal of Nutrition* 146(4): 858S–85S.

Kupka, R., F. Mugusi, S. Aboud et al. (2008). Randomized, double-blind, placebo-controlled trial of selenium supplements among HIV-infected pregnant women in Tanzania: effects on maternal and child outcomes. *American Journal of Clinical Nutrition* 87(6): 1802–8.

Kupka, R., F. Mugusi, S. Aboud, E. Hertzmark, D. Spiegelman, and W. W. Fawzi. (2009). Effect of selenium supplements on hemoglobin concentration and morbidity among HIV-1-infected Tanzanian women. *Clinical Infectious Diseases* 48(10): 1475–8.

Lodha, R., N. Shah, N. Mohari et al. (2014). Immunologic effect of zinc supplementation in HIV infected children receiving highly active antiretroviral therapy: a randomized, double blind placebo controlled trial. *Journal of Acquired Immune Deficiency Syndromes* 66(4): 386–92.

Look, M., J. Rockstroh, G. Rao et al. (1998). Sodium selenite and N-acetylcysteine in antiretroviral-naive HIV-1-infected patients: a randomized, controlled pilot study. *European Journal of Clinical Investigation* 28(5): 389–97.

Mansouri, F., A. Janbakhsh, S. Vaziri et al. (2011). Comparative study of levamisole–selenium supplementation effect on CD4 increase in HIV/AIDS patients. *Caspian Journal of Internal Medicine* 2(2): 218–21.

McComsey, G., H. Southwell, B. Gripshover, R. Salata, and H. Valdez. (2003). Effect of antioxidants on glucose metabolism and plasma lipids in HIV-infected subjects with lipoatrophy. *Journal of Acquired Immune Deficiency Syndromes* 33(5): 605–7.

Mocchegiani, E., S. Veccia, F. Ancarani, G. Scalise, and N. Fabris. (1995). Benefit of oral zinc supplementation as an adjunct to zidovudine (AZT) therapy against opportunistic infections in AIDS. *International Journal of Immunopharmacology* 17(9): 719–27.

Olmsted, L., G. N. Schrauzer, M. Flores-Arce, and J. Dowd. (1989). Selenium supplementation of symptomatic human immunodeficiency virus infected patients. *Biological Trace Element Research* 20(1–2): 59–65.

Pace, G. W. and C. D. Leaf. (1995). The role of oxidative stress in HIV disease. *Free Radical Biology and Medicine* 19(4): 523–8.

Range, N., J. Changalucha, H. Krarup, P. Magnussen, A. B. Andersen, and H. Friis. (2006). The effect of multi-vitamin/mineral supplementation on mortality during treatment of pulmonary tuberculosis: a randomised two-by-two factorial trial in Mwanza, Tanzania. *British Journal of Nutrition* 95(4): 762–70.

Reich, E. and J. Church. (1994). Oral zinc supplementation in the treatment of HIV-infected children. *Pediatric AIDS and HIV Infection* 5(6): 357–60.

Semba, R. D. and A. M. Tang. (1999). Micronutrients and the pathogenesis of human immunodeficiency virus infection. *British Journal of Nutrition* 81(3): 181–9.

Shor-Posner, G., R. Lecusay, M. J. Miguez et al. (2003). Psychological burden in the era of HAART: impact of selenium therapy. *International Journal of Psychiatry in Medicine* 33(1): 55–69.

Srinivas A. and B. F. Dias. (2008). Antioxidants in HIV positive children. *Indian Journal of Pediatriacs* 75(4): 347–50.

Srinivasan, M. G., G. Ndeezi, C. K. Mboijana et al. (2012). Zinc adjunct therapy reduces case fatality in severe childhood pneumonia: a randomized double blind placebo-controlled trial. *BMC Medicine* 10: 14.

Stephensen C. B., G. S. Marquis, R. A. Jacob, L. A. Kruzich, S. D. Douglas, and C. M. Wilson. (2006). Vitamins C and E in adolescents and young adults with HIV infection. *American Journal of Clinical Nutrition* 83(4): 870–9.

Sudfeld, C. R., S. Aboud, R. Kupka, F. M. Mugusi, and W. W. Fawzi. (2014). Effect of selenium supplementation on HIV-1 RNA detection in breast milk of Tanzanian women. *Nutrition* 30(9): 1081–4.

Tang A. M., E. Smit, R. D. Semba et al. (2000). Improved antioxidant status among HIV-infected injecting drug users on potent antiretroviral therapy. *Journal of Acquired Immune Deficiency Syndromes* 23(4): 321–6.

UNAIDS. (2013). *Global Report: UNAIDS Report on the Global AIDS Epidemic 2013*. Geneva: Joint United Nations Programme on HIV/AIDS.

Villamor, E., S. Aboud, I. N. Koulinska et al. (2006). Zinc supplementation to HIV-1-infected pregnant women: effects on maternal anthropometry, viral load, and early mother-to-child transmission. *European Journal of Clinical Nutrition* 60(7): 862–9.

WHO and FAO. (2004). *Vitamin and Mineral Requirements in Human Nutrition*, 2nd ed. Geneva: World Health Organization, Food and Agriculture Organization of the United Nations.

Zazzo J. F., J. Chalas, A. Lafont, F. Camus, and P. Chappuis P. (1988). Is nonobstructive cardiomyopathy in AIDS a selenium deficiency-related disease? *Journal of Parenteral and Enteral Nutrition* 12(5): 537–8.

Zazzo, J. F., B. Rouveix, P. Rajagopalon, M. Levacher, and P. M. Girard. (1989). Effect of zinc on the immune status of zinc-depleted AIDS related complex patients. *Clinical Nutrition* 8(5): 259–61.

6 Micronutrients and Perinatal Outcomes in HIV-Infected Pregnant Women

Julia L. Finkelstein and Saurabh Mehta

CONTENTS

INTRODUCTION

MICRONUTRIENTS IN HIV-INFECTED PREGNANT WOMEN

HIV-infected pregnant women are at higher risk of both micronutrient deficiencies and adverse pregnancy outcomes. However, there are no specific World Health Organization (WHO) guidelines for micronutrient supplementation for HIV-infected pregnant women. The current guideline from 2003 is the same for pregnant women, irrespective of HIV status, stating that pending additional information, micronutrient intakes at the recommended dietary allowance (RDA) level are recommended for HIV-infected women during pregnancy and lactation. On one hand, multivitamin supplementation with vitamins B-complex, C, and E in HIV-infected pregnant women has been shown to reduce the risk of adverse pregnancy outcomes, such as fetal loss, low birthweight, small-for-gestational-age (SGA) infants, prematurity, and mother-to-child transmission (MTCT) of HIV. However, there are concerns regarding the safety and efficacy of other micronutrient supplements, and there is limited evidence in the context of antiretroviral therapy (ART), which may have adverse effects on nutritional status (Ivers et al., 2009). Therefore, in this chapter, we review the literature to examine the existing evidence, inform clinical care, and address the unique healthcare needs of HIV-infected pregnant women.

STANDARD OF CARE

Iron and folic acid supplementation is part of standard prenatal care for the prevention of anemia and neural tube defects (WHO, 2012). Current WHO guidelines recommend daily prenatal iron–folic acid supplements (60 mg iron and 400 μg folic acid) throughout pregnancy. Iron supplementation is recommended once daily to prevent anemia (hemoglobin [Hb] < 11.0 g/dL during the first and third trimesters and Hb < 10.5 g/dL during the second trimester), and twice daily for the treatment of severe anemia (Hb < 7.0 g/dL) (WHO, 2012). To date, there is limited evidence to suggest that the dose and administration of prenatal folic acid should differ in the context of HIV/AIDS. However, there is increasing concern regarding the safety and efficacy of iron supplementation in the context of HIV. Current WHO guidelines for universal prenatal iron supplementation do not differ in settings with endemic infectious diseases, and there are no specific guidelines for HIV-infected individuals. This is discussed in detail in Chapter 3 of this volume.

OBJECTIVES

In this review, we focus on the interplay of micronutrient deficiencies and HIV in the context of pregnancy. We begin with a brief review of the role of micronutrients in pregnancy in HIV-infected women. We then examine the efficacy and safety of micronutrient supplementation in HIV-infected pregnant women, including maternal, pregnancy, and neonatal outcomes, with an emphasis on evidence from randomized clinical trials. Finally, we discuss the implications of findings for clinical care and public health practice, with an emphasis on resource-limited settings.

METHODS

SEARCH STRATEGY AND SELECTION PROCESS

We conducted a structured literature search using the MEDLINE® and Cochrane Library electronic databases. Relevant Medical Subject Heading (MeSH®) terms were used to identify published studies through January 1, 2015. The MeSH terms used are shown in Figure 6.1, which summarizes the search strategy. All randomized trials of maternal micronutrient supplementation and perinatal outcomes in HIV-infected pregnant women were included. Initial inclusion criteria for this review were the availability of an abstract and the inclusion of data on micronutrient supplementation, pregnancy, and HIV/AIDS.

Micronutrient Supplementation

The following micronutrients were considered for inclusion in this review: vitamin A carotenoids; vitamins C, D, E, and K; vitamins B_1 (thiamine), B_2 (riboflavin), B_3 (niacin), B_5 (pantothenic acid), B_6 (pyridoxine), B_7 (biotin), B_9 (folic acid), and B_{12} (cobalamin); inositol; and minerals (boron, cadmium, calcium, chromium, cobalt, copper, iodine, iron, magnesium, manganese, molybdenum, nickel, selenium, silicon, vanadium, and zinc).

Outcomes

The following maternal, pregnancy, and neonatal outcomes were included in this review: (1) *maternal outcomes,* including all-cause and AIDS-related mortality, WHO HIV disease stage progression, opportunistic infections, CD4 and CD8 T-cell counts, HIV RNA viral load, HIV viral shedding, weight gain during pregnancy, anemia and micronutrient status, preeclampsia, and depression during pregnancy; (2) *pregnancy outcomes,* including miscarriage (<28 weeks gestation), stillbirth (≥28 weeks gestation), fetal loss (miscarriage or stillbirth), gestational age at delivery, preterm birth (<37 weeks gestation), birthweight, low birthweight (<2500 g), small-for-gestational age (birthweight < 10th percentile for gestational age), mother-to-child transmission of HIV, breast milk micronutrient

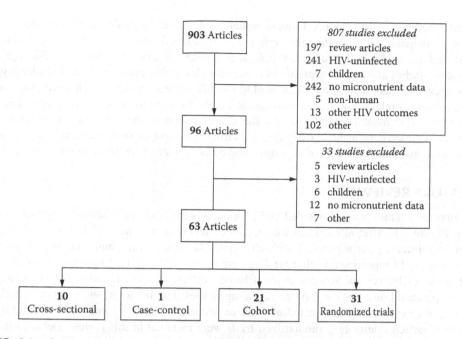

FIGURE 6.1. Study selection. Search terms: MeSH Terms: ("HIV" OR "HIV"[MeSH] OR "HIV Infections"[MeSH] OR "AIDS" OR "hiv" OR "hiv1" OR "hiv-1*" OR "hiv2" OR "hiv-2*" OR hiv infect* OR "human immunodeficiency virus" OR "human immunedeficiency virus" OR "human immune-deficiency virus" OR "human immuno-deficiency virus" OR "human immune deficiency virus" OR ((human immun*) AND (deficiency virus)) OR ((acquired immun*) AND (deficiency syndrome)) OR "acquired immunodeficiency syndrome" OR "acquired immunodeficiency syndrome"[MeSH] OR "acquired immunedeficiency syndrome" OR "acquired immune-deficiency syndrome") AND ("micronutrients" OR "micronutrients"[MeSH] OR "micronutrient" OR "trace element" OR "trace elements" OR "vitamins" OR "vitamin" OR "nutrition" OR "nutritional status" OR carotenoids OR carotenoid OR carotenes OR carotene OR "24,25-dihydroxyvitamin D 3" OR "25-hydroxyvitamin D 2" OR "4- aminobenzoic acid" OR acetylcarnitine OR alpha-tocopherol OR aminobenzoic acids OR ascorbic acid OR beta carotene OR beta-tocopherol OR biotin OR boron OR cadmium OR calcifediol OR calcitriol OR carnitine OR cholecalciferol OR chromium OR cobalt OR cobamides OR cod liver oil OR copper OR dehydroascorbic acid OR dihydrotachysterol OR dihydroxycholecalciferols OR ergocalciferols OR flavin mononucleotide OR folic acid OR formyltetrahydrofolates OR fursultiamin OR gamma-tocopherol OR hydroxocobalamin OR hydroxycholecalciferols OR inositol OR iodine OR iron OR leucovorin OR manganese OR magnesium OR molybdenum OR niacin OR niacinamide OR nickel OR nicorandil OR nicotinic acids OR palmitoylcarnitine OR pantothenic acid OR pteroylpolyglutamic acids OR pyridoxal OR pyridoxal phosphate OR pyridoxamine OR pyridoxine OR riboflavin OR selenium OR silicon OR tetrahydrofolates OR thiamine OR thiamine monophosphate OR thiamine pyrophosphate OR thiamine triphosphate OR thioctic acid OR tin OR tocopherols OR tocotrienols OR ubiquinone OR vanadium OR zinc) AND ("pregnancy" OR "pregnancy"[MeSH] OR "pregnant" OR pregnan* OR "gravidity" OR "gestation" OR "parturient" OR "pregnant women" OR "pregnant women"[MeSH] OR "maternal-fetal relations"[MeSH] OR "prenatal care"[MeSH])

composition, and mastitis; and (3) *infant outcomes*, including HIV infection, co-infections, and clinical symptoms (i.e., measles, respiratory infections, diarrhea, malaria); anthropometry and growth (i.e., weight, length, head circumference, and mid-upper arm circumference), including weight for age (WAZ), weight for length (WLZ), and length for age (LAZ) WHO z-scores (underweight, WAZ < –2; wasting, WLZ < –2; stunting, LAZ < –2); cognitive and psychomotor development; and anemia and micronutrient status.

Available abstracts of all studies were searched, full-text articles were extracted and reviewed, and the following inclusion criteria were applied: (1) human studies, (2) HIV-infected pregnant individuals, and (3) availability of data on maternal micronutrient supplementation, status, or intake and perinatal outcomes. All randomized, quasi-randomized, and uncontrolled trials and interventions that met participant and methodological criteria were included. Sources were retrieved, collected, indexed, and assessed for micronutrient supplementation and perinatal outcome data. Bibliographies of published studies and manual searches of related articles in references were used to identify additional sources. An additional search was used to identify review articles, which were examined for references to other relevant studies. A standardized table was used to extract and organize key information from experimental studies that met the abovementioned selection criteria. Extracted data included publication date, authors, study design, setting, target population, micronutrient supplement type and composition, definitions of exposures and outcomes, main findings, and limitations.

LITERATURE REVIEW

The structured literature search yielded 903 articles. Results from the search strategy are summarized in Figure 6.1. After 807 studies were excluded based on abstracts (197 reviews, 241 studies without HIV-infected participants, 7 with children, 242 without micronutrient data, 5 animal or *in vitro* studies, 13 reporting on other HIV outcomes, and 102 for other reasons), 96 studies were extracted for further review. Sources were retrieved, collected, indexed, and assessed for micronutrient and perinatal outcome data. After excluding studies that did not meet inclusion criteria (*n* = 33) and 32 observational studies, including 10 cross-sectional, 1 case-control, and 21 cohort studies, a total of 31 articles describing randomized trials were included in this review. Detailed findings from randomized trials are summarized in Table 6.1.

MICRONUTRIENT STATUS AND PREGNANCY OUTCOMES IN HIV-INFECTED WOMEN

Micronutrient deficiencies may increase the risk of adverse pregnancy outcomes among HIV-infected women via a number of biological mechanisms and have been described in earlier review articles (Mehta et al., 2008a). For example, suboptimal micronutrient status may increase the risk of MTCT of HIV by impairing systemic immune function and epithelial integrity of the maternal lower genital tract (Dreyfuss and Fawzi, 2002; Kupka and Fawzi, 2002). Micronutrient deficiencies may also accelerate maternal clinical, immunologic, and virologic HIV disease progression, and consequently increase morbidity and risk of HIV transmission (Dreyfuss and Fawzi, 2002; Fawzi et al., 2003). HIV infection itself may also affect nutrient absorption, metabolism, and excretion and contribute to the development of micronutrient deficiencies, thus perpetuating a vicious cycle (Keusch and Farthing, 1990) and increasing the risk of established nutrition-related adverse pregnancy outcomes in those who are infected.

Observational Studies

Vitamin A and Carotenoids

In some of the earliest studies conducted in Sub-Saharan Africa, low maternal vitamin A status was associated with increased risk of adverse pregnancy outcomes (Semba et al., 1994; Friis et al., 2001a). Most of these studies were cross-sectional or assessed nutrition status at enrollment and followed up HIV-infected pregnant women through delivery. For example, in a cohort study in Malawi by Semba et al. (1994), 338 HIV-infected pregnant women were enrolled and followed up every three months during pregnancy. Low maternal plasma retinol levels (<0.7 µmol/L) were associated with increased odds of low birthweight (<2500 g), infant mortality, and MTCT of HIV (odds ratio [OR], 0.56; 95% CI, 0.37–0.80; *p* = 0.0001) (Semba et al., 1994, 1995). Similar findings were reported in an observational study in Rwanda (Graham et al., 1993).

In an observational analysis that was part of the Trial of Vitamins (TOV), described later in this chapter (*n* = 1078 pregnant women, 12–27 weeks gestation), low maternal vitamin A status (serum retinol < 0.7 mmol/L) was associated with a higher risk of severe maternal anemia (Hb <

TABLE 6.1
Randomized Trials

Ref.	Location	Sample	Methods	Exposures	Outcomes	Main Findings
Multivitamins						
Fawzi et al. (1998)	Dar es Salaam, Tanzania	1078 HIV-1-infected pregnant women (subsample: 1075 women; 941 live births) ART naïve	Double-blind, placebo-controlled, 2 × 2 factorial randomized trial Enrollment: 12–27 weeks of gestation Follow-up to 24 months postpartum (mean follow-up time: 8.6 months; SD: 7.2) Daily regimens: (1) multivitamins, (2) vitamin A, (3) multivitamins + vitamin A, (4) placebo All received iron (60 mg ferrous sulfate) and folic acid (5 mg) daily and prophylactic chloroquine phosphate (500 mg) weekly.	2 × 2 factorial randomization to daily 20 mg vitamin B_1, 20 mg vitamin B_2, 100 mg B_3, 25 mg vitamin B_6, 50 mg vitamin B_{12}, 500 mg vitamin C, 30 mg vitamin E, and 0.8 mg folic acid 30 mg β-carotene plus 5000 IU of preformed vitamin A; at delivery, additional 200,000 IU vitamin A Multivitamins and vitamin A Placebo	*Birth outcomes* Miscarriage (delivery at <28 weeks of gestation) Stillbirth (delivery of a dead infant ≥28 weeks gestation) Fetal death Birthweight: low birthweight (<2500 g); very low birthweight (<2000 g) Small-size-for-gestational age (birthweight < 10th percentile gestational age) Delivery time: preterm (<37 weeks); severe preterm (<34 weeks)	Multivitamins decreased: • Risk of low birthweight by 44% (RR, 0.56; 95% CI, 0.38–0.82; $p = 0.003$) • Risk of very low birthweight by 58% (RR, 0.42; 95% CI, 0.18–1.01; $p = 0.05$) • Risk of severe preterm birth by 39% (RR, 0.61; 95% CI, 0.38–0.96; $p = 0.03$) • Risk of small-size-for-gestational-age at birth by 43% (RR, 0.57; 95% CI, 0.39–0.82; $p = 0.002$) • Risk of fetal death (RR, 0.61; 95% CI, 0.39–0.94; $p = 0.02$) Multivitamins increased: • Birthweight (mean, 3048 g; SD, 484) compared to control (mean, 2948 g; SD, 552) ($p = 0.01$) • Heavier placentas ($p = 0.02$) • Maternal hemoglobin concentrations at 6 weeks postpartum ($p < 0.0001$) • Maternal CD4, CD8, and CD3 T-cell counts between baseline and 6 weeks postpartum ($p < 0.001$) Vitamin A had no significant effects on these outcomes.

(continued)

TABLE 6.1 (continued)
Randomized Trials

Ref.	Location	Sample	Methods	Exposures	Outcomes	Main Findings
Fawzi et al. (2000)	Dar es Salaam, Tanzania	See above.	See above. HIV infection was assessed by PCR on a peripheral blood mononuclear cell specimen at delivery or 6 weeks postpartum.	See above.	MTCT of HIV (positive PCR at birth or 6 weeks of age) *Birth outcomes* As defined above: low birthweight, very low birthweight, small-size-for-gestational age	Multivitamins predicted a lower risk of fetal loss vs. no multivitamins (RR, 0.59; 95% CI, 0.39–0.91; $p = 0.02$). There were no significant effects of multivitamins (RR, 1.54; 95% CI, 0.94–2.51; $p = 0.08$) or vitamin A (RR, 1.49; 95% CI, 0.91–2.43; $p = 0.11$) on HIV infection at birth or the combined endpoint of HIV infection or death at delivery ($p > 0.05$). Multivitamins significantly increased birthweight (94 g) among infants who were not infected with HIV at delivery ($p = 0.02$ in a multivariate model adjusted for maternal age, CD4 T-cell count, income, and MUAC). There were no effects of supplements on birthweight in infants who were HIV-infected at birth.
Fawzi et al. (2002)	Dar es Salaam, Tanzania	1078 HIV-1-infected pregnant women (subsample: 898 children) ART naïve	See above. HIV infection was assessed by PCR at <18 months of age or ELISA and western blot at ≥18 months.	See above.	HIV transmission via intrauterine, intrapartum, and early breastfeeding route Death within first 2 years of life Combined endpoint of HIV infection or death	Vitamin A: • Increased the risk of breastfeeding HIV transmission (RR, 1.38; 95% CI, 1.09–1.76; $p = 0.009$) • Had no effect on child mortality by 24 months (RR, 1.03; 95% CI, 0.66–1.62; $p = 0.89$)

			See above.	HIV transmission through breastfeeding: HIV infection after 6 weeks of age among infants who were HIV-uninfected at 6 weeks	Multivitamins: • Reduced breastfeeding HIV transmission in mothers with low baseline lymphocyte counts (RR, 0.37; 95% CI, 0.16–0.85; $p = 0.02$) • Protected against HIV transmission among nutritionally or immunologically compromised mothers • Reduced the risk of death and prolonged HIV-free survival among children born to women in lowest quartile of maternal lymphocyte counts (RR, 0.30; 95% CI, 0.10–0.92; $p = 0.04$)
Villamor et al. (2002)	Dar es Salaam, Tanzania	1078 HIV-1-infected pregnant women ART naïve	See above.	Weight gain during the second and third trimesters of pregnancy: total weight gain since randomization; low total weight gain (≤100 g/week; regression slope of individual below 25th percentile at gestational week) Weight loss (negative regression slope)	Multivitamins resulted in: • Greater average weight gain in 3rd trimester by 304 g (95% CI, 17–590; $p = 0.04$) • An average of 39 g/week more weight gain by 36 weeks vs. placebo • Lower risks of low total weight gain by 3rd trimester (RR, 0.70; 95% CI, 0.55–0.90; $p = 0.005$), weight loss (RR, 0.69; 95% CI, 0.50–0.95; $p = 0.02$), and low rate of weight gain (RR, 0.73; 95% CI, 0.58–0.93; $p = 0.01$) Vitamin A decreased the risk of low rate weight gain among non-anemic women (Hb ≥ 110 g/L) in the 2nd trimester (RR, 0.31; 95% CI, 0.14–0.68; $p < 0.05$).

(continued)

TABLE 6.1 (continued)
Randomized Trials

Ref.	Location	Sample	Methods	Exposures	Outcomes	Main Findings
Fawzi et al. (2003)	Dar es Salaam, Tanzania	1078 HIV-1 infected pregnant women ART naïve	See above. 100,000 IU of vitamin A were given to infants at 6 months of age and 200,000 IU of vitamin A every 6 months thereafter. Child weight, height, MUAC, and morbidity were assessed monthly. Maternal and infant CD4, CD3, and CD8 T-cell counts were measured every 3 months and 6 months, respectively. Findings were adjusted for baseline maternal age, education level, CD4 and CD8 T-cell counts, erythrocyte sedimentation rate, hemoglobin, and plasma vitamin A and E levels.	See above.	Risk of diarrhea: ≥3 watery stools in the prior 24 hr; acute diarrhea (≥1 day and <14 days of diarrhea); dysentery (episodes of diarrhea including mucus or blood or watery diarrhea); persistent diarrhea (≥14 days) Respiratory infection: fever, cough, difficulty breathing, chest retractions, and difficulties with eating, drinking, or breastfeeding Rapid respiratory rate: ≥50 breaths/min for infants and ≥40 breaths/min for children > 1 year CD4 T-cell counts	Multivitamins reduced the risk of child diarrhea by 17% (RR, 0.83; 95% CI, 0.71–0.98; p = 0.03), particularly among preterm infants (RR, 0.53; 95% CI, 0.33–0.84; p = 0.007); there were no significant effects of vitamin A. Vitamin A reduced the risk of child cough with rapid respiratory rate (RR, 0.69; 95% CI, 0.49–0.96; p = 0.03). Multivitamins significantly increased child CD4 T-cell count (151 cells/mL; 95% CI, 64–237 cells/mL; p = 0.0006); vitamin A supplementation had no effect on child CD4 T-cell counts.
Fawzi et al. (2004a)	Dar es Salaam, Tanzania	1078 HIV-1-infected pregnant women (subsample: 393) ART naïve	See above. Cervicovaginal lavage was collected just before delivery. IL-1β was measured at 36 weeks gestation. Viral content was expressed as HIV-1 RNA copies/mL.	See above.	Genital HIV-1 shedding (continuous, dichotomous, tertiles) IL-1β (continuous, quartiles), as a cytokine marker of vaginal inflammation and promoter of HIV-1 infection	Detectable HIV-1 levels in CVL were present in more women who received vitamin A (74.8%) compared to no vitamin A (65.1%) (p = 0.04). There were no effects on median IL-1β concentrations in CVL specimens. Vitamin A significantly increased HIV-1 shedding (p = 0.04).

| Fawzi et al. (2004b) | Dar es Salaam, Tanzania | 1078 HIV-1-infected pregnant women (subsample: 1074 women, 962 live births) ART naïve | See above. | See above. | Progression of HIV status to ≥ WHO stage 3 or stage 4, or death MTCT of HIV CD4 T-cell counts Viral load | Multivitamins reduced the risk of progression to HIV stage 4 or death during follow-up (24.7% vs. 31.1%; RR, 0.71; 95% CI, 0.51–0.98; p = 0.04). Multivitamins reduced the risk of AIDS-related death (RR, 0.73; 95% CI, 0.51–1.04; p = 0.09), progression to WHO stage 4 (RR, 0.50; 95% CI, 0.28–0.90; p = 0.02), or progression to WHO stage 3 or higher (RR, 0.72; 95% CI, 0.58–0.90; p = 0.003). Multivitamins increased CD4 T-cell counts (48 cells/mm^3; 95% CI, 10–85; p = 0.01) and reduced viral load (95% CI, −0.32 to −0.03; p = 0.02). Multivitamins significantly reduced the risk of oral and gastrointestinal symptoms: oral ulcers (RR, 0.52; p < 0.001), angular cheilitis (RR, 0.44; p < 0.001), difficult or painful swallowing (RR, 0.47; p < 0.001), dysentery (RR, 0.75; p = 0.03), and fatigue (RR, 0.76; p = 0.007). Vitamin A increased the risk of angular cheilitis (RR, 1.51; p = 0.04) and reduced CD8 T-cell counts (46 cells/mm^3; p = 0.04). Multivitamins reduced the risk of progression to HIV stage 4 or AIDS-related death (RR, 0.66; p = 0.08). |

(continued)

TABLE 6.1 (continued)
Randomized Trials

Ref.	Location	Sample	Methods	Exposures	Outcomes	Main Findings
Baylin et al. (2005)	Dar es Salaam, Tanzania	1078 HIV-1-infected pregnant women (subsample: 716 mother–infant pairs) ART naïve	See above.	See above.	Infant serum vitamin A, vitamin B_{12}, and vitamin E levels in the first 6 months of life (continuous, categorical) Vitamin A deficiency: serum retinol < 0.70 and < 0.35 umol/L Vitamin E deficiency: <11.6 umol/L Vitamin B_{12} deficiency: <150 pmol/L	Maternal multivitamin supplementation significantly increased infant serum vitamin E and vitamin B_{12} ($p = 0.0008$ and $p < 0.0001$, respectively) at 6 weeks and 6 months ($p = 0.004$ and $p < 0.0001$, respectively); there were no significant effects of vitamin A. The prevalence of vitamin B_{12} deficiency was lower among infants born to mothers provided multivitamins at 6 weeks ($p < 0.0001$) and 6 months ($p < 0.0001$); the prevalence of vitamin E deficiency was significantly lower among infants born to mothers supplemented with multivitamins at 6 months ($p = 0.03$). Maternal vitamin A supplementation increased infant serum retinol at 6 weeks (mean difference, 0.09 µmol/L; $p < 0.0001$) and 6 months (mean difference, 0.06 µmol/L; $p = 0.0002$) of age. The prevalence of vitamin A deficiency was significantly lower among infants whose mothers were supplemented with vitamin A at 6 weeks ($p < 0.0001$) and 6 months ($p < 0.02$).

| Merchant et al. (2005) | Dar es Salaam, Tanzania | 1078 HIV-1-infected pregnant women ART naïve | See above. Hypertensive events were measured through 3 months postpartum. | Hypertension: systolic blood pressure ≥ 140 mmHg or diastolic blood pressure ≥ 90 mmHg at any time during pregnancy High systolic blood pressure: >120 mmHg vs. ≤120 mmHg | See above. | Multivitamins reduced the risk of hypertension during pregnancy by 38% (RR, 0.62; 95% CI, 0.40–0.94; $p = 0.03$). Vitamin A supplementation did not affect hypertension risk. Women with high baseline systolic blood pressure (RR, 6.02; 95% CI, 2.59–13.97; $p < 0.001$) or higher MUAC (RR, 1.12; 95% CI, 1.04–1.19; $p < 0.001$) were more likely to develop hypertension during pregnancy. |
| Villamor et al. (2005) | Dar es Salaam, Tanzania | 1078 HIV-1-infected pregnant women (subsample: 886 children) ART naïve | See above. Child growth monitoring was conducted at monthly visits. Children were followed up for 24 months (median 21). Vitamin A arm was terminated in September 2000 due to adverse effects of MTCT of HIV. | Growth of infants during the first 2 years of life: child weight, child length, child head circumference, MUAC WHO z-scores: weight-for-age (WAZ), weight-for-length (WLZ), and length-for-age (LAZ) Underweight (WAZ < –2), wasting (WLZ < –2), stunting (LAZ < –2) | See above. | Maternal multivitamin supplementation significantly increased child weight at 24 months (459 g; 95% CI, 35–882; $p = 0.03$). The effect of multivitamins on child weight at 24 months was greater for HIV-infected children (1332 g; 95% CI, 323–2340 g; $p = 0.01$). Multivitamins significantly increased WLZ (0.38; 95% CI, 0.07–0.68; $p = 0.01$) and WAZ scores (0.42; 95% CI, 0.07–0.77; $p = 0.02$) at 24 months. Multivitamins reduced the risk of child wasting by 47% (HR, 0.53; 95% CI, 0.32–0.88; $p = 0.01$) and reduced the risk of child underweight by 33% (HR, 0.67; 95% CI, 0.46–0.97; $p = 0.03$). Multivitamins or vitamin A had no effects on MUAC, length, LAZ, or head circumference. |

(continued)

TABLE 6.1 (continued)
Randomized Trials

Ref.	Location	Sample	Methods	Exposures	Outcomes	Main Findings
Fawzi et al. (2007)	Dar es Salaam, Tanzania	1078 HIV-1-infected pregnant women ART naïve	See above.	See above.	Hemoglobin concentrations: anemia (Hb <11.0 g/dL), severe anemia (Hb < 8.5 g/dL) Hypochromic microcytic anemia: severe (hypochromasia ≤ 2+ and microcytosis observed), moderate (hypochromasia ≤ 1+ and microcytosis observed), mild and above (hypochromasia ≤ 1+ with or without microcytosis) Macrocytosis: presence of macrocytic cells	Multivitamins increased hemoglobin concentrations ($p = 0.07$), and this was significant during the first 2 years of follow-up ($p = 0.0002$). There were no effects of supplements on risk of maternal anemia. Multivitamins reduced the risks of infant severe anemia (RR, 0.61; 95% CI, 0.38–1.00; $p = 0.004$) and macrocytic anemia (RR, 0.37; 95% CI, 0.18–0.79; $p = 0.01$).
McGrath et al. (2006)	Dar es Salaam, Tanzania	1078 HIV-1-infected pregnant women (subsample: 327) ART naïve	See above. The Bayley Scales of Infant and Toddler Development (BSID-II) was used to measure infant mental and psychomotor development at 6, 12, and 18 months of age.	See above.	Child mental and psychomotor development: MDI and PDI in BSID-II Indices (conversion of raw scores) and raw MDI and PDI scores	Multivitamin supplementation significantly increased child PDI score by an average of 2.6 points (95% CI, 0.1–5.1; $p = 0.04$) from 6 to 18 months of age (raw score, 0.8 items; 95% CI, 0.02–1.6; $p = 0.04$). At 12 months, vitamin A was associated with a 2.8-point average increase (95% CI, 0.4–5.2) in PDI and a 1.1-item average increase (95% CI, 0.3–1.9) in raw motor score in multivariate analyses ($p = 0.05$) (no effects at 6 or 18 months).

Multivitamin supplements reduced the risk of developmental delay on the motor scale (RR, 0.40; 95% CI, 0.20–0.70; $p = 0.004$), but not MDI. Maternal baseline CD4 T-cell counts modified the effect of vitamin A supplements on infant mental and psychomotor development; children of mothers taking vitamin A with baseline CD4 count of <200 cells/mm³ had a 10.2 point increase in MDI (95% CI, 4.5–15.5) and 12.1 point increase in PDI (95% CI, 4.2–20.0) vs. no vitamin A; there was no effect for women with CD4 ≥ 200 cells/mm³.

Fawzi et al. (2007) — Dar es Salaam, Tanzania — 1078 HIV-1-infected pregnant women ART naïve

See above. Median follow-up time for hemoglobin measurement was 57.3 months for mothers (IQR, 28.6–66.8) and 28.0 months for children (IQR, 5.3–41.7).

See above.

Hemoglobin levels (g/dL): anemia (hemoglobin < 11.0 g/dL), severe anemia (hemoglobin < 8.5 g/dL). Hypochromic microcytic anemia: severe (hypochromasia ≤ 2+ and microcytosis observed), moderate (hypochromasia ≤ 1+ and microcytosis observed), mild and above (hypochromasia ≤ 1+ with or without microcytosis) Macrocytosis: presence of macrocytic cells

Multivitamins increased maternal hemoglobin concentrations by 0.33 g/dL ($p = 0.07$). Multivitamins reduced the risk of child severe hypochromic microcytosis (RR, 0.60; 95% CI, 0.42–0.85; $p = 0.004$). There were no effects of vitamin A on hemoglobin concentrations.

(continued)

TABLE 6.1 (continued)
Randomized Trials

Ref.	Location	Sample	Methods	Exposures	Outcomes	Main Findings
Villamor et al. (2007)	Dar es Salaam, Tanzania	1078 HIV-1-infected pregnant women (subsample: 829) ART naïve	See above. Incidence of childhood malaria was assessed through blood smears at monthly and interim clinic visits from birth to 24 months of age.	See above.	Any parasitemia ≥ 1/μL High parasitemia: ≥ 5000/μL Clinical malaria: parasitemia ≥ 5000/μL Death from malaria: malaria as the primary cause of death, verbal autopsy	Multivitamins reduced the incidence of clinical malaria in children by 71% (95% CI, 11–91%; $p = 0.02$); vitamin A had a non-statistically significant reduction in clinical malaria by 63% (95% CI, 4–87%; $p = 0.06$). Multivitamin supplementation reduced the incidence of high parasitemia by 43% (95% CI, 2–67%; $p = 0.04$). Multivitamins reduced the risk of high parasitemia by 43% (95% CI, 2–67%; $p = 0.04$).
Webb et al. (2009)	Dar es Salaam, Tanzania	1078 HIV-1-infected pregnant women (subsample: 626) ART naïve	See above. Effects of micronutrients on breast milk concentrations were estimated at delivery and at 3, 6, and 12 months postpartum.	See above.	Concentrations of retinol, total β-carotene, α-carotene, α-tocopherol, γ-tocopherol, and δ-tocopherol in breast milk	Vitamin A supplementation significantly increased concentrations of breast milk retinol, β-carotene, and α-carotene at all time points during the first 12 months postpartum (all $p < 0.0001$). Supplementation with vitamin A did not influence concentrations of α-, β- and γ-tocopherol from delivery to 1 year postpartum. Multivitamin supplementation significantly increased concentrations of α-tocopherol at 3, 6, and 12 months postpartum; there were no changes in β-carotene or β-carotene.

						Multivitamin supplementation significantly decreased concentrations of breast milk γ-tocopherol at all time points and reduced retinol at delivery. Concentrations of breast milk retinol, β-carotene, and α-carotene decreased from 0–3 months postpartum regardless of intervention; women in the vitamin A group had higher concentrations of these nutrients during 1 year postpartum vs. no vitamin A (4549 ± 214 vs. 2210 ± 118, 465 ± 45 vs. 50 ± 6, 27 ± 3 vs. 10 ± 1, respectively).
Arsenault et al. (2010)	Dar es Salaam, Tanzania	1078 HIV-1-infected pregnant women (subsample: 674) ART naïve	See above. Women were followed during pregnancy and throughout the lactation period. Breast milk was measured every 3 months during the first 2 years postpartum; timing for breast milk collection was defined as <2 weeks and 3, 6, 9, 12, and >12 months postpartum.	Subclinical mastitis in the first 2 years postpartum Subclinical mastitis (ratio of Na/K breast milk concentrations > 0.6), moderate (Na/K > 0.6 and <1), severe (Na/K > 1)	See above.	Multivitamins without vitamin A increased the risks of subclinical mastitis by 33% ($p = 0.005$) and severe subclinical mastitis by 75% ($p = 0.0006$) vs. placebo. Vitamin A increased the risk of severe subclinical mastitis by 45% ($p = 0.03$). Multivitamins did not vary over the postpartum period for moderate (p-interaction = 0.90) or severe (p-interaction = 0.53) subclinical mastitis. Women with CD4 T-cell counts ≥ 350 cells/mL in the multivitamin group had a 49% increased risk of any subclinical mastitis vs. placebo ($p = 0.006$).

(continued)

TABLE 6.1 (continued)
Randomized Trials

Ref.	Location	Sample	Methods	Exposures	Outcomes	Main Findings
Gomo et al. (2003)	Zimbabwe	83 HIV-infected and 84 HIV-uninfected pregnant women	HIV-infected and HIV-uninfected pregnant women were randomized to multivitamins or placebo supplementation from 22–35 weeks gestation until 3 months postpartum (randomization in blocks of 4). Sociodemographic, anthropomorphic, obstetric, and medical data were assessed. Women were followed up at 3, 6, 9, 12, and 15 months postpartum; breast milk samples were collected until 4.5 months postpartum. All women received iron and folic acid according to standard of antenatal care.	Group 1: Micronutrients (10,000 IU vitamin A, 1.5 mg vitamin B_1, 1.6 mg B_2, 17 mg vitamin B_3, 2.2 mg vitamin B_6, 4.0 µg vitamin B_{12}, 80 mg vitamin C, 10 µg vitamin D, 10 mg vitamin E, 15 mg zinc, 1.2 mg copper, 65 µg selenium) Group 2: Placebo	Subclinical mastitis (ratio of Na/K breast milk concentrations > 0.6), moderate (Na/K > 0.6 and <1), severe (Na/K > 1) Birthweight (kg)	Micronutrient supplementation did not affect geometric mean Na/K ratio ($p = 0.33$); there were no differences between HIV-infected and HIV-uninfected women ($p = 0.59$). Birthweights of infants born to mothers with severe subclinical mastitis (severely raised Na/K ratio) were significantly higher (5.5 kg; SEM = 0.3; $n = 7$) than birthweights of infants with normal breast milk Na/K ratio (6.2 kg; SEM = 0.1; $n = 57$) ($p = 0.049$).
Kawai et al. (2010)	Dar es Salaam, Tanzania	1129 HIV-infected pregnant women	HIV-infected pregnant women were recruited between 12 and 27 weeks gestation. Women were randomly assigned to single- or multiple-RDA-level multivitamins from enrollment until 6 weeks postpartum.	Group 1: Single-RDA multivitamins (1.4 mg thiamine, 1.4 mg riboflavin, 18 mg niacin, 1.9 mg vitamin B_6, 2.6 mg vitamin B_{12}, 70 mg vitamin C, 10 mg vitamin E, 0.4 mg folic acid)	Birthweight, gestational age, length, head circumference, and placental weight (continuous) Low birthweight (<2500 g) Pre-term delivery (<37 weeks gestation)	There were no differences between multivitamins at single and multiple RDA levels on mean birthweight, risk of low birth (11.6% vs. 10.2%, $p = 0.75$), duration of gestation ($p = 0.85$), birth length ($p = 0.76$), head circumference ($p = 0.89$), or placental weight ($p = 0.61$).

			All women received the standard-of-care 60 mg elemental iron and 25 mg folic acid daily and malaria prophylaxis at 20 and 30 weeks gestation. All women received single-dose nevirapine (200 mg) at delivery. Sociodemographic, clinical, and anthropometric measurements were collected at baseline at monthly visits. Small subset was co-enrolled in selenium supplementation trial.	Group 2: Multiple-RDA multivitamins, 6–10 times the RDA (20 mg vitamin B_1, 20 mg vitamin B_2, 100 mg B_3, 25 mg vitamin B_6, 50 mg vitamin B_{12}, 500 mg vitamin C, 30 mg vitamin E, 0.8 mg folic acid)	Small-for-gestational-age (<10th percentile of Brenner standard weight for gestational age) Fetal death (miscarriage or stillbirths) Infant death (death during the first 6 weeks of infant life) Maternal hemoglobin (anemia, Hb <11.0 g/dL) Maternal CD4, CD8, CD3 T-cell counts, HIV viral load	There were no differences in risks of small-for-gestational-age (RR, 1.30; 95% CI, 0.89–1.90; $p = 0.18$), preterm birth (RR, 1.07; 95% CI, 0.81–1.35; $p = 0.73$), miscarriage ($p = 0.17$), stillbirths ($p = 0.52$), fetal death (RR, 1.00; 95% CI, 0.63–1.58; $p = 0.99$), perinatal death (RR, 0.75; 95% CI, 0.47–1.21; $p = 0.25$), or early infant death (RR, 0.46; 95% CI, 0.14–1.48; $p = 0.19$). There were no differences in the mean maternal CD4, CD8, or CD3 T-cell counts ($p = 0.34$, $p = 0.38$, and $p = 0.59$, respectively; among subgroup participating in selenium trial); there were no differences in mean maternal hemoglobin concentrations ($p = 0.96$) or HIV viral load ($p = 0.55$).
Vitamin A					
Villamor et al. (2010)	Dar es Salaam, Tanzania	1078 HIV-1-infected pregnant women (subsample: 594)	See above. ~10 mL breast milk were collected immediately after delivery and every 3 months thereafter for 2 years postpartum (defined as 0, 3, 6, 9, 12, and >12 months postpartum).	See above.	HIV shedding in breast milk Breast milk retinol and β-carotene (detection yes/ no and quartiles) HIV viral load in breast milk (50th, 75th, and 90th percentiles)	Vitamin A significantly increased the proportion of breast milk samples with a detectable viral load compared to no vitamin A after 6 months postpartum (51.3% vs. 44.8%; RR, 1.34; 95% CI, 1.04–1.73; $p = 0.02$).

(continued)

TABLE 6.1 (continued)
Randomized Trials

Ref.	Location	Sample	Methods	Exposures	Outcomes	Main Findings
						Vitamin A (RR, 0.93; 95% CI, 0.80–1.07; $p = 0.29$) or multivitamins (RR, 1.01; 95% CI, 0.88–1.17; $p = 0.86$) had no effects on breast milk viral load.
						Breast-milk β-carotene (not retinol) concentrations were associated with increased detectable HIV viral load in milk (95% CI, 1.03–1.41; $p = 0.02$).
Coutsoudis et al. (1999)	Durban, South Africa	728 HIV-infected pregnant women ART naïve	HIV-infected women were enrolled at 28 to 32 weeks gestation and randomized to vitamin A or placebo until delivery. Sociodemographic, clinical, and anthropometric data were collected. Follow-up: delivery, 1 week, 6 weeks, and 3 months of age until 6 months postpartum; every 3 months for maternal and infant symptoms, anthropometric data, breastfeeding practices, and infant blood samples	Group 1: Vitamin A (5000 IU retinyl palmitate and 30 mg β-carotene; additional 200,000 IU megadose of retinyl palmitate at delivery) Group 2: Placebo	Preterm birth (≤ 37 weeks gestation) Low birthweight (<2500 g) HIV infection by 3 months of age Fetal and infant mortality	Vitamin A significantly reduced the risk of preterm delivery (11.4% vs. 17.4%; $p = 0.03$) compared to placebo. MTCT of HIV was similar in both groups: vitamin A, 20.3% (95% CI, 15.7–24.9) vs. placebo, 22.3% (95% CI, 17.5–27.1). Vitamin A reduced the risk of HIV infection by 3 months of age among preterm infants: vitamin A, 17.9% (95% CI, 3.5–32.2) vs. placebo, 33.8% (95% CI, 19.8–47.8). There were no significant effects of vitamin A on early HIV transmission in other subgroups (baseline, maternal serum retinol level, hemoglobin, CD4 cell count, CD4/CD8 cell ratio, mode of delivery, feeding practices).

| Kennedy et al. (2000) | South Africa | 728 HIV-infected pregnant women (subsample: 312) ART naïve | See above. Follow-up: delivery, 1 week, 3 months, and 6 months after delivery | HIV-related symptoms: persistent swollen glands, fever > 1 week, unintentional weight loss > 10% of previous follow-up weight, fatigue, diarrhea > 1 week, oral thrush, and loss of appetite > 1 week Pregnancy-related symptoms: lower abdominal pain and nausea/vomiting | See above. | Vitamin A had no significant effects on mortality by 1 month of age (vitamin A, 2.35% vs. placebo, 3.24%), 3 months (5.52% vs. 5.44%), or 12 months (9.26% vs. 9.99%) compared to placebo. There were significant differences in symptoms at baseline: the vitamin A group had more unintentional weight loss, nausea/vomiting, and pregnancy related symptoms. At 4 weeks after treatment (or at delivery if not available), the vitamin A group was more likely to report symptoms of maternal fatigue (RR, 4.40; 95% CI, 1.56–12.38; $p = 0.02$), oral thrush ($p = 0.04$), loss of appetite for 1 week (RR, 1.40; 95% CI, 0.52–3.76; $p = 0.03$), lower abdominal pain (RR, 1.46; 95% CI, 0.75–2.84; $p = 0.05$), and HIV-related symptoms (RR, 1.60; 95% CI, 0.87–2.92; $p = 0.04$) vs. placebo. At 1 week postpartum, the vitamin A group was more likely to report headaches vs. placebo (RR, 0.43; 95% CI, 0.17–1.12; $p = 0.04$). At 3 months postpartum, there were no significant differences between arms for HIV-related symptoms. |

(continued)

TABLE 6.1 (continued)
Randomized Trials

Ref.	Location	Sample	Methods	Exposures	Outcomes	Main Findings
Kennedy-Oji et al. (2001)	South Africa	728 HIV-infected pregnant women (subsample: 312) ART naïve	See above.	See above.	Prenatal and postnatal weight (kg), weight gain, weight retention (BMI) at 3 months postpartum Prepartum weight gain (weight at delivery or 4 weeks before delivery – weight at registration) Postpartum weight retention (weight at 3 to 6 months – weight at 1 week postpartum)	Maternal vitamin A was not associated with maternal BMI at baseline ($p = 0.61$), delivery ($p = 0.74$), 1 week postpartum ($p = 0.65$), or 3–6 months postpartum ($p = 0.76$), or with prepartum weight gain ($p = 0.75$) or retention of postpartum weight. Vitamin A supplementation was associated with retention of postpartum weight from delivery to 3–6 months partum ($p = 0.02$). The vitamin A arm had higher maternal BMI 3–6 months postpartum among those with CD4 T-cells < 200 cells/μL at baseline ($p = 0.01$), serum retinol ≤ 20 μg/dL at baseline ($p = 0.03$), or Hb > 10 g/dL ($p = 0.04$).
Filteau et al. (2001)	South Africa	728 HIV-infected pregnant women (subsample: 238) ART naïve	See above. Follow-up clinic for infants at 1, 6, and 14 weeks of age Excretion of sugars was also expressed per creatinine. HIV infection by 14 weeks, birthweight, child morbidity, and maternal viral load were measured.	See above.	Intestinal permeability as measured by the ratio of concentrations of lactulose and mannitol sugars in urin: increased ratio (increased permeability or decreased integrity), decreased ratio (decreased permeability)	HIV infection status by 14 weeks significantly predicted lactulose/mannitol ratios (6 weeks: $\Delta R^2 = 0.22$, $p = 0.008$; 14 weeks: $\Delta R^2 = 0.21$, $p = 0.01$). At 1 week, history of ever having been breastfed ($\Delta R^2 = 0.22$; $p = 0.008$) and birthweight ($\Delta R^2 = 0.07$; $p = 0.02$) were significant.

Lactulose/mannitol dual sugar intestinal permeability tests were performed, blood samples collected, and infant weight and feeding history assessed.

Infant weight and maternal plasma retinol and blood lymphocyte counts did not significantly affect permeability at any time point. Maternal HIV viral load during pregnancy was significantly correlated with lactulose/mannitol ratio at 6 weeks ($r = 0.41$; $p = 0.004$) but not at 1 week ($r = 0.15$; $p = 0.30$) or 14 weeks ($r = 0.21$; $p = 0.15$).

Effects of maternal vitamin A supplementation on lactulose/mannitol ratios among HIV-uninfected infants was not significantly different from placebo. Vitamin A supplements prevented decreases in the ratio of HIV-infected infants: vitamin A, 0.17 (95% CI, 0.13–0.23) vs. placebo, 0.50% (95% CI, 0.37–0.68).

Vitamin A was associated with a lower lactulose/creatinine ratio at 1 week ($p = 0.009$) and 14 weeks ($p = 0.014$) in HIV-infected infants.

Infant HIV infection increased the lactulose/creatinine ratio at 6 weeks ($p = 0.036$).

Infant characteristics associated with undetectable lactulose at 1 week were lower birthweight ($p = 0.014$) and gestational age ($p = 0.028$).

(continued)

TABLE 6.1 (continued)
Randomized Trials

Ref.	Location	Sample	Methods	Exposures	Outcomes	Main Findings
Humphrey et al. (2006)	Harare, Zimbabwe	14,110 mother–infant pairs; 4495 infants born to HIV-infected mothers ART naive	Mother–infant pairs: singleton infants with birthweight ≥ 1500 g 2 × 2 factorial design (4 groups): (1) both mother and infant vitamin A (Aa); (2) mother alone (Ap); (3) infant alone (Pa); or (4) placebo (Pp) MUAC, HIV status, infant birthweight, gestational weight, and baseline characteristics were measured. Follow-up visits were conducted at 6 weeks, 3 months, and then every 3 months for 12–24 months. Study was shortened and pairs were assigned to 24 months, ≥18 months, and ≥12months.	Maternal vitamin A supplementation: 400,000 IU compared to placebo; ≤96 hours after delivery given supplementation or placebo Infant vitamin A supplementation: 50,000 IU compared to placebo	MTCT of HIV (PCR) Child morbidity: risk of death in the first 24 months Subgroups: Infants born to HIV-infected vs. uninfected women, infants who were PCR negative at baseline, and infants who were negative at 6 weeks	Risk of HIV infection or death was significantly different higher in Ap vs Pp (HR, 1.10; 95% CI, 1.01–1.41; $p = 0.04$). There were no significant differences in infection or death between the 4 groups at 6 weeks of age. Neither mother nor child vitamin A supplementation significantly affected MTCT of HIV via breastfeeding. Vitamin A supplementation was not significantly associated with infant mortality after adjusting for covariates. In analyses in infants born to HIV-infected mothers, maternal vitamin A supplementation (HR, 1.24; 95% CI, 1.02–1.50; $p = 0.03$) and infant vitamin A supplemented arms (HR, 1.21; 95% CI, 0.99–1.46; $p = 0.05$) had higher risk of death in the first 24 months, compared to placebo. There were no significant differences in supplemented groups in the risk of child mortality in HIV-infected infants at birth.

| Zvandasara et al. (2006) | Harare, Zimbabwe | 14,110 mother–infant pairs; 4495 infants born to HIV-infected mothers | See above. Serum retinol and Hb were measured from blood samples. | See above. Maternal CD4 counts (>400, 200–400, 100–200, <100 cells × 10^6/L), hemoglobin (>120, 70–120, <70 g/L), MUAC, cause-specific risk of death, serum retinol (deficiency, <1.05μmol/L), Maternal hospitalization, number of hospitalizations, hospitalization > 1 day Infant HIV status | For infants HIV-infected by 6 weeks, infants in the vitamin A supplemented groups had significantly lower vitamin A levels compared to the placebo arm (HR, 0.72; 95% CI, 0.57–0.92; $p = 0.01$). For infants HIV-uninfected at 6 weeks, all three vitamin A regimens were associated with a 2-fold increase in mortality ($p < 0.05$). For HIV-infected women (with baseline CD4 count <200), vitamin A supplementation increased mean serum retinol and reduced the risk of vitamin A deficiency ($p < 0.05$) but had no effect on HIV-infected women with other CD4 cell count concentrations. Vitamin A had no significant effect on mortality in either HIV group. Vitamin A supplementation had no effect on the risk of sick clinic visits (IRR, 0.95; 95% CI, 0.86–1.04; $p = 0.25$) or upper ARI, abdominal pain, or fever. Vitamin A supplementation had no effect on the proportion of women ever hospitalized (IRR, 0.98; 95% CI, 0.76–1.26), number of hospitalizations (IRR, 0.96; 95% CI, 0.66–1.40), or risk of having a hospitalization > 1 day (IRR, 0.84; 95% CI, 0.45–1.58). |

(continued)

TABLE 6.1 (continued)
Randomized Trials

Ref.	Location	Sample	Methods	Exposures	Outcomes	Main Findings
Kumwenda et al. (2002)	Blantyre, Malawi	697 HIV-infected pregnant women	Women were recruited at 18–28 weeks gestation and randomized to daily vitamin A or placebo until delivery. All women received 30 mg of elemental iron and 400 μg of folic acid daily until delivery as standard of care. Mother and child sociodemographic characteristics, blood samples, and breast milk samples were collected. Infant HIV infection was assessed via PCR at 6 weeks and 12 months of age.	Group 1: 3 mg retinol equivalent (10,000 IU) daily from enrollment until delivery. Group 2: Placebo	Low birthweight (<2500 g) Birth length Infant hemoglobin (anemia, <110 g/L) MTCT of HIV at 6 or 24 months MTCT of HIV via breastfeeding (>6 but ≤24 months) Maternal serum and breast milk vitamin A levels (<0.07 μmol/L) Infant mortality (first 24 months of life)	Vitamin A supplementation predicted lower risk of low birthweight (14.0% vs. 21.2%; $p = 0.03$). There were no significant difference in MTCT of HIV overall between groups. Risk of MTCT of HIV via breastfeeding was higher in the control group than the vitamin A group ($p = 0.04$). Maternal vitamin A supplementation increased infant mean hemoglobin concentration ($p = 0.04$) and reduced the risk of prevalence of anemia ($p = 0.001$) at 6 weeks of age.
Zinc						
Fawzi et al. (2005)	Tanzania	400 HIV-infected pregnant women	HIV-infected pregnant women were enrolled at 12–27 weeks gestation and randomized (20 block) to daily zinc or placebo through 6 weeks postpartum. All women received iron (400 mg ferrous sulfate) and folic acid (5 mg) daily and prophylactic chloroquine phosphate (500 mg) weekly as per standard of care.	Group 1: zinc (25 mg as zinc sulfate included in an effervescent citrus-flavored tablet) Group 2: Placebo	Fetal death: miscarriage (<28 weeks gestation), stillbirth (≥28 weeks) Birthweight: low birthweight (<2500 g) Small-for-gestational-age at delivery (<10th percentile by Brenner) Preterm (<37 weeks gestation), severe preterm (<34 weeks)	Zinc supplementation had no significant effects on birth outcomes or maternal CD4, CD8, or CD3 T-cell counts during the follow-up. Hemoglobin levels increased from baseline to 6 weeks postpartum in both groups; the increase in Hb was lower in the zinc group vs. placebo (11.5 ± 17.9 g/L vs. 15.2 ± 18.6 g/L; $p = 0.03$).

Study	Country	Population	Methods	Outcomes	Results
			All women received multivitamin supplements (20 mg vitamin B_1, 20 mg vitamin B_2, 25 mg vitamin B_6, 100 mg niacin, 50 µg vitamin B_{12}, 500 mg vitamin C, 30 mg vitamin E, and 0.8 mg folic acid). Sociodemographic, anthropometric, and clinical data were collected. Nevirapine was administered at delivery.	Maternal hemoglobin, red blood cell count, mean packed cell volume Maternal CD4, CD8, CD3 T-cell counts	Changes in maternal red blood cell count and packed cell volume from baseline to 6 weeks postpartum were significantly lower in the zinc group than in the placebo group: adjusted red blood cell count (95% CI, −0.35 to −0.04; $p = 0.01$), adjusted packed cell volume (95% CI, −2.29–0.12; $p = 0.03$).
Villamor et al. (2006)	Tanzania	400 HIV-infected pregnant women	See above.	See above. Wasting (MUAC < 22 cm) Weight loss: estimated regression slope (rate of weight gain) ≤ 0, low weight gain as a regression slope ≤ 200 g/wk (25th percentile) Viral load: >100,000 copies/mL MTCT of HIV: infection by 6 weeks Infant death by 6 weeks Child deaths: <21 days	Zinc supplements had no effect on maternal viral load or early MTCT ($p = 0.11$). Zinc supplementation was not associated with weight gain during pregnancy, rate of weight gain, or weight loss ($p = 0.27$, $p = 0.50$, and $p = 0.56$, respectively). The risk of high viral load was lower in women in the zinc supplementation arm of the trial (RR, 0.77; 95% CI, 0.42–1.40; $p = 0.38$). The risk of wasting was greater in the zinc group than in the placebo group (RR, 2.66; 95% CI, 1.10–6.43; $p = 0.03$).

(continued)

TABLE 6.1 (continued)
Randomized Trials

Ref.	Location	Sample	Methods	Exposures	Outcomes	Main Findings
Selenium						
Kupka et al. (2008)	Tanzania	913 HIV-infected pregnant women	All women received iron (200 mg ferrous sulfate) and folic acid (0.25 mg) daily, and sulfadoxine–pyrimethamine as malaria prophylaxis. All women received daily multivitamins (20 mg vitamin B_1, 20 mg vitamin B_2, 25 mg vitamin B_6, 100 mg niacin, 50 μg vitamin B_{12}, 500 mg of vitamin C, 30 mg of vitamin E, and 0.8 mg of folic acid). Women with WHO stage 4 HIV disease and CD4 count < 200 cells/μL or WHO stage 3 HIV disease and CD4 count < 350 cells/μL received ART. Sociodemographic, anthropometric, and clinical data were collected; blood samples and breast milk samples were collected. Participants were followed monthly until 6 months postpartum. Sample was increased to study the effects of selenium on pregnancy outcomes.	Group 1: Selenium (200 μg of elemental selenium, selenomethionine, in tablet form) Group 2: Placebo	HIV-1 viral load, CD4 cell counts, lower genital shedding of HIV-1-infected cells, mastitis HIV viral load, T-cell counts Birthweight: low birthweight (<2500 g) Preterm (<37 weeks gestation), severe preterm (<34 weeks) Small-for-gestational-age at delivery (<10th percentile) Length, head circumference Fetal death: miscarriage (<28 weeks gestation), stillbirth (≥ 28 weeks), neonatal death (42 days after delivery), infant death (first 180 days) Maternal death: <180 days postpartum	Selenium had no effects on CD4, CD8, and CD3 cell counts, or on viral load over the follow-up period ($p = 0.72$, $p = 0.86$, $p = 0.91$, and $p = 0.71$, respectively). Birthweight was not significantly different for selenium vs. placebo ($p = 0.76$). Selenium non-significantly decreased the risk of low birthweight (RR, 0.71; 95% CI, 0.49–1.05; $p = 0.09$) and risk of fetal death (RR, 1.58; 95% CI, 0.95–2.63; $p = 0.08$). Selenium had no effect on preterm birth (RR, 0.99; 95% CI, 0.73–1.34; $p = 0.93$) or small-for-gestational-age (RR, 1.10; 95% CI, 0.81–1.49; $p = 0.54$). There was no difference in maternal mortality for selenium vs. placebo ($p = 0.96$). There were no effects on risk of infant death (RR, 0.64; 95% CI, 0.36–1.13; $p = 0.12$); selenium decreased the risk of infant death after 6 week (RR, 0.43; 95% CI, 0.19–0.99; $p = 0.048$).

| Kupka et al. (2009) | Tanzania | 915 HIV-infected pregnant women (subsample: 570) | See above. Hemoglobin concentration was measured at baseline, 6 weeks, and 6 months postpartum. | Maternal hemoglobin concentrations. Infant diarrhea: ≥3 watery stools in the prior 24 hr; acute diarrhea (≥1 day and <14 days of diarrhea); dysentery (episodes of diarrhea including mucus or blood or watery diarrhea) | Selenium did not significantly increase maternal hemoglobin concentrations (95% CI, −0.07–0.16 g/dL; $p = 0.73$) or affect the risk of anemia (HR, 0.62; 95% CI, 0.22–1.74; $p = 0.36$) vs. placebo. Selenium reduced the risks of acute diarrhea (RR, 0.59; 95% CI, 0.42–0.83; $p = 0.003$) and watery diarrhea (RR, 0.56; 95% CI, 0.39–0.81; $p = 0.002$). |
| Sudfeld et al. (2014) | Tanzania | 915 HIV-infected pregnant women (subsample: 420) | See above. Breast milk HIV-1 RNA measurements were made. | Breast milk shedding of HIV-1: detection of HIV-1 RNA in breast milk 4–9 weeks postpartum | Selenium group had higher prevalence of detectable HIV-1 in breast milk (36.4% vs. 27.5%; RR, 1.32; 95% CI, 1.00–1.76; $p = 0.05$) vs. placebo. Among HAART-naïve women, selenium significantly increased the prevalence of women with detectable HIV-1 RNA in breast milk vs. placebo (37.8% vs. 27.5%; RR, 1.37; 95% CI, 1.03–1.82; $p = 0.03$). |

Note: ARI, acute respiratory infection; ART, antiretroviral therapy; BMI, body mass index; CVL, cervicovaginal lavage; ELISA, enzyme-linked immunosorbent assay; Hb, hemoglobin; HR, hazard ratio; IL-1β, interleukin-1beta; IQR, interquartile range; IRR, incidence rate ratio; MDI, Mental Development Index; MTCT, mother-to-child transmission; MUAC, mid-upper arm circumference; PCR, polymerase chain reaction; PDI, Psychomotor Development Index; RR, relative risk; SEM, standard error of the mean, WHO, World Health Organization.

8.5 g/dL) during follow-up (risk ratio [RR], 1.47; 95% CI, 1.15–1.89; $p < 0.01$) (Antelman et al., 2000) and lower maternal plasma concentrations of vitamin E (RR, 0.62; 95% CI, 0.42–0.92; $p = 0.02$), selenium (RR, 0.49; 95% CI, 0.30–0.82; $p = 0.01$) (Kupka et al., 2005), and vitamin D (RR, 0.89; 95% CI, 0.80–0.98; $p = 0.02$) (Mehta et al., 2010b). Similarly, higher breast milk β-carotene concentrations (but not retinol or α-carotene) were associated with an increased detectable HIV-1 viral load in breast milk (quartile ≥ 2 vs. quartile 1; prevalence ratio, 1.21; 95% CI, 1.03–1.41; $p = 0.02$) (Villamor et al., 2010).

Findings regarding the associations between maternal vitamin A status and risk of adverse pregnancy outcomes in the United States are divergent. In a study conducted by Burns et al. (1999), maternal plasma vitamin A concentrations were associated with lower odds of low birthweight (OR, 2.16; 95% CI, 1.00–4.65; $p = 0.05$), but were not significantly associated with MTCT of HIV (Burns et al., 1999). In a multicenter prospective cohort study in two urban areas in the United States, low vitamin A status (severe deficiency, plasma retinol < 0.70 μmol/L; mild to moderate deficiency, plasma retinol 0.70–1.05 μmol/L) was associated with increased odds of vertical HIV transmission (total infection rate; adjusted odds ratio [AOR], 5.05; 95% CI, 1.20–21.24; $p < 0.05$) among HIV-infected pregnant women (Greenberg et al., 1997).

Hematological and Iron Status

The associations between hematological status and adverse pregnancy outcomes in HIV-infected women have been examined in several observational studies. In a cross-sectional study in Zimbabwe, HIV infection was associated with increased prevalence of anemia (Hb < 11.0 g/dL; prevalence of anemia, 54%; 95% CI, 49–58%; $p < 0.00001$) and folate deficiency (serum folate < 6.7 nmol/L; prevalence of folate deficiency, 16%; 95% CI, 13–20%; $p = 0.001$), and lower serum ferritin levels (β, 0.93; 95% CI, 0.86–0.99; $p = 0.03$) (Friis et al., 2001a,b). Additionally, haptoglobin phenotype (2–2; β, 2.34; 95% CI, 1.38–3.98; $p = 0.002$), severe iron deficiency (serum ferritin < 6.0 μg/L; β, 0.13; 95% CI, 0.13–0.53; $p = 0.013$), α1-antichymotrypsin (ACT; 0.3–0.4 g/L; β, 1.74; 95% CI, 1.17–2.63; $p = 0.007$), and Hb concentrations (β, 0.97; 95% CI, 0.96–0.99; $p = 0.001$) were significant predictors of HIV RNA viral load ($\log_{10}$ genome equivalents per mL) (Friis et al., 2003). HIV-infected pregnant women with depleted iron stores (serum ferritin < 12.0 μg/L) had significantly lower HIV RNA viral load compared to HIV-infected pregnant women with replete iron stores (serum ferritin > 24.0 μg/L).

Similarly, in a prospective observational analysis of 584 HIV-infected pregnant women participating in the TOV, maternal serum ferritin concentrations were significantly correlated with higher maternal HIV viral load ($p < 0.05$) (Kupka et al., 2007a). In an observational analysis in the same trial ($n = 840$), maternal anemia (Hb < 11.0 g/dL) was also associated with a greater risk of the combined outcome of MTCT of HIV or child mortality (HR, 2.58; 95% CI, 1.66–4.01; p-value for trend < 0.0001) (Isanaka et al., 2012). In an analysis of data from four randomized trials from Tanzania, Zambia, and Malawi, with a sample of 2126 HIV-infected pregnant women, severe maternal anemia (Hb < 8.5 g/dL) was associated with increased odds of fetal loss or stillbirth (OR, 3.67; 95% CI, 1.16–11.66; $p = 0.02$), preterm birth (<37 weeks gestation; OR, 2.08; 95% CI, 1.39–3.10; $p < 0.01$), low birthweight (<2500 g; OR, 1.76; 95% CI, 1.07–2.90; $p = 0.04$), and MTCT of HIV at birth (OR, 2.26; 95% CI, 1.18–4.34; $p = 0.01$) and in the first six weeks of life (OR, 2.33; 95% CI, 1.15–4.73; $p = 0.02$) (Mehta et al., 2008b).

Similar findings were observed in a cohort study of 1084 HIV-infected pregnant women in Thailand (Traisathit et al., 2009). Pregnant women were recruited at 28 to 35 weeks of gestation and administered different zidovudine regimens. Higher baseline Hb levels were associated with increased odds of preterm birth (>11.5 vs. ≥11.5 g/dL; OR, 1.9; 95% CI, 1.2–3.1; $p = 0.01$) compared to lower Hb levels. In a cross-sectional study of 483 HIV-infected pregnant women on ART in Malawi, higher Hb concentrations were correlated with lower plasma HIV RNA viral load (r, –0.104; $p < 0.03$) (Semba et al., 2001).

Zinc

In a cross-sectional study in Gondar, Ethiopia, the prevalence of zinc deficiency (serum zinc < 75.0 μg/L) was higher in HIV-infected pregnant women compared to HIV-uninfected pregnant women (76.2% vs. 65.5%) (Kassu et al., 2008). The Cu/Zn (copper/zinc) ratio was also higher in HIV-infected individuals (HIV-infected, 4.7 μg/dL vs. HIV-uninfected, 3.8 μg/dL; $p < 0.05$) compared to HIV-uninfected individuals (Kassu et al., 2008). In a study in Haiti among HIV-infected pregnant women, there were no significant associations between maternal serum zinc levels and risk of MTCT of HIV (Ruff, 1997).

Selenium

In a cross-sectional study in Gondar, Ethiopia, the prevalence of selenium deficiency (serum selenium < 7.0 μg/L) was higher in HIV-infected pregnant women than in HIV-uninfected pregnant women (45.2% vs. 18.9%) (Kassu et al., 2008). In a cohort study among HIV-infected pregnant women in Tanzania, low baseline selenium status (plasma selenium < 114 μg/L; 12–27 weeks gestation) was associated with a significantly increased risk of maternal mortality over a median follow-up period of 5.7 years ($p = 0.01$) (Kupka et al., 2004). Higher maternal selenium concentrations were also associated with higher maternal CD4 T-cell counts in the first two years of follow-up ($p = 0.02$). In an analysis of the TOV, low maternal selenium status (plasma selenium < 114 μg/L) was also associated with increased risks of fetal death (RR, 1.94; 95% CI, 1.08–3.49; $p = 0.03$), child mortality (RR, 1.46; 95% CI, 1.03–2.06; $p = 0.03$), and HIV transmission during the intrapartum and early breastfeeding period (RR, 2.51; 95% CI, 1.19–5.30; $p = 0.01$) compared to higher plasma selenium concentrations (Kupka et al., 2005). Low maternal selenium status (<114 μg/L) was also associated with a lower risk of small-for-gestational-age infants (<10th percentile for gestational age; RR, 0.56; 95% CI, 0.32–0.97; p-value for trend = 0.03); however, no significant associations were noted between maternal selenium status and risks of low birthweight or preterm birth ($p > 0.05$) (Kupka et al., 2005). Women with plasma selenium concentrations in the middle tertile (114–131 μg/L) had higher HIV-1 RNA viral loads compared to the lowest tertile (<114 μg/L) (RR, 1.21; 95% CI, 1.02–1.44; $p = 0.03$). Women in the middle (114–131 μg/L) and highest (>131 μg/L) tertiles of plasma selenium also had higher risk of HIV viral shedding compared to the lowest tertile (<114 μg/L) (71% vs. 50%; RR, 1.46; 95% CI, 1.10–1.92; $p = 0.01$; and 69% vs. 50%; RR, 1.39; 95% CI, 1.05–1.84; $p = 0.02$, respectively) (Kupka et al., 2007b).

Vitamin D

The associations of maternal vitamin D status with perinatal outcomes in HIV-infected pregnant women have been investigated in several observational studies. A case-control study in Botswana found no associations between maternal vitamin D insufficiency at delivery and odds of child morbidity or mortality (AOR, 1.17; 95% CI, 0.70–1.98; $p = 0.55$), after adjusting for maternal CD4 T-cell counts and pretreatment HIV-1 RNA levels (Powis et al., 2014). In prospective observational studies, low maternal vitamin D status (serum 25-hydroxy vitamin D < 80.0 μmol/L) at baseline (12–27 weeks of gestation) was associated with increased risk of severe anemia (Hb < 8.5 g/dL; RR, 1.46; 95% CI, 1.09–1.96; $p = 0.01$) (Mehta et al., 2010a) and severe microcytosis (RR, 3.20; 95% CI, 1.04–9.85; $p = 0.04$) (Finkelstein et al., 2012b) compared to higher vitamin D status. Low maternal vitamin D status has also been associated with increased risks of adverse pregnancy and infant outcomes, including increased risks of overall MTCT of HIV by 6 weeks of age (i.e., *in utero*, intrapartum, and via breastfeeding) (RR, 1.50; 95% CI, 1.23–1.83; $p < 0.01$), stillbirth (RR, 1.49; 95% CI, 1.07–2.09; $p = 0.02$), MTCT of HIV at 6 weeks of age (RR, 1.50; 95% CI, 1.02–2.20; $p = 0.04$), and the combined endpoint of HIV infection or death at 2 years of age (RR, 1.46; 95% CI, 1.11–1.91; $p < 0.01$) (Mehta et al., 2009). Finally, low maternal vitamin D status was also associated with increased risk of pediatric cough (RR, 1.11; 95% CI, 1.02–1.21; $p = 0.01$), stunting (RR, 1.29; 95% CI, 1.05–1.59; $p = 0.02$), and underweight (RR, 1.33; 95% CI, 1.03–1.71; $p = 0.03$) in offspring at 2 years of age (Finkelstein et al., 2012a).

Randomized Trials

The findings from the observational studies noted here informed the development of several randomized trials to examine the effects of micronutrient supplementation on pregnancy outcomes in HIV-infected pregnant women. These are all summarized in Table 6.1.

Vitamin A and β-Carotene

In Malawi, 697 HIV-infected pregnant women were randomized to receive either daily vitamin A (10,000 IU) supplementation with iron–folic acid or iron–folic acid supplementation alone, from enrollment (18–28 weeks gestation) until delivery (Kumwenda et al., 2002). Maternal vitamin A supplementation significantly reduced the risk of low birthweight (<2500 g; 14.0% vs. 21.2%; $p = 0.03$) and infant anemia (Hb < 11.0 g/dL; 23.4% vs. 40.6%; $p < 0.001$) at six weeks postpartum; however, vitamin A supplementation did not decrease the risk of other adverse pregnancy outcomes, including MTCT of HIV, prematurity, fetal death, or infant mortality ($p > 0.05$) (Kumwenda et al., 2002).

In a trial in South Africa, Coutsoudis et al. (1999) examined the effects of vitamin A supplementation on the risk of adverse perinatal outcomes in HIV-infected pregnant women. Investigators randomized 728 HIV-infected pregnant women to receive either vitamin A supplements or placebo. The vitamin A intervention consisted of a daily dose of 5000 IU of vitamin A and 30 milligrams of β-carotene during the third trimester and a 200,000-IU dose of vitamin A at delivery. This vitamin A regimen significantly reduced the risk of preterm delivery (11.4% vs. 17.4%; $p = 0.03$). However, vitamin A had no significant effects on the risks of MTCT of HIV, low birthweight, small-for-gestational-age infants, or fetal death ($p > 0.05$) (Coutsoudis et al., 1999).

In a randomized trial in Zimbabwe, Humphrey et al. (2006) evaluated the efficacy of vitamin A supplementation in preventing adverse pregnancy outcomes in HIV-infected women. The vitamin A intervention consisted of a single postpartum dose of vitamin A administered to women (400,000 IU) and/or infants (50,000 IU) at delivery. Vitamin A supplementation to either the mother or infant significantly increased the risk of vertical HIV transmission and infant mortality compared to placebo. However, vitamin A administered to both the mother and infant did not increase the risk of these outcomes compared to the placebo. Additionally, all three vitamin A regimens resulted in a twofold increase in the risk of mortality among infants who were not infected with HIV at six weeks postpartum ($p < 0.05$) compared to the placebo (Humphrey et al., 2006).

Zinc

The effect of maternal zinc supplementation on pregnancy outcomes was examined in HIV-infected women in a randomized trial in Tanzania (Villamor et al., 2006). Investigators enrolled 400 HIV-infected pregnant women and randomized them to receive daily zinc supplementation (25 mg) or placebo until six weeks postpartum. All women also received iron (60 mg) and folic acid (400 µg), in accordance with national and international guidelines. There were no significant differences in the risk of MTCT of HIV or maternal HIV-1 viral load ($p > 0.05$) between the zinc- and placebo-supplemented groups. However, maternal zinc supplementation significantly increased the risk of maternal wasting (mid-upper arm circumference [MUAC] < 22 cm) compared to placebo, with a 2.7 times greater risk during the follow-up period (mean, 22 weeks; RR, 2.7; 95% CI, 1.1–6.4; $p = 0.03$) and a 4-mm mean reduction in MUAC during the second trimester ($p = 0.02$) (Villamor et al., 2006). Furthermore, zinc supplementation had no significant effects on maternal CD4, CD8, or CD3 T-cell counts or the risks of low birthweight, preterm delivery, fetal death, or neonatal mortality compared to placebo ($p > 0.05$). Maternal Hb concentrations increased in both the zinc and control groups, although this effect was blunted in the zinc-supplemented group (mean increase, zinc: 11.5 ± 17.9 g/L vs. placebo: 15.2 ± 18.6 g/L). This finding may be attributable to zinc's interference with enteric iron absorption (via DMT1 and ferroportin-1) (Fawzi et al., 2005; Villamor et al., 2006).

Selenium

The effect of selenium supplementation on maternal HIV disease progression and adverse pregnancy outcomes was investigated in a trial in Tanzania (Kupka et al., 2008). A total of 913 women were enrolled at 12 to 27 weeks of gestation and randomized to receive daily supplements of selenium (200 μg elemental selenium, selenomethionine) or placebo until six months after delivery. All women also received iron (60 mg) and folic acid (400 μg), in accordance with national and international guidelines. Selenium did not significantly reduce maternal HIV disease progression or the risks of low birthweight, preterm delivery, fetal death, or neonatal mortality compared to the placebo ($p > 0.05$). However, infants born to mothers who received selenium supplements had significantly lower risk of death by 6 weeks of age (RR, 0.43; 95% CI, 0.19–0.99; $p = 0.048$) (Kupka et al., 2008). Selenium supplements had no significant effects on maternal hemoglobin concentrations during follow-up (mean difference, 0.05 g/dL; 95% CI, −0.07–0.16 g/dL; $p > 0.05$) compared to placebo. However, compared to the placebo, selenium supplementation significantly reduced the risk of maternal diarrheal morbidity by 40% (RR, 0.60; 95% CI, 0.42–0.84; $p < 0.05$) for both acute diarrhea (≥1 day and <14 days; RR, 0.59; 95% CI, 0.42–0.83; $p = 0.003$) and watery diarrhea (diarrheal episodes without mucus or blood) (RR, 0.56; 95% CI, 0.39–0.81; $p = 0.002$) during the follow-up period (Kupka et al., 2008, 2009). In a subsequent analysis, investigators examined the effects of maternal selenium supplementation on the presence of HIV-1 in breast milk among 420 HIV-infected lactating women who were participating in the aforementioned selenium trial (Sudfeld et al., 2014). The proportion of women with detectable HIV-1 in breast milk was not significantly higher in the selenium group than in the placebo group (36.4% vs. 27.5%; RR, 1.32; 95% CI, 1.00–1.76; $p = 0.05$). However, in secondary analyses among HAART-naïve women, the prevalence of detectable HIV-1 viral load in breast milk was significantly higher in the selenium group than in the placebo group (37.8% vs. 27.5%; RR, 1.37; 95% CI, 1.03–1.82; $p = 0.03$) (Sudfeld et al., 2014).

Multiple Micronutrients

The TOV was conducted to investigate the effects of maternal micronutrient supplementation on HIV disease progression, MTCT of HIV, and risk of adverse pregnancy outcomes among ART-naïve, HIV-infected pregnant women and their children in Tanzania. In this randomized, double-blind, placebo-controlled trial, 1078 HIV-infected pregnant women were enrolled at 12 to 27 weeks gestation and randomized to receive daily doses of (1) vitamin A alone, (2) multivitamins alone, (3) vitamin A and multivitamins, or (4) placebo, using a 2 × 2 factorial design. The multivitamin supplement included vitamins B-complex, C, and E in doses at 6 to 10 times the RDA level (20 mg vitamin B_1, 20 mg vitamin B_2, 100 mg vitamin B_3, 25 mg vitamin B_6, 0.8 mg folic acid, 50 mg vitamin B_{12}, 500 mg vitamin C, and 30 mg vitamin E). The vitamin A intervention consisted of 5000 IU of preformed vitamin A and 30 mg of β-carotene daily, with an additional 200,000 IU of vitamin A administered at delivery. All women also received iron (60 mg) and folic acid (400 μg) daily during pregnancy in accordance with WHO and Tanzania Ministry of Health guidelines.

Pregnancy Outcomes   Maternal multivitamin supplements significantly decreased the risks of severe preterm birth (<34 weeks gestation) by 39% (RR, 0.61; 95% CI, 0.38–0.96; $p = 0.03$), low birthweight (<2500 g) by 44% (RR, 0.56; 95% CI, 0.38–0.82; $p = 0.003$), small-for-gestational-age infants by 43% (RR, 0.57; 95% CI, 0.39–0.82; $p = 0.002$), and fetal death by 39% (RR, 0.61; 95% CI, 0.39–0.94; $p = 0.02$) compared to no multivitamins. Vitamin A supplementation had no significant effects on these pregnancy outcomes ($p > 0.05$) (Fawzi et al., 1998). Multivitamin supplementation did not affect the risk of MTCT of HIV in the overall population; however, multivitamins significantly reduced the risk of HIV transmission through breastfeeding in a subgroup of women who were nutritionally and/or immunologically compromised at baseline, defined as low T-cell lymphocyte counts (<1340/mm³; RR, 0.37; 95% CI, 0.16–0.85; $p = 0.02$), severe anemia (Hb < 8.5g/dL; p-for-interaction = 0.06), or high erythrocyte sedimentation rate (≥81 mm/hr; p-for-interaction

= 0.06) (Fawzi et al., 2002). In contrast to *a priori* hypotheses, vitamin A supplementation signifi-cantly increased the presence of detectable HIV in the genital tract (vitamin A, 74.8% vs. no vitamin A, 65.1%; $p = 0.04$) compared to no multivitamins (Fawzi et al., 2004a). Vitamin A supplementation also increased the risk of severe subclinical mastitis (Na/K > 1.0) by 45% ($p = 0.03$) (Arsenault et al., 2010) and increased HIV viral shedding in breast milk (proportion of breast milk samples with a detectable viral load at six months postpartum; RR, 1.34; 95% CI, 1.04–1.73; $p = 0.02$) compared to no multivitamins (Villamor et al., 2010). Vitamin A supplementation also significantly *increased the risk of HIV transmission* through breastfeeding by 38% (RR, 1.38; 95% CI, 1.09–1.76; $p = 0.009$) (Fawzi et al., 2002).

Maternal Outcomes   Multivitamin (B-complex, C, and E) supplementation significantly increased maternal CD4 and CD8 T-cell counts (mean difference, 385 cells/µL; $p < 0.001$) (Fawzi et al., 1998) and Hb concentrations (mean difference, 0.33 g/dL; $p = 0.07$) (Fawzi et al., 2007) and increased maternal weight gain during pregnancy by 304 g (95% CI, 17–590; $p = 0.04$) (Villamor et al., 2002). Multivitamins also reduced the incidence of clinical malaria by 71% (95% CI, 11–91; $p = 0.02$) com-pared to no multivitamins (Villamor et al., 2007). Prenatal multivitamin supplementation signifi-cantly reduced the risk of developing hypertension during pregnancy (RR, 0.62; 95% CI, 0.40–0.94; $p = 0.03$) compared to no multivitamins (Merchant et al., 2005). Vitamin A supplementation had no effects on any of these maternal outcomes (Villamor et al., 2002; Fawzi et al., 2004b; Merchant et al., 2005). Vitamin A supplementation significantly increased the risk of severe subclinical mas-titis ($p = 0.03$) (Arsenault et al., 2010). Women who received multivitamins (B-complex, C, and E) also had a 33% greater risk of subclinical mastitis (Na/K > 0.6; $p = 0.005$) and a 75% greater risk of severe subclinical mastitis (Na/K > 1.0; $p = 0.0006$) compared to women who did not receive multivitamins. A second Trial of Vitamins (TOV2) was conducted to examine the efficacy of multi-vitamin B-complex, C, and E supplementation at multiples of the RDA level compared to the single RDA level in decreasing the risk of adverse pregnancy outcomes among HIV-infected pregnant women in Tanzania (Kawai et al., 2010). In this double-blind, randomized controlled trial, a total of 1,129 HIV-infected pregnant women were enrolled at 12 to 27 weeks of gestation and randomized to receive daily oral supplements of multivitamins B-complex, C, and E through six weeks post-partum. The multiple RDA level regimen included vitamins B-complex, C, and E at 6 to 10 times the RDA level (i.e., 20 mg vitamin B_1, 20 mg vitamin B_2, 100 mg vitamin B_3, 25 mg vitamin B_6, 0.8 mg folic acid, 50 mg vitamin B_{12}, 500 mg vitamin C, and 30 mg vitamin E) or the same composi-tion used in the original TOV. In addition, all women received iron (60 mg ferrous sulfate) and folic acid (400 µg) in accordance with WHO and Tanzanian standard of care guidelines. There were no significant differences in the effects of multivitamins at the multiple RDA level on the risk of low birthweight (11.0% vs. 10.2%; $p = 0.75$), gestation duration, birth length, head circumference, pla-cental weight, risk of small-for-gestational-age infants, or risk of preterm birth ($p > 0.05$) compared to multivitamins at the single RDA level (Kawai et al., 2010). Findings from randomized trials on micronutrient supplementation in HIV-infected pregnant women are summarized in Table 6.1.

DISCUSSION

In summary, micronutrient deficiencies are prevalent in HIV-infected pregnant women and asso-ciated with increased risk of adverse health outcomes for both the mother and infant. Multivitamin supplementation (including vitamins B-complex, C, and E) has consistently demonstrated ben-eficial effects on the risk of adverse pregnancy outcomes among HIV-infected women, includ-ing prematurity, low birthweight, small-for-gestational-age infants, and fetal death. For vitamin A, the evidence from observational studies of a potential beneficial association with pregnancy outcomes in HIV-infected women has either not been supported or has been directly contra-dicted by randomized controlled trials. This is probably partially explained by the limitations of the observational study design. The observed associations between micronutrient deficiencies and HIV-related outcomes may be due to reverse causation; that is, HIV infection may lead to decreased nutrient absorption, impaired metabolism, and increased excretion, resulting in lower serum micronutrient concentrations and an apparent deficiency, whereas altered concentrations of micronutrients may be attributable to the acute phase response to infection, rather than actual micronutrient status. Micronutrient concentrations were also often assessed at a single time-point and associated with HIV-related outcomes, which may obscure findings between both HIV and host nutritional status, which change over time. Several vitamin A-specific mechanisms may also explain the increased risk of vertical HIV transmission in vitamin A trials in Tanzania and Zimbabwe (discussed in Chapter 1 of this volume), as well as controversies regarding infant feeding and HIV (see Chapter 7 of this volume) and pediatric health in HIV/AIDS (see Chapter 8 of this volume). Based on these findings, vitamin A supplementation at doses above the single RDA level is not recommended for HIV-infected pregnant women. In addition, findings from a trial of selenium supplementation had no significant effects on HIV disease progression and pregnancy outcomes and may even increase HIV-1 viral load in breast milk in women who are not receiving ART. There is currently no strong epidemiological evidence to support the use of selenium or other micronutrient supplements, such as zinc or vitamin D, to prevent adverse perinatal outcomes in HIV-infected pregnant women.

MICRONUTRIENT DOSE AND ADMINISTRATION

Current epidemiological evidence supports the use of multivitamin supplements B-complex, C, and E (in addition to iron–folic acid) in HIV-infected pregnant women to reduce the risk of adverse pregnancy outcomes. However, to date, there is limited evidence of an additional benefit of higher dose multivitamins (above the single RDA level) on these outcomes. Further studies on the specific effects of micronutrients in different combinations, doses, and administration are required to inform micronutrient interventions in HIV-infected pregnant women.

To date, there is limited evidence on the effects of micronutrient supplementation among HIV-infected pregnant women on ART or MTCT of HIV. Although some trials have been conducted among women receiving a single dose of nevirapine at delivery or among a subsample of women with advanced HIV disease stages receiving ART, the majority of trials included in this review were conducted among ART-naïve women. It is not clear if the observed effects of multivitamin supplementation in HIV-infected pregnant women can be generalized to non-pregnant women or individuals on ART. The importance of ensuring universal access to ART cannot be overemphasized. Further research is urgently needed to examine the role of micronutrient supplementation as an adjunct to essential ART and to elucidate potential micronutrient–ART interactions and their implications for health outcomes in the mother and infant. Randomized trials of the effects of micronutrient supplementation on perinatal outcomes in HIV-infected pregnant women have not been sufficiently powered to elucidate the specific effects of micronutrients in the context of ART, potential interactions of micronutrients and ART, and effects on maternal and child health outcomes. The safety and efficacy of micronutrient supplementation among HIV-infected pregnant women on HAART—as an adjunct to essential antiretroviral therapy—must be examined, including effects on longer term maternal and child health outcomes.

Micronutrient supplementation is unlikely to be a stand-alone mantra for success in preventing adverse pregnancy outcomes in HIV-infected women. Vulnerable groups such as HIV-infected women are likely to have multiple micronutrient deficiencies, particularly in resource-limited settings. The fact that micronutrients can have either synergistic or antagonistic interactions further complicates the interpretation of the current evidence. Therefore, further attention is needed for complementary public health approaches, such as food fortification and dietary diversification, and to establish the role of nutritional interventions as an adjunct to essential ART.

REFERENCES

Antelman, G., G. I. Msamanga, D. Spiegelman et al. (2000). Nutritional factors and infectious disease contribute to anemia among pregnant women with human immunodeficiency virus in Tanzania. *Journal of Nutrition* 130(8): 1950–7.

Arsenault, J. E., S. Aboud, K. P. Manji, W. W. Fawzi, and E. Villamor. (2010). Vitamin supplementation increases risk of subclinical mastitis in HIV-infected women. *Journal of Nutrition* 140(10): 1788–92.

Baylin, A., E. Villamor, N. Rifai, G. Msamanga, and W. W. Fawzi. (2005). Effect of vitamin supplementation to HIV-infected pregnant women on the micronutrient status of their infants. *European Journal of Clinical Nutrition* 59(8): 960–8.

Burns, D. N., G. FitzGerald, R. Semba et al.; Women and Infants Transmission Study Group. (1999). Vitamin A deficiency and other nutritional indices during pregnancy in human immunodeficiency virus infection: prevalence, clinical correlates, and outcome. *Clinical Infectious Diseases* 29(2): 328–34.

Coutsoudis, A., K. Pillay, E. Spooner, L. Kuhn, and H. M. Coovadia; South African Vitamin A Study Group. (1999). Randomized trial testing the effect of vitamin A supplementation on pregnancy outcomes and early mother-to-child HIV-1 transmission in Durban, South Africa. *AIDS* 13(12): 1517–24.

Dreyfuss, M. L. and W. W. Fawzi. (2002). Micronutrients and vertical transmission of HIV-1. *American Journal of Clinical Nutrition* 75(6): 959–70.

Fawzi, W. (2003). Micronutrients and human immunodeficiency virus type 1 disease progression among adults and children. *Clinical Infectious Diseases* 37(Suppl. 2): S112–6.

Fawzi, W. W., G. I. Msamanga, D. Spiegelman et al. (1998). Randomised trial of effects of vitamin supplements on pregnancy outcomes and T cell counts in HIV-1-infected women in Tanzania. *Lancet* 351(9114): 1477–82.

Fawzi, W. W., G. Msamanga, D. Hunter et al. (2000). Randomized trial of vitamin supplements in relation to vertical transmission of HIV-1 in Tanzania. *Journal of Acquired Immune Deficiency Syndromes* 23(3): 246–54.

Fawzi, W. W., G. I. Msamanga, D. Hunter et al. (2002). Randomized trial of vitamin supplements in relation to transmission of HIV-1 through breastfeeding and early child mortality. *AIDS* 16(14): 1935–44.

Fawzi, W. W., G. I. Msamanga, R. Wei et al. (2003). Effect of providing vitamin supplements to human immunodeficiency virus-infected, lactating mothers on the child's morbidity and CD4+ cell counts. *Clinical Infectious Diseases* 36(8): 1053–62.

Fawzi, W., G. Msamanga, G. Antelman et al. (2004a). Effect of prenatal vitamin supplementation on lower-genital levels of HIV type 1 and interleukin type 1 beta at 36 weeks of gestation. *Clinical Infectious Diseases* 38(5): 716–22.

Fawzi, W. W., G. I. Msamanga, D. Spiegelman et al. (2004b). A randomized trial of multivitamin supplements and HIV disease progression and mortality. *New England Journal of Medicine* 351(1): 23–32.

Fawzi, W. W., E. Villamor, G. I. Msamanga et al. (2005). Trial of zinc supplements in relation to pregnancy outcomes, hematologic indicators, and T cell counts among HIV-1-infected women in Tanzania. *American Journal of Clinical Nutrition* 81(1): 161–7.

Fawzi, W. W., G. I. Msamanga, R. Kupka et al. (2007). Multivitamin supplementation improves hematologic status in HIV-infected women and their children in Tanzania. *American Journal of Clinical Nutrition* 85(5): 1335–43.

Filteau, S. M., N. C. Rollins, A. Coutsoudis, K. R. Sullivan, J. F. Willumsen, and A. M. Tomkins. (2001). The effect of antenatal vitamin A and beta-carotene supplementation on gut integrity of infants of HIV-infected South African women. *Journal of Pediatric Gastroenterology and Nutrition* 32(4): 464–70.

Finkelstein, J. L., S. Mehta, C. Duggan et al. (2012a). Maternal vitamin D status and child morbidity, anemia, and growth in human immunodeficiency virus-exposed children in Tanzania. *Pediatric Infectious Disease Journal* 31(2): 171–5.

Finkelstein, J. L., S. Mehta, C. P. Duggan et al. (2012b). Predictors of anaemia and iron deficiency in HIV-infected pregnant women in Tanzania: a potential role for vitamin D and parasitic infections. *Public Health Nutrition* 15(5): 928–37.

Friis, H., E. Gomo, P. Koestel et al. (2001a). HIV and other predictors of serum beta-carotene and retinol in pregnancy: a cross-sectional study in Zimbabwe. *American Journal of Clinical Nutrition* 73(6): 1058–65.

Friis, H., E. Gomo, P. Koestel et al. (2001b). HIV and other predictors of serum folate, serum ferritin, and hemoglobin in pregnancy: a cross-sectional study in Zimbabwe. *American Journal of Clinical Nutrition* 73(6): 1066–73.

Friis, H., E. Gomo, N. Nyazema et al. (2003). Iron, haptoglobin phenotype, and HIV-1 viral load: a cross-sectional study among pregnant Zimbabwean women. *Journal of Acquired Immune Deficiency Syndromes* 33(1): 74–81.

Gomo, E., S. M. Filteau, A. M. Tomkins, P. Ndhlovu, K. F. Michaelsen, and H. Friis. (2003). Subclinical mastitis among HIV-infected and uninfected Zimbabwean women participating in a multimicronutrient supplementation trial. *Transactions of the Royal Society of Tropical Medicine and Hygiene* 97(2): 212–6.

Graham, N., M. Bulterys, A. Chao et al. (1993). Effect of Maternal Vitamin A Deficiency on Infant Mortality and Perinatal HIV Transmission, paper presented at the National Conference on Human Retroviruses and Related Infection, Johns Hopkins University, Baltimore, MD, December 12–16.

Greenberg, B. L., R. D. Semba, P. E. Vink et al. (1997). Vitamin A deficiency and maternal-infant transmissions of HIV in two metropolitan areas in the United States. *AIDS* 11(3): 325–32.

Humphrey, J. H., P. J. Iliff, E. T. Marinda et al. (2006). Effects of a single large dose of vitamin A, given during the postpartum period to HIV-positive women and their infants, on child HIV infection, HIV-free survival, and mortality. *Journal of Infectious Diseases* 193(6): 860–71.

Isanaka, S., D. Spiegelman, S. Aboud et al. (2012). Post-natal anaemia and iron deficiency in HIV-infected women and the health and survival of their children. *Maternal and Child Nutrition* 8(3): 287–98.

Ivers, L. C., K. A. Cullen, K. A. Freedberg, S. Block, J. Coates, and P. Webb. (2009). HIV/AIDS, undernutrition and food insecurity. *Clinical Infectious Diseases* 49(7): 1096–102.

Kassu, A., T. Yabutani, A. Mulu, B. Tessema, and F. Ota. (2008). Serum zinc, copper, selenium, calcium, and magnesium levels in pregnant and non-pregnant women in Gondar, Northwest Ethiopia. *Biological Trace Element Research* 122(2): 97–106.

Kawai, K., R. Kupka, F. Mugusi et al. (2010). A randomized trial to determine the optimal dosage of multivitamin supplements to reduce adverse pregnancy outcomes among HIV-infected women in Tanzania. *American Journal of Clinical Nutrition* 91(2): 391–7.

Kennedy, C. M., A. Coutsoudis, L. Kuhn et al. (2000). Randomized controlled trial assessing the effect of vitamin A supplementation on maternal morbidity during pregnancy and postpartum among HIV-infected women. *Journal of Acquired Immune Deficiency Syndromes* 24(1): 37–44.

Kennedy-Oji, C., A. Coutsoudis, L. Kuhn et al. (2001). Effects of vitamin A supplementation during pregnancy and early lactation on body weight of South African HIV-infected women. *Journal of Health, Population and Nutrition* 19(3): 167–76.

Keusch, G. T. and M. J. Farthing. (1990). Nutritional aspects of AIDS. *Annual Review of Nutrition* 10(1): 475–501.

Kumwenda, N., P. G. Miotti, T. E. Taha et al. (2002). Antenatal vitamin A supplementation increases birth weight and decreases anemia among infants born to human immunodeficiency virus-infected women in Malawi. *Clinical Infectious Diseases* 35(5): 618–24.

Kupka, R. and W. Fawzi. (2002). Zinc nutrition and HIV infection. *Nutrition Reviews* 60(3): 69–79.

Kupka, R., G. I. Msamanga, D. Spiegelman et al. (2004). Selenium status is associated with accelerated HIV disease progression among HIV-1-infected pregnant women in Tanzania. *Journal of Nutrition* 134(10): 2556–60.

Kupka, R., M. Garland, G. Msamanga, D. Spiegelman, D. Hunter, and W. Fawzi. (2005). Selenium status, pregnancy outcomes, and mother-to-child transmission of HIV-1. *Journal of Acquired Immune Deficiency Syndromes* 39(2): 203–10.

Kupka, R., G. I. Msamanga, F. Mugusi, P. Petraro, D. J. Hunter, and W. W. Fawzi. (2007a). Iron status is an important cause of anemia in HIV-infected Tanzanian women but is not related to accelerated HIV disease progression. *Journal of Nutrition* 137(10): 2317–23.

Kupka, R., G. I. Msamanga, C. Xu, D. Anderson, D. Hunter, and W. W. Fawzi. (2007b). Relationship between plasma selenium concentrations and lower genital tract levels of HIV-1 RNA and interleukin type 1beta. *European Journal of Clinical Nutrition* 61(4): 542–7.

Kupka, R., F. Mugusi, S. Aboud et al. (2008). Randomized, double-blind, placebo-controlled trial of selenium supplements among HIV-infected pregnant women in Tanzania: effects on maternal and child outcomes. *American Journal of Clinical Nutrition* 87(6): 1802–8.

Kupka, R., F. Mugusi, S. Aboud, E. Hertzmark, D. Spiegelman, and W. W. Fawzi. (2009). Effect of selenium supplements on hemoglobin concentration and morbidity among HIV-1-infected Tanzanian women. *Clinical Infectious Diseases* 48(10): 1475–8.

McGrath, N., D. Bellinger, J. Robins, G. I. Msamanga, E. Tronick, and W. W. Fawzi. (2006). Effect of maternal multivitamin supplementation on the mental and psychomotor development of children who are born to HIV-1-infected mothers in Tanzania. *Pediatrics* 117(2): e216–25.

Mehta, S., J. L. Finkelstein, and W. W. Fawzi. (2008a). Micronutrient status and pregnancy outcomes in HIV-infected women. In: *Nutrition and Health: Handbook of Nutrition and Pregnancy* (Lammi-Keefe, C.J., Couch, S. C., and Philipson, E. H., Eds.), pp. 355–365. Totowa, NJ: Humana Press.

Mehta, S., K. P. Manji, A. M. Young et al. (2008b). Nutritional indicators of adverse pregnancy outcomes and mother-to-child transmission of HIV among HIV-infected women. *American Journal of Clinical Nutrition* 87(6): 1639–49.

Mehta, S., D. J. Hunter, F. M. Mugusi et al. (2009). Perinatal outcomes, including mother-to-child transmission of HIV, and child mortality and their association with maternal vitamin D status in Tanzania. *Journal of Infectious Diseases* 200(7): 1022–30.

Mehta, S., E. Giovannucci, F. M. Mugusi et al. (2010a). Vitamin D status of HIV-infected women and its association with HIV disease progression, anemia, and mortality. *PLoS One* 5(1): e8770.

Mehta, S., D. Spiegelman, S. Aboud et al. (2010b). Lipid-soluble vitamins A, D, and E in HIV-infected pregnant women in Tanzania. *European Journal of Clinical Nutrition* 64(8): 808–17.

Merchant, A. T., G. Msamanga, E. Villamor et al. (2005). Multivitamin supplementation of HIV-positive women during pregnancy reduces hypertension. *Journal of Nutrition* 135(7): 1776–81.

Powis, K., S. Lockman, L. Smeaton et al. (2014). Vitamin D insufficiency in HIV-infected pregnant women receiving antiretroviral therapy is not associated with morbidity, mortality or growth impairment in their uninfected infants in Botswana. *Pediatric Infectious Disease Journal* 33(11): 1141–7.

Ruff, A. (1997). Zinc deficiency and transmission and progression of HIV infection. In: *Zinc for Child Health* (Kelley, L. and Black, R. E., Eds.), p. 10. Bethesda, MD: American Society for Clinical Nutrition.

Semba, R. D., P. G. Miotti, J. D. Chiphangwi et al. (1994). Maternal vitamin A deficiency and mother-to-child transmission of HIV-1. *Lancet* 343(8913): 1593–7.

Semba, R. D., P. G. Miotti, J. D. Chiphangwi et al. (1995). Infant mortality and maternal vitamin A deficiency during human immunodeficiency virus infection. *Clinical Infectious Diseases* 21(4): 966–72.

Semba, R. D., T. E. Taha, N. Kumwenda et al. (2001). Iron status and indicators of human immunodeficiency virus disease severity among pregnant women in Malawi. *Clinical Infectious Diseases* 32(10): 1496–9.

Sudfeld, C. R., S. Aboud, R. Kupka, F. M. Mugusi, and W. W. Fawzi. (2014). Effect of selenium supplementation on HIV-1 RNA detection in breast milk of Tanzanian women. *Nutrition* 30(9): 1081–4.

Traisathit, P., J. Y. Mary, S. Le Coeur et al. (2009). Risk factors of preterm delivery in HIV-infected pregnant women receiving zidovudine for the prevention of perinatal HIV. *Journal of Obstetrics and Gynaecology Research* 35(2): 225–33.

Villamor, E., G. Msamanga, D. Spiegelman et al. (2002). Effect of multivitamin and vitamin A supplements on weight gain during pregnancy among HIV-1-infected women. *American Journal of Clinical Nutrition* 76(5): 1082–90.

Villamor, E., E. Saathoff, R. J. Bosch et al. (2005). Vitamin supplementation of HIV-infected women improves postnatal child growth. *American Journal of Clinical Nutrition* 81(4): 880–8.

Villamor, E., S. Aboud, I. N. Koulinska et al. (2006). Zinc supplementation to HIV-1-infected pregnant women: effects on maternal anthropometry, viral load, and early mother-to-child transmission. *European Journal of Clinical Nutrition* 60(7): 862–9.

Villamor, E., G. Msamanga, E. Saathoff, M. Fataki, K. Manji, and W. W. Fawzi. (2007). Effects of maternal vitamin supplements on malaria in children born to HIV-infected women. *American Journal of Tropical Medicine and Hygiene* 76(6): 1066–71.

Villamor, E., I. N. Koulinska, S. Aboud et al. (2010). Effect of vitamin supplements on HIV shedding in breast milk. *American Journal of Clinical Nutrition* 92(4): 881–6.

Webb, A. L., S. Aboud, J. Furtado et al. (2009). Effect of vitamin supplementation on breast milk concentrations of retinol, carotenoids and tocopherols in HIV-infected Tanzanian women. *European Journal of Clinical Nutrition* 63(3): 332–9.

WHO. (2012). *Guideline: Daily Iron and Folic Acid Supplementation in Pregnant Women*. Geneva: World Health Organization.

Zvandasara, P., J. W. Hargrove, R. Ntozini et al. (2006). Mortality and morbidity among postpartum HIV-positive and HIV-negative women in Zimbabwe: risk factors, causes, and impact of single-dose post-partum vitamin A supplementation. *Journal of Acquired Immune Deficiency Syndromes* 43(1): 107–16.

7 HIV and Infant Feeding

Ameena Goga and Anna Coutsoudis

CONTENTS

GENERAL OVERVIEW AND INTRODUCTION

Over the last 10 to 15 years, significant advances have been made in implementing comprehensive policies to prevent HIV transmission from mother to child (MTCT) (Table 7.1). This has culminated in the population-level reduction of MTCT (Table 7.2) even in high HIV-prevalence settings (Goga et al., 2015). Consequently, the global agenda has shifted from the *prevention* of MTCT (PMTCT) to the *elimination* of MTCT (EMTCT). In resource-limited settings where breastfeeding is a critical child survival strategy, EMTCT was initially defined as a reduction in MTCT to <2% by six weeks postpartum and <5% by 18 months postpartum (UNAIDS, 2011). More recently, the World Health Organization (WHO) introduced specific criteria to measure the elimination of MTCT (WHO, 2014):

- New pediatric HIV infections due to MTCT of HIV are ≤50 cases per 100,000 live births.
- The MTCT rate of HIV is less than 5% in breastfeeding populations or less than 2% in non-breastfeeding populations.

These two impact indicators must be achieved for at least one year.
The following process indicators must be achieved for at least two years:

- At least 95% of pregnant women have received at least one antenatal visit, regardless of their HIV status.
- At least 95% of pregnant women know their HIV status.
- At least 90% of HIV-positive pregnant women receive antiretroviral drugs.

The United Nations recommends a four-pronged approach to PMTCT (UNAIDS, 2011):

1. Primary prevention of incident HIV infections in women of childbearing age
2. Prevention of unplanned pregnancies in HIV-infected women
3. Specific drug and intrapartum interventions to prevent MTCT
4. Care, treatment, and support to mothers and their families living with HIV

TABLE 7.1

Summary of WHO PMTCT Guidelines: 2000 to Date

2000–2006[a]	2006–May 2010[b]	June 2010–March 2012[c]	April 2012 to Date[d]
AZT, AZT + 3TC, or sdNVP[e] or combinations (as ART) Choice should consider feasibility, efficacy, and cost	*Treatment for mother* ART [AZT + 3TC + NVP (or EFV) for stage 3 or 4 disease, or stages 1 and 2 disease with CD4 cell count < 200 cells/mm³ *Post-exposure prophylaxis for infant* AZT × 7 days *or* *Prophylaxis for mother* Antepartum: AZT from 28 weeks gestation Intrapartum: sdNVP + AZT/3TC Postpartum: AZT/3TC × 7 days *Post-exposure prophylaxis for infant* sdNVP + AZT × 7 days (or 28 days if no maternal prophylaxis)	*Treatment for mother* ART if CD4 ≤ 350 cells/mm³ or stage 3 or 4 disease: AZT + 3TC + NVP (or EFV)[e] *or* TDF + 3TC (or FTC) + NVP (or EFV)[e] *Post-exposure prophylaxis for infant* Daily NVP or twice daily AZT × 4–6 weeks *or* **Option A** *Prophylaxis for mother* If CD4 count ≤ 350 cells/mm³, triple ART starting as soon as diagnosed and continue for life. If CD4 count > 350 cells/mm³, antepartum AZT from 14 weeks gestation; intrapartum sdNVP and AZT + 3TC; postpartum AZT + 3TC × 7 days *Post-exposure prophylaxis for infant* Daily sdNVP for 6 weeks in non-breastfed infants or if mother on ART, or daily sdNVP until 1 week after BF stops if mother is breastfeeding and not on ART **Option B** *Prophylaxis for mother* All pregnant women will be started on ART regardless of CD4 cell count: AZT + 3TC + LPV/r (or ABC or EFV) *or* TDF + 3TC (or FTC) + EFV If CD4 count ≤ 350 cells/mm³, ART will be continued for life If CD4 count >350 cells/mm³, ART will be started as early as 14 weeks gestation, continue intrapartum and through childbirth, and then stopped if not breastfeeding or continued until 1 week after complete cessation of breastfeeding *Post-exposure prophylaxis for infant* Daily NVP or AZT from birth to 4–6 weeks	During this period, maternal treatment evolved from Option A to Option B and then to Option B+. B+ includes lifelong ART for all pregnant and lactating women. *Treatment for mother* AZT + 3TC + NVP (or EFV)[e] *or* TDF + 3TC (or FTC) + NVP (or EFV)[e] *Post-exposure prophylaxis for infant* Daily NVP or twice daily AZT × 4–6 weeks; treatment may continue to 12 weeks if mother started ART late or is not virally suppressed

Note: 3TC, lamivudine; ABC, abacavir; ART, triple antiretroviral therapy; AZT, azidothymidine; BF, breastfeeding; EBF, exclusive breastfeeding; EFV, efavirenz; FF, formula feeding; FTC, emtricitabine; LPV/r, lopinavir/ritonavir; NVP, nevirapine; sdNVP, single-dose nevirapine.

[a] UNFPA et al. (2000).

[b] WHO (2006).

[c] WHO (2010).

[d] WHO (2012).

[e] At the time, guidelines recommended avoiding EFV in the first trimester and using NVP instead.

TABLE 7.2

Estimated Timing and Risk of Mother-to-Child Human Immunodeficiency Type 1 Transmission without Antiretroviral Interventions and with Minimal Antiretroviral Prophylaxis

| Timing | Without Antiretroviral Cover | | | | With Minimal Antiretroviral Cover | |
| | No Breastfeeding | | Breastfeeding through 18–24 Months | | | |
	Relative Proportion	Absolute Risk	Relative Proportion	Absolute Risk	Breastfeeding Absolute Risk	No Breastfeeding Absolute Risk
Intrauterine	25–35%	5–10%	20–25%	5–10%	2.6%[a]	<0.5%[c]
Intrapartum	65–75%	10–20%	35–50%	10–15%		
Breastfeeding	0	0	25–45%	15–20%	Cumulative risk 4% (3–6%) on triple ART or infant prophylaxis by 48 weeks[b]	0
Overall	Not applicable	15–30%	0	30–45%	3–6%	<0.5%

Source: De Cock, K.M. et al., *JAMA*, 283(9), 1175–82, 2000.

[a] Goga et al. (2016).
[b] Jamieson et al. (2012).
[c] Forbes et al. (2012), Townsend et al. (2014).

In the absence of antiretroviral interventions, the absolute risk of MTCT is 5 to 10% during the intrauterine period, 10 to 20% during the intrapartum period (De Cock et al., 2000), and 15 to 20% through 18 to 24 months of breastfeeding, or approximately 0.89% per month of breastfeeding (Table 7.2) (BHITS Study Group et al., 2004). With antiretroviral interventions, the risk of MTCT has been reduced significantly (Table 7.2).

The main risk factors for MTCT are maternal viral load (which is closely related to disease stage, type of antiretroviral regimen, duration of regimen, and adherence) and infant exposure to infectious fluids (amniotic, cervical, vaginal, and breast milk). The infectivity of amniotic, cervical, and vaginal fluids is closely related to co-infections and type of delivery; breast milk infectivity is closely associated with breastfeeding pattern and duration.

In utero infection is thought to occur mainly in the last trimester, as the placenta seems to block transmission of free HIV-1 virus (by unknown mechanisms) (Dolcini et al., 2003). Thus, *in utero* infection depends on breaks in the placental barrier or transcytosis of infected cells (Lagaye et al., 2001). In recent years, research has demonstrated that early and long-term dual and triple antiretroviral therapy (ART) among HIV-positive women with higher CD4 cell counts (250 to 500 cells/mm³) has HIV-free survival benefits for their infants (Kumwenda et al., 2008; SWEN Study Team, 2008; Shapiro et al., 2010). This resulted in the adoption of policies that recommend ART for all HIV-positive pregnant or lactating women, regardless of their health status, viral load, and CD4 cell count, thus strengthening the third of the four PMTCT prongs (National Department of Health and SANAC, 2010; WHO, 2010; National Department of Health, 2013). Coverage of more efficacious antiretroviral regimens leading toward lifelong ART use at population level has increased substantially over the past two to five years. For example, between 2011 and 2012, coverage of more advanced antiretroviral regimens (i.e., not single-dose nevirapine) for PMTCT increased from 57% (95% CI, 51–64%) to 62% (95% CI, 57–70%) (UNAIDS, 2013a). By 2014, the absolute risk of MTCT was reduced to less than 1% in many developed countries (Lallemant et al., 2004;

TABLE 7.3

Percentage Decline in New HIV Infections among Children from 2009 to 2015 in 20 Global Plan Priority Countries

>66% Decline	33%–66% Decline	<33% Decline
Burundi (84%)	Botswana (63%)	Angola (24%)
Malawi (71%)	Cameroon (49%)	Nigeria (21%)
Mozambique (75%)	Chad (49%)	
Namibia (79%)	Côte d'Ivoire (36%)	
South Africa (84%)	Democratic Republic of the Congo (66%)	
Swaziland (80%)	Ghana (46%)	
Uganda (86%)	Kenya (55%)	
United Republic of Tanzania (69%)	Lesotho (44%)	
Zambia (69%)	Zimbabwe (65%)	

Source: UNAIDS, *On the Fast-Track to an AIDS-Free Generation: The Increadible Journey of the Global Plan Towards the Elimination of New HIV Infections Among Children by 2015 and Keeping Their Mothers Alive,* Joint United Nations Programme on HIV/AIDS, Geneva, 2016 (http://www.aidsdatahub.org/fast-track-aids-free-generation-unaids-2016).

Forbes et al., 2012; WHO, 2012) where breastfeeding is avoided. Between 2009 and 2015, the number of children newly infected with HIV declined in most of the 22 countries where 90% of the world's HIV-positive pregnant women live (Global Plan priority countries), though at varying rates (Table 7.3) (UNAIDS, 2013b).

Data on the population-level impact of interventions to prevent MTCT in resource-limited settings are scanty. We define population-level impact as impact at a national level, which is different from impact in one facility or district. In South Africa, at the population level, early MTCT was reduced to 3.5% by eight weeks postdelivery when PMTCT interventions included maternal prophylaxis (AZT from 28 weeks gestation with a single dose of nevirapine to mother and baby peripartum, and 7 to 28 days AZT) or ART if maternal CD4 cell count ≤ 250 cells/μL (Goga et.al. 2013, 2015). Population-level early MTCT was further reduced to 2.6% by eight weeks postdelivery when the national PMTCT policy was WHO Option A (Table 7.1) (Goga et al., 2016).

As more intensive antiretroviral regimens reduce the risk of intrauterine and intrapartum MTCT, the attributable risk of MTCT through breastfeeding increases, necessitating more focused, advanced, and intensive interventions to achieve the goal of EMTCT. This refers to potentially identifying key high-risk target populations (focused), developing more potent drugs (advanced), and increasing the duration of maternal ART used to reduce maternal viral load and prevent MTCT (intensive) during this and subsequent pregnancies. By 2016, all global plan priority countries had shifted to WHO Option B+, which is a public health approach to reduce vertical and horizontal transmission of HIV (BLC and UNICEF, 2012). Several concerns have been raised around PMTCT Option B+ (Coutsoudis et al., 2013), and some of these have been demonstrated at the country level. A recent national assessment of retention in "Option B+ care" among HIV-infected women in Malawi found that 17% were lost to follow-up six months after ART initiation; most losses occurred in the first three months of initiation (Tenthani et al., 2014). Option B+ pregnant women with CD4 cell count > 350 cells/mL were five times more likely to be lost to follow-up than women who started ART in WHO stage 3 or 4 or with a CD4 cell count ≤ 350 cells/mL (odds ratio [OR], 5.0; 95% CI, 4.2–6.1). Option B+ patients who started therapy postnatally were twice as likely to miss their first follow-up visit (OR, 2.2; 95% CI, 1.8–2.8). Loss to follow-up was highest in pregnant Option B+ patients who initiated ART at large clinics on the day they were diagnosed with HIV (Tenthani et al., 2014).

ROLE OF BREAST MILK IN HIV-FREE SURVIVAL, WAYS TO OPTIMIZE BREASTFEEDING PRACTICES, AND THE PATHOGENESIS OF BREAST MILK HIV TRANSMISSION

Malnutrition predisposes to infection, and infection commonly aggravates malnutrition, resulting in a vicious cycle (Scrimshaw et al., 1968; Scrimshaw, 2003). In resource-limited settings, common childhood infections are the main causes of infant and under-5 mortality. This vicious cycle among malnutrition, infection, and mortality necessitates close attention to nutrition to reduce under-5 mortality (United Nations, 2012) and to meet the post-2015 Sustainable Development Goals (United Nations, 2014). Post-2015 Goal 2 aims to end hunger, improve nutrition, and promote sustainable agriculture (to end all forms of malnutrition by 2020, with special attention to stunting and wasting in children under 5 years of age, and to address the nutritional needs of pregnant and lactating women). Goal 3 aims to attain healthy lives for all (end preventable newborn, infant, and under five deaths by 2030 and end the epidemics of HIV/AIDS, tuberculosis, malaria, and neglected tropical diseases). Pattern of feeding is a significant predictor of malnutrition and consequent child morbidity and mortality (Victora et al., 1987, 1989; WHO Collaborative Study Team, 2000; Black et al., 2008). Following are the WHO definitions of infant feeding (Labbok and Krasovec, 1990):

- *Exclusive breastfeeding* (EBF) means giving the infant breast milk only and any minerals, vitamins, or prescribed medicines as needed for the first six months.
- *Mixed breastfeeding* (MBF) means giving the infant breast milk and other fluids and solids. MBF may be further classified into predominant breastfeeding and partial breastfeeding:
  - *Predominant breastfeeding* (PredBF) means giving the infant breast milk and non-nutritive liquids.
  - *Partial breastfeeding* (ParBF) means feeding breast milk and non-nutritive and nutritive liquids and solids.
- *Exclusive formula feeding* (EFF) means giving the infant only commercial infant formula milk for the first six months of life.
- *Replacement feeding* (RF) refers to the process of feeding a child who is not receiving any breast milk a diet that provides all the nutrients the child needs until the child is fully fed on family foods. During the first six months a suitable breast milk substitute should be used, and, subsequently, complementary foods made from appropriately prepared and nutrient-enriched family foods should be added. This can also been referred to as not breastfeeding (NBF).

Compared with exclusive breastfeeding, predominant breastfeeding, partial breastfeeding, and not breastfeeding are associated with adverse child outcomes (Black et al., 2008):

- A higher overall mortality risk in general—EBF risk ratio [RR] 1.48 (95% CI, 1.13–1.92), PredBF RR 2.85 (95% CI, 1.59–5.10), and ParBF RR 14.40 (95% CI, 6.09–34.05) at 0 to 5 months and NBF RR 3.86 (95% CI, 1.49–9.29) at 6 to 23 months
- A higher mortality risk from diarrhea—EBF RR 2.28 (95% CI, 0.85–6.11), PredBF RR 4.62 (95% CI, 1.81–11.77), and ParBF RR 10.53 (95% CI, 2.80–39.64) at 0 to 5 months and NBF RR 2.83 (95% CI, 0.15–54.82) at 6 to 23 months
- A higher mortality risk from pneumonia—EBF RR 1.75 (95% CI, 0.48–6.43), PredBF RR 2.49 (95% CI, 1.03–6.04), and ParBF RR 15.13 (95% CI, 0.61–373.84) at 0 to 5 months and NBF RR 1.52 (95% CI, 0.09–27.06) at 6 to 23 months

Globally, universal coverage with EBF for six months and continued breastfeeding up to one year may prevent 13% of under-5 deaths globally, even in the context of HIV (Jones et al., 2003).

Although exclusive breastfeeding is not commonly practiced, three seminal papers, published in *The Lancet* between 1999 and 2011, reported results of clinical trials in Mexico, Bangladesh, and Africa that demonstrated improvements in exclusive breastfeeding practices after well-designed, home-based interventions. In a randomized controlled trial conducted in Dhaka, Bangladesh, local mothers who received 10 days of training and graduated as peer counselors implemented a peer counseling intervention for breastfeeding (Haider et al., 2000). Fifteen home-based counseling visits were scheduled between pregnancy and five months postpartum: two visits were in the last trimester, three in the first two weeks postdelivery (within 48 hours, on day 5, and between days 10 and 14), and one visit every two weeks thereafter until five months postpartum. Peer counseling significantly improved breastfeeding practices: the prevalence of exclusive breastfeeding at five months was 202/228 (70%) for the intervention group and 17/285 (6%) for the control group (difference = 64%; 95% CI, 57–71%); $p > 0.0001$). Mothers in the intervention group initiated breastfeeding earlier than control mothers and were less likely to give prelacteal and postlacteal foods.

A similar trial in peri-urban Mexico compared three-month breastfeeding practices among three groups: (1) six peer counseling visits between pregnancy and early postpartum, (2) three peer counseling visits, or (3) a "no visit" control group (Morrow et al., 1999). Peer counselors were recruited from the same community and trained by La Leche League. At three-months postpartum, EBF was practiced by 67% of mothers receiving six visits, 50% of those receiving three visits, and 12% of control mothers (intervention groups vs. controls, $p < 0.001$; six visits vs. three visits, $p = 0.02$). Duration of breastfeeding was significantly ($p = 0.02$) longer in intervention groups than in controls, and fewer infants of mothers in the intervention group, compared with the control group, had episodes of diarrhea (12% vs. 26%; $p = 0.03$).

A cluster randomized trial from Africa, conducted among 24 communities in Burkina Faso, 24 in Uganda, and 34 in South Africa, compared five home visits (one antenatally and four subsequent visits up to 10 to 20 weeks postdelivery) with a control group (Tylleskar et al., 2011). At 12 weeks postdelivery, the reported EBF prevalence (based on 24-hour recall) was higher in the intervention arm compared to the control arm in all countries:

- In Burkina Faso, 79.1% for the intervention arm vs. 34.6% for the control (prevalence ratio [PR] adjusted for cluster and site, 2.29; 95% CI, 1.33–3.92)
- In Uganda, 81.6% for the intervention arm vs. 43.9% for the control (PR, 1.89; 95% CI, 1.70–2.11)
- In South Africa, 10.5% for the intervention arm vs. 6.2% for the control (PR, 1.72; 95% CI, 1.12–2.63)

The prevalence ratios based on seven-day recall results were similar. At 24 weeks, the overall prevalences were lower, but the prevalence ratios remained similar.

HIV transmission through breast milk potentially begins with the first exposure to breast milk. The main portal of entry is the infant's gastrointestinal tract, starting from the mouth. There is general agreement that MTCT through breast milk is surprisingly inefficient, considering the large volumes of HIV-1-contaminated breast milk ingested by infants born to untreated HIV-1 infected mothers (Lohman-Payne et al., 2012). Although the average six-month old ingests more than 100 liters of milk from birth to six months, on average only 15 to 20% of infants will be infected through breastfeeding even without any antiretroviral (ARV) interventions.

Understanding the stages of lactogenesis, as well as physiology and immunology, helps to guide the interventions necessary to prevent HIV transmission through breast milk. Lactogenesis is divided into three stages:

1. Lactogenesis I, which occurs from mid-to-late pregnancy until days 2 to 3 postpartum
2. Lactogenesis II, which occurs from days 2 to 3 postpartum until day 8 postpartum
3. Lactogenesis III, which occurs after day 8 postpartum

During lactogenesis I, mammary alveolar epithelial cells differentiate into secretory cells, fat droplets accumulate, and the concentration of lactose and lactalbumin increases in alveolar cells. During this predominantly antenatal stage, the pregnant woman is primed for milk production and breastfeeding. The main source of infant nutrition during days 0 to 3 is colostrum, packed with lactalbumin and other immune molecules that play a role in inhibiting viral replication. Any disruption to lactogenesis I could affect the concentration of immune protection in breast milk. This, coupled with inadequate antenatal antiretroviral cover (less than four weeks of maternal ART), which increases plasma and thus, breast milk viral load, thereby increases early (peripartum) MTCT through breast milk.

During lactogenesis II there is onset of copious milk secretion. Triggered by delivery of the placenta and a reduction in serum progesterone and estrogen, milk volume increases rapidly from 36 to 96 hours postpartum and then abruptly levels off. This is accompanied by closure of the tight intracellular junction complexes between alveolar cells, reduction in the concentration of breast milk sodium chloride and protein, and an increase in lactose and lipids. Oxytocin and prolactin are released, and there is an increase in maternal metabolism and mammary blood flow. Any circumstance that prevents the closure of tight intracellular junctions, such as non-exclusive breastfeeding and inflammation (subclinical or clinical mastitis), increases the risk of MTCT during days 2 to 8 (Semba et al., 1999). During lactogenesis III there is autocrine regulation of milk production (galactopoesis). Factors that increase the risk of MTCT during lactogenesis II also play a role in increasing MTCT during this phase.

The population attributable fraction (PAF) of viral load and CD4 cell count to late postnatal MTCT in Malawi, Tanzania, and Zambia varies from 16 to 37%, depending on CD4 cell count and viral load (see Table 7.4). Thus, a substantial proportion of late postnatal transmission (LPT) is accounted for in high-risk women with low CD4 and high viral load (VL). Treating these high-risk women with antiretroviral therapy is essential. There is evidence that low viral load is protective against transmission; however, not all transmission occurs among women with high viral loads (see Table 7.4) (Townsend et al., 2014).

Data on the role of breast milk immunological factors in the prevention of MTCT are increasingly emerging (Rowland-Jones et al., 1993; Lohman-Payne et al., 2012; Hicar, 2013). Data from South Africa and Europe suggest that HIV-exposed, uninfected infants can develop HIV-1 specific T-cell responses (Cheynier et al., 1992; Rowland-Jones et al., 1993; Aldhous et al., 1994; Kuhn et al., 2001). A study in Nairobi demonstrated that resistance to postnatal HIV transmission correlated with the magnitude of the HIV-1 specific T-cell response (John-Stewart et al., 2009). This provides optimism that enhancing the immune response to HIV-1 using immunotherapeutic strategies could confer protection against later infection. Table 7.5 lists these protective properties and their role.

TABLE 7.4

Population Attributable Fractions for Late Postnatal Transmission in Sub-Saharan Africa

RF	Late Postnatal Period	Total Incidences	Expected Incidences	Population Attributable Fraction	95% CI
CD4 ≥ 200 cells/mm³ and viral load > 50,000 copies/mL	42–365 days	78	49.5	37	22–51
CD4 < 200 cells/mm³	42–365 days	77	57.2	26	12–36
CD4 < 200 cells/mm³ and viral load > 50,000 copies/mL	42–365 days	73	61.1	16	6–25

Source: Chen, Y.Q. et al., *Journal of Acquired Immune Deficiency Syndromes*, 54(3), 311–316, 2010.

TABLE 7.5
Immunologic Properties in Breast Milk and Infant Responses to HIV Exposure May Protect Against MTCT

Immunologic Property of Breast Milk	Protection Conferred
Secretory immunoglobulin A (sIgA)	Local immunity against entry of HIV, although some studies have shown that sIgA does not appear to be a protective factor against HIV transmission through breast milk (Kuhn et al., 2006)
T and B cells	Antiviral activity
Oligosaccharides	Form viral ligands to prevent mucosal entry of free HIV
	A higher concentration of human milk oligosaccharides (HMOs) was associated with a reduced odds of breastfeeding transmission after adjusting for CD4 cell count and breast milk HIV viral load (OR, 0.45; 95% CI, 0.21–0.97; $p = 0.06$).
	The proportion of 3′-sialyllactose was higher among transmitting women than among non-transmitting women ($p = 0.003$) and correlated with higher plasma and breast milk HIV RNA and lower CD4 cell counts (Bode et al., 2012).
Glycoconjugates	Form viral ligands to prevent mucosal entry of free HIV
α-Defensins	α-Defensins have been associated with a reduction in the risk of intrapartum and postnatal mother-to-child transmission.
IFN-γ cellular immune responses	HIV-specific IFN-γ-secreting cells present in the breast milk of the majority of HIV-1-infected mothers confer a 70% reduction in the likelihood of early mother-to-child transmission.
	Breast milk IFN-γ responses were associated with an approximately 70% reduction in infant HIV infection (adjusted odds ratio, 0.29; 95% CI, 0.092–0.91) (Lohman-Payne et al., 2012).
	Research in Kenya demonstrated a correlation between HIV antigenic exposure and infant IFN-γ responses in HIV-exposed, uninfected infants (Liu et al., 2015).
Immunologic responses in infants: specific T-cell responses	Some data suggest that infants exposed to HIV can develop HIV-1-specific T-cell responses. It is unclear whether this contributes to protection against HIV infection; however, it has been found that resistance to postnatal mother-to-child transmission correlates with the magnitude of HIV-1-specific T-cell responses in a Kenyan study.

Source: Lohman-Payne, B. et al., *Advances in Experimental Medicine and Biology*, 743, 185–195, 2012.

HIV transmission through breast milk is thus a balance between the protection offered by the immune system (natural immunity and host responses within the mother and infants) and the following characteristics:

- Plasma viral load
- Breast milk viral load
- Maternal co-infections
- Leaky alveolar cell junctions
- HIV-1 subtype
- Maternal/infant genetic factors

BREAST MILK HIV TRANSMISSION BEFORE THE ERA OF ANTIRETROVIRAL INTERVENTIONS

Studies conducted in African settings before antiretroviral (ARV) interventions were available made the main recommendations shown below (Table 7.6).

TABLE 7.6
Breast Milk HIV Transmission When No Antiretroviral Interventions Were Available

Year, Study, Location, Study Design, Characteristics of Population	Regimens Mother	Baby	Results and Major Contribution
1997 Ekpini et al. (1997) Abidjan, Côte d'Ivoire Prospective observational study (POC) All breastfeeding	None	None	HIV transmission rate until 6 months: 28% (19–39%) for children born to HIV-1-infected women and 18% (9–30%) for children born to HIV-2-infected women. HIV transmission rate after 6 months: 12% (3–23%) for children born to HIV-1-infected women and 6% (0–14%) for children born to HIV-2-infected women, adjusting for loss to follow-up. *Main messages:* The risk of transmission continues throughout the breastfeeding period. Early cessation of breastfeeding at 6 months of age is a possible intervention to reduce postnatal HIV transmission.
1999 Miotti et al. (1999) Malawi Prospective observational study (POC) All breastfeeding	None	None	Of 672 infants, 7% became HIV infected while breastfeeding; none became HIV-positive after breastfeeding stopped. Cumulative risks of infection for infants continuing to breastfeed after 1 month to the end of months 5, 11, 17, and 23 were 3.5%, 7%, 8.9%, and 10.3%, respectively. HIV infection rates per person per month were 0.7% in months 1–5, 0.6% in months 6–11, 0.3% in months 12–17, and 0.2% in months 18–23 (*p* = 0.01), suggesting that HIV transmission decreases significantly as the child gets older 12–17, and 0.2% in months 18–23 (*p* = 0.01), suggesting that HIV transmission decreases significantly as the child gets older. *Main messages:* Breast milk transmission continues throughout the breastfeeding period but decreases as the child gets older and stops when breastfeeding stops.
1999 Semba et al. (1999) Blantyre, Malawi Prospective observational study (POC) All breastfeeding	None	None	Mothers of HIV-infected infants have significantly greater breast milk viral load than mothers of uninfected infants. Mastitis (probably as a result of poor breastfeeding technique) and breast milk viral load were independently associated with mother-to-child transmission of HIV-1 at 6 months (AOR, 2.38; 95% CI, 1.26–4.42) and (AOR, 2.97; 95% CI, 1.23–7.18), respectively. *Main messages:* Higher breast milk viral load increases transmission risk through breast milk. Mastitis also increases risk of HIV transmission, independently of breast milk viral load.
2000 Nduati et al. (2000) Nairobi, Kenya Randomized controlled trial (RCT) Women randomized to breastfeeding or formula feeding (clean water available and formula subsidized)	None	None	The cumulative probability of HIV-1 infection at 23 months was 36.7% (95% CI, 29.4–44%) in the breastfeeding arm and 20.5% (95% CI, 14–27%) in the formula-feeding arm (*p* = 0.001). The estimated rate of transmission (excess risk of transmission) was 16.2% (95% CI, 6.5–25.9%). 44% of HIV-1 infection was attributable to breast milk. Kaplan–Meier estimates of the 2-year mortality rate were similar in the breastfeeding arm: 24.4% (95% CI, 18.2–30.7%) and 20.0% (95% CI, 14.4–25.6%; *p* = 0.30). The 2-year HIV-free survival rate was significantly lower in the breastfeeding arm (58%) compared with the formula feeding arm (70%) (*p* = 0.02). *Main messages:* Most breast milk transmission seemed to occur early during breastfeeding; however, transmission risk difference continued to increase throughout the breastfeeding period. HIV-free survival at 2 years was better in the formula-feeding arm.
2003 Richardson et al. (2003) Nairobi, Kenya Prospective RCT; nested case-control study within RCT of breastfeeding and formula feeding	None	None	Mothers with HIV-1 RNA plasma viral load above the median (>43, 120 copies/mL) had a sixfold significantly higher risk of MTCT per liter of breastmilk ingested by the infant and per day of breastfeeding (separately, *p* = 0.01). Mothers' CD4 count <400 × 10⁶/L was associated with 3-fold higher breast milk infectivity per liter of breast milk ingested and per day of breastfeeding by the infant compared with CD4 cell count <400 × 10⁶/L. *Main messages:* Breast milk infectivity remains high throughout the breastfeeding period. Lowering breast milk viral load during breastfeeding is a potential strategy to reduce breast milk infectivity.

1. Breastfeeding should be avoided or stopped early to prevent MTCT through breast milk. The rationale was that most MTCT through breast milk occurred early. A Kenyan study found that HIV-free survival at two years of age was better among infants who avoided breastfeeding; however, findings were contradictory, and some later studies suggested that breast milk infectivity remains high and constant throughout breastfeeding (see Table 7.6).
2. Better breastfeeding technique is necessary (exclusive breastfeeding with good attachment) to prevent mastitis.
3. Lowering plasma and breast milk viral load and increasing CD4 cell count are critical interventions to reduce postnatal MTCT.

BREAST MILK HIV TRANSMISSION WITH MINIMAL VS. MULTI-DRUG ANTIRETROVIRAL INTERVENTIONS

Table 7.7 shows how knowledge of postnatal MTCT evolved between 1999 and 2005 when:

- The pattern of breastfeeding was found to influence the risk of MTCT.
- The risk of MTCT through breastfeeding remained high and constant throughout breastfeeding.
- Early cessation of breastfeeding was found to increase the risk of HIV infection or death.
- Replacement feeding (avoiding breastfeeding and feeding infants commercial infant formula) was found to increase infant morbidity and mortality by six months postpartum although these differences were attenuated by two years postpartum.

Recent studies on prophylaxis during breastfeeding consistently show that maternal ART alone (Kilewo et al., 2009) or with one week (Kesho Bora Study Group and de Vincenzi, 2011), four weeks (Shapiro et al., 2010), or 24 weeks infant prophylaxis (Jamieson et al., 2012) or infant prophylaxis alone (with limited maternal prophylaxis; no ART) for six weeks (SWEN Study Team, 2008), 14 weeks (Kumwenda et al., 2008), or 24 weeks (Afolabi et al., 2013) reduces postnatal HIV transmission (i.e., breast milk transmission; see Table 7.8). Maternal postnatal regimens appear to be just as efficacious as infant postnatal regimens, although the BAN study suggests that at 28 weeks there was a trend favoring infant nevirapine over maternal ART (both used from one week to six months postdelivery) (Jamieson et al., 2012). The Post-Exposure Prophylaxis in Infants (PEPI) trial showed that, adjusting for risk factors (maternal CD4 cell count, maternal presentation <4 vs. ≥4 hours before delivery, sex of infant, and infant birthweight), nine-month HIV-free survival was higher among infants who received 14 weeks postnatal prophylaxis compared with control infants who only received one week of ARV cover (Table 7.8) (Kumwenda et al., 2008). Both PEPI (Kumwenda et al., 2008) and SWEN (2008) show that the protective effect of infant postnatal prophylactic ARV regimens on breast milk HIV transmission stops once the regimens stop (Kumwenda et al., 2008; SWEN, 2008).

KNOWLEDGE GAPS AND FUTURE INTERVENTIONS AND RESEARCH

Immune therapy and vaccination are current innovations being investigated to reduce postnatal MTCT though breastfeeding. The main question is whether this should be administered to mother or baby. The immunotherapeutic trials applicable to MTCT are summarized in Table 7.9. The third row (PACTG 230) highlights the agents that are currently most promising. A mucosal vaccine for infants could exploit the common mucosa-associated lymphoid tissue through oral or nasal delivery. Attenuated canary pox vector (vCP 205) and *Salmonella* vaccine vector (CKS257) vaccine platforms have been well tolerated. A modified vaccinia virus Ankara (MVA)-vectored vaccine is also currently under evaluation in an open randomized phase I/II study. Apart from these innovations, the only other intervention being considered is maternal antiretroviral therapy throughout the breastfeeding period. This will be covered in the sections that follow.

POLICIES ON HIV AND INFANT FEEDING

Policies on HIV and infant feeding have been based on the child survival benefits of breastfeeding, which have been well documented and appreciated for several decades. Even early records from the Middle Ages showed the poor outcome of abandoned infants being fed artificial milk compared to those fed human milk (Matthews-Grieco, 1991). Increases in technological prowess encouraged the baby food industry to produce what they were convinced was equivalent to human milk. Despite the labeling that "breast is best," the underlying concept communicated was "but formula milk is not bad; it is just a different choice," thereby leading the public and policymakers to forget some of the earlier well-established risks of formula feeds (Jelliffe and Jelliffe, 1978). This subtle communication also portrayed the food companies as protectors of mothers' rights in an age where women might want to overcome the need to provide human breast milk to their children and the supposed restrictive barriers imposed by breastfeeding. HIV and infant feeding policies must be understood against the backdrop of this swing against breastfeeding by modern women and society. In 1985, when HIV was first reported, it was no surprise that very soon the U.S. Centers for Disease Control (CDC) issued guidelines that recommended avoidance of all breastfeeding by HIV-infected women (CDC, 1985). These recommendations created a huge dilemma: On the one hand, it would be difficult for poorer countries to justify following this guidance without putting infants at risk of mortality, but, on the other hand, international agencies did not want to be accused of double standards. Eventually, the World Health Organization (WHO) and other agencies navigated their way through this conundrum by encouraging avoidance of breastfeeding in well-developed countries, where it was assumed that the environmental conditions and health systems adequately ameliorated the risks of formula feeding. Initially, this was supported by research (see Table 7.6). In resource-limited settings where this was clearly not the case, the WHO/United Nations Children's Fund (UNICEF) consensus statement advocated breastfeeding with early cessation (by three to four months postdelivery) among HIV-positive women as the safest option or avoiding breastfeeding altogether, if safe to do so (WHO, 1992).

The next milestone to be met was the need to quantify the risk of HIV transmission through breastfeeding in order to better inform policy. One of the first key studies was a randomized controlled trial (RCT) of breastfeeding vs. formula feeding from Kenya (Nduati et al., 2000), which reported postnatal transmission of HIV of 16% (95% CI, 17–26%) (see Table 7.6). This prevalence was consistent with a previous prevalence estimated through a meta-analysis conducted by Dunn et al. (1992). This Kenyan study, which reported good outcomes on formula feeding, was criticized for methodological flaws and limitations of generalizability (Bulterys, 2000), and these findings were never replicated even in some of the large studies (WHO Collaborative Study Team, 2000; Thior et al., 2006; Becquet et al. 2007; Coovadia et al., 2007). Nevertheless, because this study was an RCT and therefore categorized as high-quality evidence, it became instrumental in the WHO policy shift in 2000 toward support of formula feeding. This shift in policy implied that formula feeding was, under the circumstances, the best option for HIV-positive women and should be supported. In order to be sure that no women in poor communities were put at unnecessary risk, WHO introduced a caveat to their policy: Formula feeding would only be encouraged when it was

- Acceptable and
- Feasible and
- Affordable and
- Sustainable and
- Safe

TABLE 7.7

HIV Transmission through Breastfeeding with Minimal ARV Interventions

Year, Study, Location, Study Design, Characteristics of Population	Antiretroviral Interventions Mother	Antiretroviral Interventions Baby	Results and Comments
2004 BHITS Study Group et al. (2004) Meta-analysis 9 randomized, placebo-controlled trials	None	None	Overall estimated risk of late postnatal (negative at or before 4 weeks followed by positive results) HIV transmission was 8.9 transmissions per 100 child-years of breastfeeding. The cumulative probability of late postnatal transmission at 18 months was 9.3%. *Main messages:* Cases of postnatal transmission continued to occur throughout the breastfeeding period. Breast milk transmission remained fairly constant throughout the breastfeeding period.
2001 Coutsoudis et al. (2001) Cato Manor, Durban, South Africa (urban area) Unexpected findings from a vitamin A RCT Women self-selected to EBF or EFF	None	None	Cumulative probabilities of HIV infection were similar among those never breastfeeding (0.19; CI, 0.14–0.26) and exclusive breastfeeders (0.19; 95% CI, 0.13–0.27) up to 6 months. Probabilities among mixed breastfeeders surpassed both groups, reaching 0.26 (95% CI, 0.21–0.32) by 6 months. Cumulative probability of HIV infection by 15 months was 0.25 (95% CI, 0.16–0.34) among infants who exclusively breastfed for at least 3 months. This was still lower than MTCT among other (mixed) breastfeeders, which was 0.36 (95% CI, 0.27–0.45). In multivariate analysis, EBF was associated with a significantly lower risk of HIV infection (adjusted HR, 0.56; 95% CI, 0.22–1.42) than mixed breastfeeding (adjusted HR, 0.87; 95% CI, 0.33–2.33). *Main messages:* Pattern of infant feeding affects transmission. EBF was associated with a lower risk of HIV transmission than mixed feeding.
2005 Iliff et al. (2005) Zimbabwe RCT Mothers randomized to 1 of 4 vitamin A treatment groups All mothers breastfeeding	None	None	Compared with EBF early mixed feeding was associated with a 4.03 (95% CI, 0.98–16.61), 3.79 (95% CI, 1.40–10.29), and 2.60 (95% CI, 1.21–5.55) greater risk of postnatal HIV transmission at 6, 12, and 18 months, respectively. Predominant breastfeeding was associated with a 2.63 (95% CI, 0.59–11.66), 2.69 (95% CI, 0.95–7.63), and 1.61 (95% CI, 0.72–3.64) trend toward greater postnatal transmission risk at 6, 12, and 18 months, respectively, compared with EBF. *Main messages:* EBF was associated with a lower risk of HIV transmission compared with mixed feeding. Predominant breastfeeding also tended to carry higher risks of transmission compared with EBF.
2006 MASHI study Thior et al. (2006) Botswana RCT	AZT for 6 months; FF	Infant AZT; BF	With the exception of grade 3/4 pneumonia and in the context of weaning at 6 months by the BF arm, differences by feeding arm were attenuated by 24 months. The 24-month HIV-free survival did not differ between arms. *Main messages:* FF was associated with significantly higher rates of infant mortality and severe pneumonia and diarrhea by 6 months, particularly among HIV-infected children.

Study			Findings
2007 Coovadia et al. (2007) Hlabisa, South Africa (rural area) POC AFASS criteria-guided feeding	sdNVP	sdNVP	14.1% (95% CI, 12.0–16.4) of exclusively breastfed infants were infected with HIV-1 by age 6 weeks and 19.5% (95% CI, 17.0–22.4) by 6 months. Transmission risk was significantly associated with maternal CD4 cell counts below 200 cells per μL (adjusted HR, 3.79; 95% CI, 2.35–6.12) and birthweight less than 2500 g (1.81; 95% CI, 1.07–3.06). Kaplan–Meier estimated risk of acquisition of infection at 6 months of age was 4.04% (95% CI, 2.29–5.76). Breastfed infants who also received solids were significantly more likely to acquire infection than exclusively breastfed children (HR, 10.87; 95% CI, 1.51–78.00; $p = 0.018$), as were infants who at 12 weeks received both breast milk and formula milk (1.82; 95% CI, 0.98–3.36; $p = 0.057$). Cumulative 3-month mortality in exclusively breastfed infants was 6.1% (95% CI, 4.74–7.92%) vs. 15.1% (95% CI, 7.63–28.73%) in infants given replacement feeds (HR, 2.06; 95% CI, 1.00–4.27; $p = 0.051$). *Main messages*: Early introduction of solids increases transmission risks, as does mixed feeding. Three-month mortality was highest in infants receiving no breast milk as compared with infants who were EBF; low maternal CD4 cell count increased risk of infant HIV acquisition.
2007 Zambia Exclusive Breastfeeding Study (ZEBS) Kuhn et al. (2007) Zambia Epidemiologic study nested within a RCT evaluating the safety and efficacy of early weaning	sdNVP	sdNVP	Post-natal HIV transmission before 4 months was significantly lower ($p = 0.004$) among EBF (0.040; 95% CI, 0.024–0.055) than non-EBF infants (0.102; 95% CI, 0.047–0.157); time-dependent RH of transmission due to non-EBF was 3.48 (95% CI, 1.71–7.08). There were no significant differences in the severity of disease between EBF and non-EBF mothers, and the association remained significant (RH, 2.68; 95% CI, 1.28–5.62) after adjusting for maternal CD4 count, plasma viral load, syphilis screening results, and low birthweight. *Main messages*: Non-EBF more than doubles the risk of early postnatal (by 4 months) HIV transmission. Early cessation of breastfeeding increases morbidity and mortality risks.

Note: BF, breastfeeding; EBF, exclusive breastfeeding; EFF, exclusive formula feeding; FF, formula feeding; HR, hazard ratio; POC, prospective observational study; RCT, randomized controlled trial; RH, relative hazard; sdNVP, single-dose nevirapine.

TABLE 7.8
HIV Transmission through Breastfeeding in the Era of Maternal or Infant ARV Prophylaxis/Treatment

Year, Study, Location, Study Design, Characteristics of Population	Antiretroviral Interventions		Results and Comments
	Mother	Baby	
2008 SWEN Study Team (2008) Ethiopia, Uganda, and India Three similar RCTs All BF	C: sdNVP Int: sdNVP	C: sdNVP Int: sdNVP + extended daily NVP until 6 weeks	There was a 46% decrease in postnatal HIV infection at age 6 weeks in infants uninfected at birth and receiving extended nevirapine compared with the control arm. There was a continued risk of postnatal HIV transmission after the regimens were discontinued in infants who continued to be breastfed; however, this risk was similar in both arms. *Main messages:* Postnatal infant NVP for 6 weeks reduced transmission compared with sdNVP and improved 6-month HIV-free survival. Transmission risk continued after NVP was stopped.
2008 Kumwenda et al. (2008) Post-Exposure Prophylaxis of Infant (PEPI) trial Malawi RCT All BF	C: sdNVP Int1: sdNVP Int2: sdNVP	C: sdNVP + 1 week AZT Int1: sdNVP + 14weeks daily NVP Int2: sdNVP + 14 weeks NVP and AZT	At 9 months, the estimated rate of HIV-1 infection (the primary endpoint) was 10.6% in the control group, compared with 5.2% in the extended-nevirapine group ($p < 0.001$) and 6.4% in the extended-dual-prophylaxis group ($p = 0.002$). There were no significant differences between the two extended prophylaxis groups. There was a continued risk of postnatal HIV transmission after the regimens were discontinued in infants who continued to be breastfed; however, this risk was similar in both arms. *Main messages:* Extended prophylaxis with NVP, or with NVP and AZT, for the first 14 weeks of life significantly reduced postnatal HIV-1 infection in 9-month-old infants. 9-month HIV-free survival was higher among infants who received 14 weeks postnatal prophylaxis compared with control infants who only received 1 week ARV cover (adjusted HR = 0.001 for the 14-week postnatal infant NVP prophylaxis group, and adjusted HR = 0.004 for the 14-week postnatal infant NVP + AZT prophylaxis group—both compared with control).
2008 MITRA study Kilewo et al. (2008) Dar es Salaam, Tanzania POC All BF	AZT/3TC to mothers from 36 weeks gestation to 1 week postpartum	1 weeks AZT/3TC to infants for 1 week followed by daily 3TC to infants for a maximum of 6 months	Cumulative HIV transmission was 3.8% at 6 weeks and 4.9% at 6 months of age. The risk of postnatal infection from 6 weeks to 6 months was 1.1%. *Main messages:* Infant prophylaxis for 6 months resulted in a low risk of HIV transmission through breast milk.

Study	Intervention	Infant prophylaxis	Results
2011 Data collection ended in August 2009 Kesho Bora Study Group and de Vincenzi Five sites in Burkina Faso, Kenya, and South Africa HIV-infected women with 200–500 CD4 cells/μL randomized RCT All BF	C: AZT started 28–36 weeks + sdNVP at labor + 1 week postnatal AZT/3TC Int: ART started 28–36 weeks pregnancy through 6 months postpartum	sdNVP + 1 week AZT in both arms	The rates of HIV infection at birth were similar in both arms: 1.8% in the ART arm vs. 2.2% in short-course AZT arm. At age 6 months, cumulative HIV infection rates were 4.9% in the maternal ART arm compared with 8.5% in the short-course AZT arm. Between 6 weeks and 6 months, the postnatal infection rate was 1.6% in the maternal ART arm compared with 3.7% in the short-course AZT arm without extended prophylaxis. The rate of infection after the prophylaxis/ART was discontinued was similar in both arms. *Main message:* A maternal ART arm was more efficacious than short-course regimens.
2010 Data collection ended in 2009 Mma Bana Study Shapiro et al. (2010) Botswana RCT HIV-infected pregnant women with CD4 cell counts > 200 cells/μL randomized All BF	Int1: Triple nucleoside ART regimen Int2: Protease inhibitor containing ART regimen started 26–34 weeks through 6 months of BF	sdNVP + 4 weeks AZT	The rates of viral suppression at delivery and during breastfeeding were similar between the two ART regimens. The cumulative infant HIV infection rate at age 6 months was 1% (95% CI, 0.5–2%), with only two infections (0.4% transmission) in 553 infants and no difference between the two arms. *Main message:* Maternal ART regimens were efficacious in reducing postnatal transmission in mothers with CD4 cell count > 200 cells/μL.
2009 Mitra Plus Study Kilewo et al. (2009) Dar es Salaam, Tanzania POC All BF	ART to pregnant women starting at 34 weeks and continuing through 6 months of breastfeeding	—	Cumulative risk of HIV-infection was 5% at 6 months and 6% at 18 months of age. The risk of postnatal infection between 6 weeks and 6 months was only 1%. *Main message:* Maternal ART during breastfeeding reduced postnatal transmission through breast milk.

(continued)

TABLE 7.8 (continued)
HIV Transmission through Breastfeeding in the Era of Maternal or Infant ARV Prophylaxis/Treatment

Year, Study, Location, Study Design, Characteristics of Population	Antiretroviral Interventions		Results and Comments
	Mother	Baby	
South Africa PMTCT Evaluation Team Goga et al. (2015) South Africa Breastfeeding population	Observational study using ART if CD4 ≤ 250 cells/mL or stage 4 disease AZT from 28 weeks for all other mothers with single dose maternal nevirapine in labor, nevirapine to infant at delivery, and infant AZT for 7–28 days		Early MTCT by 4–8 weeks postpartum was highest amongst breastfeeding mothers: 11.50% (95% CI, 4.67–18.33%) for exclusive breastfeeding; 11.45% (95% CI, 7.45–16.35%) for mixed breastfeeding; and 3.45% (95% CI, 0.53–6.35%) for no-breastfeeding, but ART or >10 weeks prophylaxis negated this difference (MTCT: 3.94% [95% CI, 1.98–5.90], 2.07% [95% CI, 0.55–3.60], and 2.11% [95% CI, 1.28–2.95], respectively). Main message: Antiretroviral cover negates the early transmission difference between feeding groups.

Note: 3TC, lamivudine; ART, antiretroviral therapy; AZT, zidovudine; BF, breastfeeding; C, control group; CI, confidence interval; Int, intervention group; MTCT, mother-to-child transmission; NVP, nevirapine; POC, prospective observational study; RCT, randomized controlled trial; sdNVP, single-dose nevirapine.

This guidance became known as the AFASS criteria (see Figure 7.1) (WHO Collaborative Study Team, 2000; WHO et al., 2003). This new mantra enabled policymakers and healthcare workers to inject renewed confidence into formula feeding, leading to several countries and beneficent agencies providing HIV-infected mothers with free commercial infant formula milk in the belief that, if the affordability and sustainability criteria of the AFASS mantra were satisfied, then formula feeding with the avoidance of breastfeeding would automatically be safe. Despite several calls to reconsider the policy of free formula distribution (Coutsoudis et al., 2002, 2008), countries were slow to give up their renewed confidence and instead concentrated on a narrow view of attempting to minimize the risks of environmental contamination among formula-feeding mothers. Countries attempted to make situations and settings AFASS compliant but in doing so clouded two important realities:

1. Implementing the AFASS criteria was not simple and depended on the counseling skills and perspectives of healthcare personnel and infant feeding counselors; of concern is that very few settings have trained infant feeding counselors to optimize the correct implementation of the AFASS criteria.
2. No matter how "clean" and safe a setting is, excluding breast milk from the diet of an infant also excludes the important immune components in breast milk that confer the well-documented benefits of breastfeeding (Goldman, 1993; Labbok et al., 2004; Morrow and Rangel, 2004; Hanson, 2007).

The years that followed were littered with anecdotal personal stories and evidence from several studies that either encouraged no or a shorter duration (three to four months) of breastfeeding and found marked increases in diarrheal morbidity—in some settings, even increased early mortality (Phadke et al., 2003; Kagaayi et al., 2008; Peltier et al., 2009; Homsy et al., 2010; Kafulafula et al., 2010; Nyandiko et al., 2010; Onyango-Makumbi et al., 2010). During this time, it was not surprising that even in developed countries where formula feeding was supposedly AFASS compliant and mothers were predominately HIV uninfected, the increased morbidity associated with formula feeding was also documented (Chantry et al., 2006; Quigley et al., 2007; Bartick and Reinhold, 2010).

With hindsight, it is unfortunate that policymakers forged ahead with anti-breastfeeding policies in the context of HIV. This is indeed the dilemma we face often in public health—the need for action is usually far more urgent than the need for hard data to justify specific actions (Figure 7.2). It is not usually clear when the best time is to move ahead with policies. Is one RCT enough? The decision is usually based on a risk/benefit analysis. In this case, there is a possibility that the pressure to save infants from HIV infection outweighed the pressure to save infants from other infectious diseases; consequently, less attention was given to the risk/benefit analysis. This is not surprising, given the backdrop of very effective marketing conducted by formula milk companies, which seduced countries into thinking that commercial infant formula is a safe alternative for the majority of people.

Gradually, as a result of a variety of events, the death knell of the free formula milk program was felt in many resource-limited settings, including South Africa, the country with the largest PMTCT and free formula milk distribution program:

1. A South African evaluation of the safety of preparation of formula feeds documented that even women who had been well trained on formula milk preparation and who had met the AFASS criteria experienced problems with incorrect preparation. This South African evaluation reported that 63% of the bottles collected from mothers during their PMTCT clinic visits were found to be heavily contaminated by *Escherichia coli* (Andresen et al., 2007).
2. Healthcare workers were reporting that, despite receiving counseling, mothers were experiencing difficulties in making an informed decision as to whether their circumstances met the AFASS criteria. Their decisions were made all the more complex by the fact that

TABLE 7.9
Immunotherapeutic (Vaccine) Trials Applicable to MTCT

Trial	Vaccine/ Immunotherapy	Cohort	Phase	Safe?	Outcomes	Comments
AVEG 104	HIV MN gp120	Pregnant women	I	Safe	No difference in MTCT between groups	Not powered to address MTCT as an outcome
PACTG 185	HIV immunoglobulin (HIV-IG) in the context of nevirapine and AZT prophylaxis	Pregnant mothers and their infants received HIV-IG	III	Safe	No difference between the two arms	Low transmission rate overall
PACTG 230	MN or SF2 gp120	HIV-exposed children	I/II	Safe	9.2% MTCT in infants who did not receive AZT, which was lower than MTCT in the untreated PACTG 076 AZT trial Maternal antibodies did not appear to affect immunogenicity	Not powered for subgroup analysis but partial efficacy demonstrated
PACTG 326	ALVAC vCP205, Vcp 1452, Canary pox ± MN gp120	HIV-exposed infants	I/II	Safe	A significant minority of patients did not demonstrate a significant immune response. Among responders, the breadth of response was limited and did not cover specific strains outside those included in the vaccine.	Aimed to increase cytotoxic T-lymphocyte responses

Study	Intervention	Phase	Participants	Safety	Results	Comments
RV-144 (Rerks-Ngarm et al., 2009) Vaccination with ALVAC™ and AIDSVAX®	Canary pox virus prime–ALVAC vCP205 compared with recombinant gp120 AIDSVAX (clade B and E)	III	8000 participants per arm; 60% males	Safe	31% reduction in risk but only statistically significant in 1 of 3 analyses. Protective effect was most prominent in the lowest risk cohort. Infected adults were no different in viral load, CD4 cell count, or T-cell functional indices. Studies are ongoing, particularly with regard to efficacy and effect on strain variation.	Unclear whether maternal partial vaccination will affect strain compartmentalization or passage to the fetus
HIVIGLOB Phase II/III Study	Nevirapine ± immunoglobulin	III	Pregnant mother/child pairs in Uganda with pooled analysis from Ethiopia and India	Safe	This has demonstrated safety. No effect on transmission.	—
HPTN 027	ALVAC vCP 1521	I	60 infants	No results	Results not yet available	—
PedVacc 001 and 002	MVA.HIVA	I/II	Pregnant mother/child pairs	No results	Did not induce sufficient HIV-1 antibody responses (Afolabi et al., 2013)	—

Source: Hicar, M.D., *Current HIV Research*, 11(2), 137–43, 2013.

Note: AZT, zidovudine; MTCT, mother-to-child transmission.

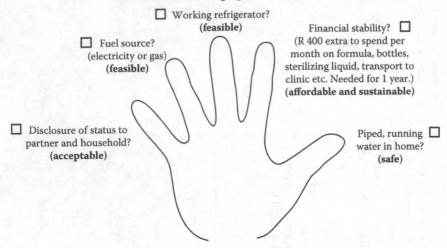

Antenatal Infant Feeding Options Counseling

☐ Working refrigerator?
(feasible)

☐ Fuel source?
(electricity or gas)
(feasible)

Financial stability? ☐
(R 400 extra to spend per
month on formula, bottles,
sterilizing liquid, transport to
clinic etc. Needed for 1 year.)
(affordable and sustainable)

☐ Disclosure of status to
partner and household?
(acceptable)

Piped, running ☐
water in home?
(safe)

If **ALL FIVE** of the boxes are **NOT ticked**, please *do not* recommend replacement feeding and *do* **recommend six months of exclusive breastfeeding** for this mother and her infant.

Feeding recommendation made to mother:_____

Maternal feeding choice:_____

• I have explained the risks and benefits of this feeding choice to my client

**Note: general safety point – where IMR is > 25/1000 formula feeding in
the first 6 months is not safe.**

**(From Anna Coutsoudis, Department of Paediatrics and Child Health, University of
KwaZulu Natal, South Africa)**

*"Please note that in the HIV/infant feeding guidelines we normally talk about non-breastfeeding as
replacement feeding and this basically means anything other than breastmilk so it could be commercially
prepared powdered formula milk or animal milk which has been diluted (and modified at home)
to make it more suitable for infants.*

*In South Africa most women who will replacement feed will use formula milk as the difference in cost
between formula milk and animal milk is not that large whereas in other parts of Africa the cost of
formula milk is very high."*

FIGURE 7.1 Example of an algorithm used to apply the AFASS Criteria in South Africa. (Courtesy of A. Coutsoudis, Department of Paediatrics and Child Health, University of KwaZulu Natal, South Africa.)

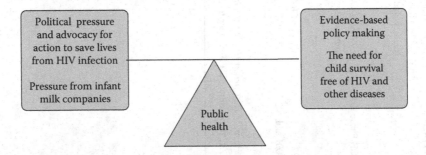

Political pressure
and advocacy for
action to save lives
from HIV infection

Pressure from infant
milk companies

Public
health

Evidence-based
policy making

The need for
child survival
free of HIV and
other diseases

FIGURE 7.2 Dilemma faced by public health.

free formula was being distributed by the healthcare workers themselves, resulting in an inadvertent message: "Surely, if healthcare workers are distributing it, then it must be a good choice similar to the other good things they provide, such as immunizations and family planning."

3. A study examining choices that mothers made documented that many mothers were making inappropriate choices: 67% of women who did not meet AFASS criteria actually used formula feeding, and infants of these women who chose to formula feed without fulfilling the AFASS criteria had the highest risk of HIV transmission/death (HR, 3.63) (Doherty et al., 2007).

4. Finally, problems with sustained access due to the mobility of populations, as well as clinics running out of formula milk supplies, were documented in an evaluation of the South African program (Chopra and Rollins, 2008).

During this period of strong promotion of formula feeding for HIV infected mothers, a surprising result from a South African observational study caused controversy. This report documented that mothers who exclusively breastfed for three months compared to mothers who mixed-breastfed during this period were less likely to transmit HIV to their infants during breastfeeding (Coutsoudis et al., 1999, 2001) (see Table 7.7). This finding seemed counterintuitive at a time when people considered the paradigm taken from bloodborne infections, that greater exposure made infection more likely. Now this breastfeeding study was suggesting that the more exposure the lower the transmission. Upon deeper investigation it became clear that there were sufficient physiological mechanisms to give biological credence to this finding (Smith and Kuhn, 2000). Understandably, WHO would not change its 2000 policy based on this single study, especially because it was not an RCT. WHO did, however, concede that the guidelines should be tweaked to suggest that when mothers breastfed they should exclusively breastfeed, and the reason given in the gray material was not because it would reduce transmission but because of the known morbidity and mortality benefits of exclusive breastfeeding. WHO called on scientists to test these South African findings, and many groups then proceeded to do. Despite the different settings, all of the studies (Coutsoudis et al., 2001; Illif et al., 2005; Coovadia et al., 2007; Kuhn et al., 2007) reached the same conclusion that exclusive breastfeeding resulted in a significant reduction in HIV transmission. The results of these studies led WHO to revise its infant feeding policies in 2006 (WHO, 2006). The new guidelines strongly recommended six months of exclusive breastfeeding. Although this was a welcome step in the right direction, unfortunately it was misinterpreted to mean that when exclusive breastfeeding became no longer possible (i.e., at six months), then all breastfeeding should stop. A Zambian study was specifically set up to test this guideline by means of an RCT that randomized mothers to stop breastfeeding at four months or to continue breastfeeding (see Table 7.7). The study reported very high rates of exclusive breastfeeding; nevertheless, the results were rather shocking, as they showed no benefit of early cessation of breastfeeding in terms of HIV-free survival and increased mortality in all infants resulted, especially those who were HIV infected (Kuhn et al., 2008) (see Table 7.7).

What was also notable at this time was the need for *support* for HIV-infected women, regardless of infant feeding choice (Table 7.10). Clearly, the scene was set, and researchers and policymakers clearly understood that the next agenda was to find ways of protecting breastfeeding further and making breastfeeding safer by raising CD4 cell count and reducing viral load, as most postnatal transmission occurred in those mothers with high viral load and low CD4 (Kuhn et al., 2010). The challenge then was to find strategies to reduce viral load in mothers and thereby reduce HIV transmission. Originally, studies tested a variety of ARVs on mothers for six months of breastfeeding (Kesho Bora Study Group and de Vincenzi, 2011), and then several studies tested nevirapine prophylaxis given to infants for six weeks (SWEN Study Team, 2008) and 14 weeks, and one study tested it for 24 weeks of breastfeeding (Kumwenda et al., 2008). All of the studies

TABLE 7.10

Support for Infant Feeding among HIV-Infected Women Based on the 2000 WHO Guidelines

Support	Action
S	Screen all women for HIV.
	Send off CD4 cell counts on all HIV-positive women.
	Screen all HIV-positive women for the six WHO AFASS criteria.
U	Understand the mother's personal and sociocultural context.
P	Promote exclusive or predominant breastfeeding if all six criteria are not met.
	Start postnatal prophylactic regimens to minimize postnatal HIV transmission.
P	Promote exclusive formula feeding if all the criteria are met.
O	Organize supplies of formula milk if mothers meet the criteria and choose to formula feed; of cotrimoxazole for infants from 6 weeks of age; of prophylactic antiretroviral if mothers do not meet the six criteria.
R	Review mothers and infants in the first 3 days postnatally, in the first 2 weeks postnatally, and monthly thereafter.
	Review mothers' and infants' health, and infant feeding practices and techniques, regardless of feeding choice.
	Review adherence to antiretroviral regimens.
T	Treat all mothers and children with antiretroviral therapy according to updated recommendations.

Source: Goga, A., *South African Journal of Child Health*, 4(3), 66–69, 2010.

showed a reduction in transmission. A Malawian study (the BAN study) conducted a three-arm RCT during six months of breastfeeding; one control arm was compared with a second arm that gave infants nevirapine prophylaxis and a third arm with mothers receiving ART (Jamieson et al., 2012). Both experimental arms were shown to significantly reduce breastfeeding transmission compared to the control. These studies, inevitably, once again necessitated a call for revision of the guidelines; thus, in 2009 WHO revised its guidelines (WHO, 2009). These guidelines made two important points:

1. In view of the result of previous guidelines that were known to be difficult for mothers to interpret, they recommended that, "National or sub-national health authorities should decide whether health services will principally counsel and support mothers known to be HIV-infected to either: breastfeed and receive ARV interventions, or avoid all breast-feeding, as the strategy that will most likely give infants the greatest chance of HIV-free survival." They further recommended that this decision should be based on international recommendations and consideration of the socio-economic and cultural contexts of the populations served by maternal, newborn and child health services; the availability and quality of health services; local epidemiology, including HIV prevalence among pregnant women; the main causes of maternal and child undernutrition; and the main causes of infant and child mortality (WHO, 2009).
2. The guidelines stated that breastfeeding should be encouraged for up to 12 months, and that mothers who were eligible for ART (CD4 count ≤ 350) should be prioritized for treatment. Infants of mothers who are not prioritized for treatment should receive nevirapine prophylaxis for the duration of the breastfeeding period (referred to as Option A), or the mothers should receive ARVs (referred to as Option B) (see Table 7.1).

At the end of 2012, the WHO guidelines were again changed in an attempt to operationalize policies by simplifying the processes and getting as many women as possible onto effective PMTCT with a streamlined process from antenatal to postpartum care. Furthermore, based on evidence that mothers with low CD4 counts who started ART had improved health, it was also argued that all pregnant women regardless of CD4 counts should be started on treatment (ART) so their health could be improved. Therefore, WHO recommended that countries who were using Option A should switch to Option B (WHO, 2012) (see Table 7.1). When UNICEF published a business case produced by the Clinton Health Access Initiative (BLC and UNICEF, 2012), there was a concerted push for countries to go even further and switch to Option B+, which would entail that all HIV-infected pregnant women be started on ART for life regardless of CD4 count and stage of HIV. There is concern that once again policies developed with a well-meaning passion for zero transmissions may be moving more swiftly than the evidence justifies—a bit reminiscent of the policies around free formula milk. This may be especially true for countries such as South Africa that carry the greatest burden of HIV. Can they really afford to invest in so many ARVs when they have other important gaps in their health services? Would the money not be better spent (Mayosi et al., 2012)? A group from South Africa (Coutsoudis et al., 2013) and other researchers issued a warning that this push was premature. Furthermore, the group at highest risk for MTCT (88%) and maternal mortality (92%) is comprised of women with CD4 counts < 350 cells/mm^3 (Kuhn et al., 2010). Under Options A and B, these women are already receiving lifelong ART; therefore, Option B+ adds very little additional benefit to this group of women.

In the absence of current conclusive evidence, many argued that it would be prudent to wait for the results of a large international study, which is investigating the difference in effectiveness of Option A vs. Option B and examining the benefits and side-effects of long-term ARVs in mothers with CD4 counts above 350 (IMPAACT Network PROMISE studies, 1077BF). Preliminary findings, presented at the 8th International Workshop on HIV Pediatrics in Durban, South Africa, in 2016 demonstrated that the risk of MTCT was similar between breastfed infants on postnatal prophylaxis throughout breastfeeding and mothers receiving ART during breastfeeding. All 2431 mothers enrolled in this RCT had a CD4 cell count > 350 cells/mL (median, 686); median duration of breastfeeding was 15 months and cumulative postnatal MTCT at 18 months was 0.6% (95% CI, 0.4–1.1%) (Taha et al., 2016).

In 2016, WHO and UNICEF updated their recommendations on infant feeding in the context of HIV (see textbox on next page). All mothers living with HIV should receive lifelong ART to support their health and to ensure the well-being of their infants. In countries that have opted to promote and support breastfeeding with ART, HIV+ mothers who are on ART and adherent to therapy should practice EBF for 6 months, and then add complementary feeding until 12 months. Breastfeeding and complementary feeding may continue until 24 months of age or beyond. These revised recommendations were based on scientific evidence or expert consensus and synchronize feeding recommendations for HIV-negative infants and HIV-exposed infants whose mothers receive and are adherent to ART (WHO and UNICEF, 2016).

CURRENT STRATEGIES TO OPERATIONALIZE POLICIES ON HIV AND INFANT FEEDING AND THEIR EFFECTS

This is indeed a promising time for HIV-infected mothers with new guidelines based on scientific evidence that encourages women to breastfeed. The challenge now is to implement these guidelines by providing ART for HIV-infected mothers and supporting exclusive breastfeeding in the first six months and continued breastfeeding for at least 12 months for the majority of women, with the possibility of extending breastfeeding for up to 24 months regardless of maternal HIV status, and in the presence of fully suppressed maternal HIV infection. How can we operationalize these policies and increase uptake? One of the most important strategies is to ease the pill burden. The move toward a fixed-dose combination drug that includes all three of the ARV drugs in one tablet to be taken only once daily has simplified treatment, which will facilitate adherence. Adherence is vital to prevent

WHO UPDATED INFANT FEEDING AND HIV GUIDELINES: 2016

- All mothers living with HIV should receive lifelong triple antiretroviral therapy (ART) to support their health and to ensure the well-being of their infants.
- In countries that have opted to promote and support breastfeeding with ART, HIV+ mothers on ART and adherent should practice EBF for 6 months and continue breastfeeding for at least 12 months, and may continue breastfeeding for up to 24 months (recommendation 1). As per previous recommendations, complementary feeding should be added at around 6 months.
- National and local authorities should actively coordinate and implement services in health facilities and activities in workplaces, communities, and homes to promote support and protect breastfeeding among women living with HIV (recommendation 2).
- Although exclusive breastfeeding is recommended, practicing mixed feeding is not a reason to stop breastfeeding in the presence of ARV drugs (guiding practice statement).

Source: WHO and UNICEF (2016)

the development of resistance; thus, strategies that encourage adherence are critical, especially in the context of PMCTC Option B+. Frequent maternal CD4 cell count testing and especially viral load monitoring are also vital to ensure that patients are not failing on treatment and also serve as an early warning system for failing adherence. Wherever possible, point-of-care testing must be encouraged. Point-of-care testing of infant HIV status at six weeks is also important for timely initiation of treatment in HIV-positive infants. At this time, several diagnostic companies are testing such point-of-care technologies that should soon be readily available and cost effective. To sustain adherence, attention must be given to finding alternative places to collect drugs to prevent the need for women to travel long distances to clinics to access their drugs. Many countries are considering alternatives such as local pharmacies, post offices, and small local stores, which offer easier access for communities. However, such a decentralized collection system will require very strict controls, and this is where electronic databases using personal identification systems will be vital to prevent abuse of the system.

How do we increase uptake of the policy of exclusive breastfeeding in the first six months? Obvious strategies include the following:

- Ensure that all health facilities are accredited for the Baby-Friendly Hospital Initiative (UNICEF, 2007).
- Ensure that all healthcare workers in the PMTCT programs and HIV care and treatment programs are trained in breastfeeding counseling and its promotion.
- Include communities in supporting mothers; there is a need to engage communities to find out constraints and ways to support mothers (Sibeko et al., 2009).
- Increase access to donor milk among mothers with difficult deliveries or who are unable to breastfeed in the first few vulnerable days postdelivery until the mothers are able to supply breast milk or until other alternatives are available. Donor human milk banks are common in Brazil, Europe, Canada, and the United States, but there is a desperate need for such facilities to be scaled up to resource-limited settings that have high HIV prevalence among pregnant women. South Africa is one such country that has begun making important moves to scale up human milk banks in neonatal intensive care units (Coutsoudis et al., 2011a,b). The Bill and Melinda Gates Foundation, recognizing the importance of this strategy for improving breastfeeding and thus child survival, recently funded the Program for Appropriate Technology in Health (PATH) to convene an international Milk Bank Technical Advisory Group meeting to develop a framework for countries to set up human milk banks (PATH, 2013).

Another way for countries to operationalize policies for HIV-infected women and their children is obviously to simplify as much as possible. A single tablet per day is a huge step, and if we could also eliminate programs that are not essential in order to ease the burden on the child and caregiver this would be another important step. One such HIV-related policy that is currently receiving attention is whether the policy of providing cotrimoxazole (CTX) prophylaxis to breastfeeding HIV-exposed but uninfected infants should continue (WHO et al., 2004). Current WHO guidelines currently recommend daily CTX prophylaxis for HIV-exposed uninfected infants for as long as the infant is being breastfed. These guidelines are based on evidence of the effectiveness of CTX prophylaxis in protecting HIV-infected infants; therefore, the guidelines were extended to include HIV-exposed infants during breastfeeding, in case they became infected. In this new era, because early infant HIV diagnosis is significantly more accessible, HIV-infected infants can be identified early on and placed on lifelong antiretroviral treatment and CTX prophylaxis. Furthermore, PMTCT regimens are now vastly more effective and accessible, such that only 1 to 2% of infants may become infected through breastfeeding. Given the dangers of antibiotic resistance and the impact of antibiotics on the gut, there have been calls to reconsider these guidelines (Coutsoudis et al., 2010), and a current study in South Africa is conducting an RCT testing the current validity of these guidelines (Coutsoudis et al., 2016). The study is registered with the Pan African Clinical Trials Registry (PACTR201311000621110).

Finally, an important piece that can play a big role in preventing transmission during breastfeeding is primary prevention, long recognized by WHO as one of the pillars of PMTCT. It is vital that a concerted effort be made to assist women who test negative during pregnancy to remain uninfected; they should be given intensive counseling and support and linked with appropriate community groups. It is also important for HIV-uninfected women to have frequently repeated testing during pregnancy and breastfeeding, given the high risk of HIV transmission for new infections.

What about the minority of women who find themselves in settings where they feel they can provide formula feeding to their infants safely and feel prepared to provide optimal follow-up infant care to prevent and treat common childhood infections, in exchange for a 100% guarantee that they will not infect postnatally their infants through breastfeeding? The door is open and the choice is still there, provided mothers understand their choices and are given sufficient guidance to ameliorate the risks.

SUMMARY AND CONCLUSIONS

The field of infant feeding and HIV has changed considerably since the 1990s, with the pendulum now swinging in favor of breastfeeding with ART for HIV-infected mothers, as breastfeeding is a critical child survival strategy. Although avoiding breastfeeding eliminates all postnatal transmission, it has been associated with adverse infant outcomes and poor survival in settings where avoiding breastfeeding cannot be sustained or practiced safely. Infant feeding and HIV must be viewed within the broader context of child survival and not just in terms of the prevention or elimination of vertical HIV transmission. In resource-limited settings, there is sufficient evidence to justify exclusive breastfeeding for six months among all HIV-exposed infants and continued breastfeeding thereafter for at least 12 months, with the possibility of extending breastfeeding to 24 months, under ART cover. New data show that antiretroviral cover during breastfeeding reduces the risk of postnatal MTCT in research settings, and early findings suggest that these successes remain at the population level.

REFERENCES

Afolabi, M. O., J. Ndure, A. Drammeh et al. (2013). A phase I randomized clinical trial of candidate human immunodeficiency virus type 1 vaccine MVA.HIVA administered to Gambian infants. *PLoS One* 8(10): e78289).

Aldhous, M. C., K. C. Watret, J. Y. Mok, A. G. Bird, and K. S. Froebel. (1994). Cytotoxic T lymphocyte activity and CD8 subpopulations in children at risk of HIV infection. *Clinical & Experimental Immunology* 97(1): 61–7.

Andresen, E., N. C. Rollins, A. W. Sturm, N. Conana, and T. Griener. (2007). Bacterial contamination and over-dilution of commercial infant formula prepared by HIV-infected mothers in a prevention of mother-to-child transmission (PMTCT) programme in South Africa. *Journal of Tropical Pediatrics* 53(6): 410–4.

Bartick, M. and A. Reinhold. (2010). The burden of suboptimal breastfeeding in the United States: a pediatric cost analysis. *Pediatrics* 125(5): e1048–56.

Becquet, R., L. Bequet, D. K. Ekouevi et al.; ANRS 1201/1202 Ditrame Plus Study Group. (2007). Two-year morbidity-mortality and alternatives to prolonged breastfeeding among children born to HIV-infected mothers in Côte d'Ivoire. *PLoS Medicine* 4(1): e17.

BHITS Study Group, A. Coutsoudis, F. Dabis, W. Fawzi et al. (2004). Late postnatal transmission of HIV-1 in breast-fed children: an individual patient data meta-analysis. *Journal of Infectious Diseases* 189(12): 2154–66.

Black, R. E., L. H. Allen, Z. A. Bhutta et al., for the Maternal and Child Undernutrition Study Group. (2008). Maternal and child undernutrition: global and regional exposures and health consequences. *Lancet* 371(9608): 243–60.

BLC and UNICEF. (2012). *A Business Case for Options B and B+ to Eliminate Mother to Child Transmission of HIV by 2015*. New York: Business Leadership Council and United Nations Children's Fund (http://www.unicef.org/aids/files/DISCUSSION_PAPER.A_BUSINESS_CASE_FOR_OPTIONS_B.pdf)

Bode, L., L. Kuhn, H. Y. Kim et al. (2012). Human milk oligosaccharide concentration and risk of postnatal transmission of HIV through breastfeeding. *American Journal of Clinical Nutrition* 96(4): 831–9.

Bulterys, M. (2000). Breastfeeding in women with HIV. *JAMA* 284(8): 956–7.

CDC. (1985). Recommendations for assisting in the prevention of perinatal transmission of human T-lymphotropic virus type III/lymphadenopathy-associated virus and acquired immunodeficiency syndrome. *Morbidity and Mortality Weekly Report (MMWR)* 34(48): 721–6, 731–2.

Chantry, C. J., C. R. Howard, and P. Auinger. (2006). Full breastfeeding duration and associated decrease in respiratory tract infection in US children. *Pediatrics* 117(2): 425–32.

Chen, Y. Q., A. Young, E. R. Brown et al. (2010). Population attributable fractions for late postnatal mother-to-child transmission of HIV-1 in Sub-Saharan Africa. *Journal of Acquired Immune Deficiency Syndromes* 54(3): 311–6.

Cheynier, R., P. Langlade-Demoyen, M.-R. Marescot et al. (1992). Cytotoxic T-lymphocyte responses in the peripheral blood of children born to HIV-infected mothers. *European Journal of Immunology* 22(9): 2211–7.

Chopra, M. and N. Rollins. (2008). Infant feeding in the time of HIV: rapid assessment of infant feeding policy and programmes in four African countries scaling up prevention of mother to child transmission programmes. *Archives of Disease in Childhood* 93(4): 288–91.

Coovadia, H. M., N. C. Rollins, R. M. Bland et al. (2007). Mother-to-child transmission of HIV-1 infection during exclusive breastfeeding in the first 6 months of life: an intervention cohort study. *Lancet* 369(9567): 1107–16.

Coutsoudis, A., K. Pillay, E. Spooner, L. Kuhn, and H. M. Coovadia, for the South African Vitamin A Study Group. (1999). Influence of infant feeding patterns on early mother-to-child transmission of HIV-1 in Durban, South Africa. *Lancet* 354(9177): 471–6.

Coutsoudis, A., K. Pillay, L. Kuhn, E. Spooner, W.-Y. Tsaic, and H. M. Coovadia; South African Vitamin A Study Group. (2001). Method of feeding and transmission of HIV-1 from mothers to children by 15 months of age: prospective cohort study from Durban, South Africa. *AIDS* 15(3): 379–87.

Coutsoudis, A., A. E. Goga, N. Rollins, and H. M. Coovadia; Child Health Group. (2002). Free formula milk for infants of HIV-infected women: blessing or curse? *Health Policy and Planning* 17(2): 154–60.

Coutsoudis, A, H. M. Coovadia, and C. M. Wilfert. (2008). HIV, infant feeding and more perils for poor people: new WHO guidelines encourage review of formula milk policies. *Bulletin of the World Health Organization* 86(3): 210–4.

Coutsoudis, A., H. M. Coovadia, and G. Kindra. (2010). Time for new recommendations on cotrimoxazole prophylaxis for HIV-exposed infants in developing countries? *Bulletin of the World Health Organization* 88: 949–50.

Coutsoudis, I., M. Adhikari, N. Nair, and A. Coutsoudis. (2011a). Feasibility and safety of setting up a donor breast milk bank in a neonatal prem unit in a resource limited setting: an observational, longitudinal cohort study. *BMC Public Health*. 11: 356.

Coutsoudis, I., A. Petrites, and A. Coutsoudis. (2011b). Acceptability of donated breast milk in a resource limited South African setting. *International Breastfeeding Journal* 6: 3.

Coutsoudis, A., A. Goga, C. Desmond, P. Barron, V. Black, and H. Coovadia. (2013). Is Option B+ the best choice? *Lancet* 381(9863): 269–71.

Coutsoudis, A., B. Daniels, E. Moodley-Govender et al. (2016). Randomised controlled trial testing the effect of cotrimoxazole prophylaxis on morbidity and mortality outcomes in breastfed HIV-exposed uninfected infants: study protocol. *BMJ Open* 6(7): e010656.

De Cock, K. M., M. G. Fowler, E. Mercier et al. (2000). Prevention of mother-to-child HIV transmission in resource-poor countries: translating research into policy and practice. *JAMA* 283(9): 1175–82.

Doherty, T., M. Chopra, D. Jackson, A. Goga, M. Colvin, and L. A. Persson. (2007). Effectiveness of the WHO/UNICEF guidelines on infant feeding for HIV-positive women: results from a prospective cohort study in South Africa. *AIDS* 21(13): 1791–7.

Dolcini, G., M. Derrien, G. Chaouat, F. Barré-Sinoussi, and E. Menu. (2003). Cell-free HIV type 1 infection is restricted in the human trophoblast choriocarcinoma BeWo cell line, even with expression of CD5, CXCR4 and CCR5. *AIDS Research and Human Retroviruses* 19(10): 857–64.

Dunn, D. T., M. L. Newell, A. E. Ades, and C. S. Peckham. (1992). Risk of human immunodeficiency virus type 1 transmission through breastfeeding. *Lancet* 340 (8819): 585–8.

Ekpini, E. R., S. Z. Wiktor, G. A. Satten et al. (1997). Late postnatal mother-to-child transmission in Abidjan, Côte d'Ivoire. *Lancet* 349(9058): 1054–9.

Forbes, J. C., A. M. Alimentia, J. Singer et al.; Canadian Pediatric AIDS Research Group (PARG). (2012). A national review of vertical HIV transmission. *AIDS* 26(6): 757–63.

Goga, A. (2010). The new WHO recommendations on HIV and infant feeding—care for the mother, and in resource-limited settings let breast milk care for the baby. *South African Journal of Child Health* 4(3): 66–69.

Goga, A. E., T. H. Dinh, and D. J. Jackson (2013). *2011 SAPMTCTE Report: Early (4–8 Weeks Postdelivery) Population-Level Effectiveness of WHO PMTCT Option A, South Africa, 2011.* South African Medical Research Council, National Department of Health South Africa and PEPFAR/U.S. Centers for Disease Control and Prevention (http://www.mrc.ac.za/healthsystems/SAPMTCTE2011.pdf).

Goga, A. E., T. H. Dinh, D. J. Jackson et al.; South Africa PMTCT Evaluation Team. (2015). First population-level effectiveness evaluation of a national programme to prevent HIV transmission from mother to child, South Africa. *Journal of Epidemiology and Community Health* 69(3): 240–8.

Goga, A. E., T. H. Dinh, D. J. Jackson et al.; South Africa PMTCT Evaluation Team. (2016). Population-level effectiveness of maternal antiretroviral treatment initiation before or during the first trimester and infant antiretroviral prophylaxis on early mother-to-child transmission of HIV, South Africa: implications for eliminating MTCT. *Journal of Global Health* 6(2): 020405 (https://www.ncbi.nlm.nih.gov/pmc/articles/PMC5032343/).

Goldman, A. S. (1993). The immune system of human milk: antimicrobial, antiinflammatory and immuno-modulating properties. *Pediatric Infectious Disease Journal* 12(8): 664–71.

Haider, R., A. Ashworth, I. Kabir, and S. Huttly. (2000). Effect of community-based peer counsellors on exclusive breastfeeding practices in Dhaka, Bangladesh: a randomised controlled trial. *Lancet* 356(9242): 1643–7.

Hanson, L. A. (2007). Session 1: feeding and infant development: breast-feeding and immune function. *Proceedings of the Nutrition Society* 66(3): 384–96.

Hicar, M. D. (2013). Immunotherapies to prevent mother-to-child transmission of HIV. *Current HIV* 11(2): 137–43.

Homsy, J., D. Moore, A. Barasa et al. (2010). Breastfeeding, mother-to-child HIV transmission, and mortality among infants born to HIV-infected women on highly active antiretroviral therapy in rural Uganda. *Journal of Acquired Immune Deficiency Syndromes* 53(1): 28–35.

Illif, P.J., E. G. Piwoz, N. V. Tavengwa et al.; ZVITAMBO Study Group. (2005). Early exclusive breastfeeding reduces the risk of postnatal HIV-1 transmission and increases HIV-free survival. *AIDS* 19(7): 699–708.

Jamieson, D. J., C. S. Chasela, M. G. Hudgens et al.; BAN Study Team. (2012). Maternal and infant antiretroviral regimens to prevent postnatal HIV-1 transmission: 48-week follow-up of the BAN randomised controlled trial. *Lancet* 379(9835): 2449–58.

Jelliffe, D. B. and E. F. P. Jelliffe. (1978). *Human Milk in the Modern World.* New York: Oxford University Press.

John-Stewart, G. C., D. Mbori-Ngacha, B. L. Payne et al. (2009). HIV-1 specific cytotoxic T lymphocytes and human breast milk HIV-1 transmission. *Journal of Infectious Diseases* 199(6): 189–98.

Jones, G., R. W. Steketee, R. E. Black, Z. A. Bhutta, S. S. Morris, and Bellagio Child Survival Study Group. (2003). How many child deaths can we prevent this year? *Lancet* 362(9377): 65–71.

Kafulafula, G., D. R. Hoover, T. E. Taha et al. (2010). Frequency of gastroenteritis and gastroenteritis-associated mortality with early weaning in HIV-1-uninfected children born to HIV-infected women in Malawi. *Journal of Acquired Immune Deficiency Syndromes* 53(1): 6–13.

Kagaayi, J., R. H. Gray, H. Brahmbhatt et al. (2008). Survival of infants born to HIV-positive mothers, by feeding modality, in Rakai, Uganda. *PLoS One* 3(12): e3877.

Kesho Bora Study Group and I. de Vincenzi. (2011). Triple antiretroviral compared with zidovudine and single-dose nevirapine prophylaxis during pregnancy and breastfeeding for prevention of mother-to-child transmission of HIV-1 (Kesho Bora study): a randomised controlled trial. *Lancet Infectious Diseases* 11(3): 171–80.

Kilewo, C., K. Karlsson, A. Massawe et al.; Mitra Study Team. (2008). Prevention of mother-to-child transmission of HIV-1 through breastfeeding by treating infants prophylactically with lamivudine in Dar es Salaam. *Journal of Acquired Immune Deficiency Syndromes* 48(3): 315–23.

Kilewo, C., K. Karlsson, M. Ngarina et al.; Mitra Plus Study Team. (2009). Prevention of mother-to-child transmission of HIV-1 through breastfeeding by treating mothers with triple antiretroviral therapy in Dar es Salaam, Tanzania: the Mitra Plus study. *Journal of Acquired Immune Deficiency Syndromes* 52(3): 406–16.

Kuhn, L., A. Coutsoudis, D. Moodley, D. Trabattoni, and N. Mngqundaniso. (2001). T-helper cell responses to HIV envelope peptides in cord blood: protection against intrapartum and breastfeeding transmission. *AIDS* 15(1): 1–9.

Kuhn, L., D. Trabattoni, C. Kankasa et al. (2006). HIV-specific secretory IgA in breast milk of HIV-positive mothers is not associated with protection against HIV transmission among breast-fed infants. *Journal of Pediatrics* 149(5): 611–6.

Kuhn, L., M. Sinkala, C. Kankasa et al. (2007). High uptake of exclusive breastfeeding and reduced early post-natal HIV transmission. *PLoS One* 2(12): e1363.

Kuhn, L., G. Aldrovandi, M. Sinkala et al.; Zambia Exclusive Breastfeeding Study. (2008). Effects of early, abrupt weaning on HIV-free survival of children in Zambia. *New England Journal of Medicine* 359(2): 130–41.

Kuhn, L., G. M. Aldrovandi, M. Sinkala, C. Kankasa, M. Mwiya, and D. M. Thea. (2010). Potential impact of new WHO criteria for antiretroviral treatment for prevention of mother-to-child HIV transmission. *AIDS* 24(9): 1374–7.

Kumwenda, N. I., D. R. Hoover, L M. Mofenson et al. (2008). Extended antiretroviral prophylaxis to reduce breast milk HIV-1 transmission. *New England Journal of Medicine* 359(2): 119–29.

Labbok, M. and K. Krasovec. (1990). Toward consistency in breastfeeding definitions. Studies in Family Planning 21(4): 226–30. Labbok, M. H., D. Clark, and A. Goldman. (2004). Breastfeeding: maintaining an irreplaceable immunological resource. *Nature Reviews Immunology* 4(7): 565–72.

Lagaye, S., M. Derrien, E. Menu et al.; European Network for the Study of In Utero Transmission of HIV-1. (2001). Cell-to-cell contact results in a selective translation of maternal human immunodeficiency virus type 1 quasispecies across a trophoblastic barrier by both trancytosis and infection. *Journal of Virology* 75(10): 4780–91

Lallemant, M., G. Jourdain, S. Le Coeur et al.; Perinatal HIV Prevention Trial (Thailand) Investigators. (2004). Single-dose perinatal nevirapine plus standard zidovudine to prevent mother-to-child transmission of HIV-1 in Thailand. *New England Journal of Medicine* 351(3): 217–28.

Liu, A. Y., B. Lohman-Payne, M. H. Chung et al. (2015). Maternal plasma and breastmilk viral loads are associated with HIV-1-specific cellular immune responses among HIV-1-exposed, uninfected infants in Kenya. *Clinical & Experimental Immunology* 180 (3): 509–19.

Lohman-Payne, B., J. Slyker, and S. Rowland-Jones. (2012). Immune approaches for prevention of breast milk transmission of HIV-1. *Advances in Experimental Medicine and Biology* 743: 185–95.

Matthews Grieco, S. F. (1991). Breastfeeding, wet nursing and infant mortality in Europe (1400–1800). In: *Historical Perspectives on Breastfeeding: Two Essays*, pp. 15–60. Florence, Italy: UNICEF.

Mayosi, B. M., J. E. Lawn, A. van Niekerk, D. Bradshaw, S. Abdool Karim, and H. M. Coovadia. (2012). Health in South Africa: changes and challenges since 2009. *The Lancet* 380(9858): 2029–43.

Miotti, P. G., T. E. Taha, N. I. Kumwenda et al. (1999). HIV transmission through breastfeeding: a study in Malawi. *JAMA* 282(8): 744–9.

Morrow, A. L., M. L. Guerrero, J. Shults et al. (1999). Efficacy of home-based peer counselling to promote exclusive breastfeeding: a randomised controlled trial. *The Lancet* 353(9160): 1226–31.

Morrow, A. L. and J. M. Rangel. (2004). Human milk protection against infectious diarrhea: implications for prevention and clinical care. *Seminars in Pediatric Infectious Diseases* 15(4): 221–8.

National Department of Health. (2013). *The South African Antiretroviral Treatment Guidelines 2013*. Republic of South Africa: Health Department (http://www.sahivsoc.org/Files/2013%20ART%20Treatment%20 Guidelines%20Final%2025%20March%202013%20corrected.pdf).

National Department of Health, South Africa, and South African National AIDS Council (SANAC). (2010). *Clinical Guidelines: PMTCT (Prevention of Mother-to-Child Transmission).* Republic of South Africa: Health Department (http://www.sahivsoc.org/Files/NDOH_PMTCT%20Apr%202008.pdf).

Nduati, R., G. John, D. Mbori-Ngacha et al. (2000). Effect of breastfeeding and formula feeding on transmission of HIV-1: a randomized clinical trial. *JAMA* 283(9): 1167–74.

Nyandiko, W. M., B.Otieno-Nyunya, B. Musick et al. (2010). Outcomes of HIV-exposed children in western Kenya: efficacy of prevention of mother to child transmission in a resource-constrained setting. *Journal of Acquired Immune Deficiency Syndromes* 54(1): 42–50.

Onyango-Makumbi, C., D. Bagenda, A. Mwatha et al. (2010). Early weaning of HIV-exposed uninfected infants and risk of serious gastroenteritis: findings from two perinatal HIV prevention trials in Kampala, Uganda. *Journal of Acquired Immune Deficiency Syndromes* 53(1): 20–7.

PATH. (2013). *Strengthening Human Milk Banking: A Global Implementation Framework, Version 1.1.* Seattle, WA: Bill & Melinda Gates Foundation Grand Challenges Initiative (http://www.path.org/publications/detail.php?i=2433).

Peltier, C. A., G. F. Ndayisaba, P. Lepage et al. (2009). Breastfeeding with maternal antiretroviral therapy or formula feeding to prevent HIV postnatal mother-to-child transmission in Rwanda. *AIDS* 23(18): 2415–23.

Phadke, M. A., B. Gadgil, K. E. Bharucha et al. (2003). Replacement-fed infants born to HIV-infected mothers in India have a high early postpartum rate of hospitalization. *Journal of Nutrition* 133(10): 3153–7.

Quigley, M. A., Y. J. Kelly, and A. Sacker. (2007). Breastfeeding and hospitalization for diarrheal and respiratory infection in the United Kingdom Millennium Cohort Study. *Pediatrics* 119(4): e837–42.

Rerks-Ngarm, S., P. Pitisuttithum, S. Nitayaphan et al.; MOPH-TAVEG Investigators. (2009). Vaccination with ALVAC and AIDSVAX to prevent HIV-1 infection in Thailand. *New England Journal of Medicine* 361(23): 2209–20.

Richardson, B. A., G. C. John-Stewart, J. P. Hughes et al. (2003). Breast-milk infectivity in human immunodeficiency virus type 1-infected mothers. *Journal of Infectious Diseases* 187(5): 736–40.

Rowland-Jones, S. I., D. F. Nixon, F. Gotch et al. (1993). HIV-specific cytotoxic T-cell activity in an HIV-exposed but uninfected infant. *Lancet* 341(8849): 860–1.

Scrimshaw, N. S. (2003). Historical concepts of interactions, synergisms and antagonism between nutrition and infection. *Journal of Nutrition* 133(1): 316S–321S.

Scrimshaw, N. S., C. E. Taylor, and J. E. Gordon. (1968). *Interactions of Nutrition and Infection,* Monograph Series No. 57. Geneva: World Health Organization.

Semba, R. D., N. Kumwenda, D. R. Hoover et al. (1999). Human immunodeficiency virus load in breast milk, mastitis, and mother-to-child transmission of human immunodeficiency virus type 1. *Journal of Infectious Diseases* 180(1): 93–8.

Shapiro, R. L., M. D. Hughes, A. Ogwu et al. (2010). Antiretroviral regimens in pregnancy and breast-feeding in Botswana. *New England Journal of Medicine* 362: 2282–94.

Sibeko, L., A. Coutsoudis, S. Nzuza, and K. Gray-Donald. (2009). Mothers' infant feeding experiences: constraints and supports for optimal feeding in an HIV-impacted urban community in South Africa. *Public Health Nutrition* 12(11): 1983–90.

Smith, M. M. and L. Kuhn. (2000). Exclusive breast-feeding: does it have the potential to reduce breast-feeding transmission of HIV-1? *Nutrition Reviews* 58(11): 333–40.

SWEN (Six Week Extended-Dose Nevirapine) Study Team. (2008). Extended dose nevirapine at 6 weeks of age for infants to prevent HIV transmission via breastfeeding in Ethiopia, India and Uganda: an analysis of 3 randomised controlled trials. *Lancet* 372(9635): 300–13.

Taha, T., P. Flynn, M. Cababasay et al.; PROMISE Team. (2016). Maternal Triple Antiretrovirals (mART) and Infant Nevirapine (iNVP) Prophylaxis for the Prevention of Mother-to-Child Transmission of HIV during Breastfeeding (BF), paper presented at 21st International AIDS Conference, Durban, South Africa, July 19.

Tenthani, L., A. D. Haas, H. Tweya et al. (2014). Retention in care under universal antiretroviral therapy for HIV-infected pregnant and breastfeeding women ("Option B+") in Malawi. *AIDS* 28(4): 589–98.

Thior, I., S. Lockman, L. M. Smeaton et al.; Mashi Study Team. (2006). Breastfeeding plus infant zidovudine prophylaxis for 6 months vs. formula feeding plus infant zidovudine for 1 month to reduce mother-to-child HIV transmission in Botswana: a randomized trial: the Mashi Study. *JAMA* 296(7): 794–805.

Townsend, C. L., L. Byrne. M. Cortina-Borja et al. (2014). Earlier initiation of ART and further decline in mother-to-child HIV transmission rates, 2000–2011. *AIDS* 28(7): 1049–57.

Tylleskär, T., D. Jackson, N. Meda et al.; PROMISE-EBF Study Group. (2011). Exclusive breastfeeding promotion by peer counsellors in sub-Saharan Africa (PROMISE-EBF): a cluster-randomised trial. *The Lancet* 378(9789): 420–7.

UNAIDS. (2011). *Global Plan Towards the Elimination of New HIV Infections among Children by 2015 and Keeping Their Mothers Alive*. Geneva: Joint United Nations Programme on HIV/AIDS (http://www. unaids.org/sites/default/files/media_asset/20110609_JC2137_Global-Plan-Elimination-HIV-Children_ en_1.pdf).

UNAIDS. (2013a). *Global Report: UNAIDS Report on the Global AIDS Epidemic 2013*. Geneva: Joint United Nations Programme on HIV/AIDS (http://www.unaids.org/sites/default/files/en/media/unaids/ contentassets/documents/epidemiology/2013/gr2013/UNAIDS_Global_Report_2013_en.pdf).

UNAIDS. (2013b). *2013 Progress Report on the Global Plan Towards the Elimination of New HIV Infections among Children by 2015 and Keeping Their Mothers Alive*. Geneva: Joint United Nations Programme on HIV/AIDS (http://www.unaids.org/sites/default/files/media_asset/20130625_progress_global_ plan_en_0.pdf).

UNAIDS. (2016). *On the Fast-Track to an AIDS-Free Generation: The Increadible Journey of the Global Plan Towards the Elimination of New HIV Infections Among Children by 2015 and Keeping Their Mothers Alive*. Geneva: Joint United Nations Programme on HIV/AIDS (http://www.aidsdatahub.org/ fast-track-aids-free-generation-unaids-2016).

UNFPA (United Nations Population Fund), UNICEF (United Nations Children's Fund), WHO (World Health Organization), and UNAIDS (Joint United Nations Programme on HIV/AIDS). (2000). *New Data on the Prevention of Mother-to-Child Transmission of HIV and Their Policy Implications: Conclusions and Recommendations*. Technical Consultation UNFPA, UNICEF, WHO, and UNAIDS Inter-Agency Team on Mother-to-Child Transmission of HIV, Geneva, October 11–13.

UNICEF. (2007). *The Baby-Friendly Hospital Initiative*. New York: United Nations Children's Fund (http:// www.unicef.org/programme/breastfeeding/baby.htm).

United Nations. (2012). *Millennium Development Goals Report, 2012*. New York: United Nations (http:// www.un.org/millenniumgoals/pdf/MDG%20Report%202012.pdf).

United Nations. (2014). *Open Working Group Proposal for Sustainable Development Goals*. New York: United Nations (http:// alive sustainabledevelopment.un.org/content/documents/1579SDGs%20Proposal.pdf).

Victora, C. G., P. G. Smith, J. P. Vaughan et al. (1987). Evidence for protection by breastfeeding against infant death from infectious diseases in Brazil. *Lancet* 2(8554): 319–22.

Victora, C. G., P. G. Smith, J. P. Vaughan et al. (1989). Infant feeding and deaths due to diarrhea: a case-control study. *American Journal of Epidemiology* 129(5): 1032–41.

WHO. (1992). *Consensus Statement from the WHO/UNICEF Consultation on HIV Transmission and Breast-Feeding*, Report No WHO/GAPA/INF/92 1. Geneva: Global Programme on AIDS, World Health Organization (http://apps.who.int/iris/bitstream/10665/61014/1/WHO_GPA_INF_92.1.pdf).

WHO. (2006). *Antiretroviral Drugs for Treating Pregnant Women and Preventing HIV Infection in Infants: Towards Universal Access: Recommendations for a Public Health Approach*. Geneva: World Health Organization (http://www.who.int/hiv/pub/mtct/antiretroviral/en/).

WHO. (2009). *HIV and Infant Feeding: Revised Principles and Recommendations: Rapid Advice*. Geneva: World Health Organization (http://apps.who.int/iris/bitstream/10665/44251/1/9789241598873_eng. pdf).

WHO. (2010). *Antiretroviral Drugs for Treating Pregnant Women and Preventing HIV Infection in Infants: Towards Universal Access: Recommendations for a Public Health Approach, Revised*. Geneva: World Health Organization (http://apps.who.int/iris/bitstream/10665/75236/1/9789241599818_eng.pdf).

WHO. (2012). *Use of Antiretroviral Drugs for Treating Pregnant Women and Preventing HIV Infection in Infants: Programmatic Update*. Geneva: World Health Organization (http://www.who.int/hiv/pub/mtct/ programmatic_update2012/en/).

WHO. (2014). *Global Guidance on Criteria and Processes for Validation: Elimination of Mother-to-Child Transmission of HIV and Syphilis*. Geneva: World Health Organization (http://apps.who.int/iris/bitstr eam/10665/112858/1/9789241505888_eng.pdf).

WHO Collaborative Study Team on the Role of Breastfeeding on the Prevention of Infant Mortality. (2000). Effect of breastfeeding on infant and child mortality due to infectious diseases in less developed countries: a pooled analysis. *Lancet* 355(9202): 451–5.

WHO (World Health Organization) and UNICEF (United Nations Children's Fund). (2016). *Guideline: Updates on HIV and Infant Feeding*. Geneva: World Health Organization (http://apps.who.int/iris/bitstr eam/10665/246260/1/9789241549707-eng.pdf?ua=1).

WHO (World Health Organization), UNICEF (United Nations Children's Fund), UNAIDS (Joint United Nations Programme on HIV/AIDS), and UNFPA (United Nations Population Fund). (2003). *HIV and Infant Feeding: Guidelines for Decision-Makers*. Geneva: World Health Organization (http://www.who. int/maternal_child_adolescent/documents/9241591226/en/).

WHO (World Health Organization), UNAIDS (Joint United Nations Programme on HIV/AIDS), and UNICEF (United Nations Children's Fund). (2004). *Joint Statement on Use of Cotrimoxazole as Prophylaxis in HIV Exposed and HIV Infected Children*, press statement. Geneva: World Health Organization (http:// www.unaids.org/sites/default/files/web_story/ps_cotrimoxazole_22nov04_en_2.pdf).

8 Micronutrients and HIV in Pediatric Populations

*Julia L. Finkelstein, Haritha Aribindi,
Heather S. Herman, and Saurabh Mehta*

CONTENTS

INTRODUCTION

In 2015, approximately 1.8 million children (<15 years; 1.5–2.0 million) were living with HIV, and 150,000 children (110,000–190,000) were newly infected with HIV (UNAIDS, 2016). An estimated 90% of HIV-infected children contract the disease perinatally during pregnancy (*in utero*), delivery (intrapartum), or postpartum periods. Effective preventive interventions—including HIV screening, essential antiretroviral therapy (ART), safe delivery and caesarean section, and optimal infant feeding practices—can reduce the risk of mother-to-child transmission of HIV to less than 2%. The number of new HIV infections per year among children has decreased by nearly 50% since 2010 due to increased availability of and access to essential ART (UNAIDS, 2016); however, the burden of HIV/AIDS among children remains unacceptably high, disproportionately affecting children in resource-limited settings. Over 90% of new HIV infections and AIDS-related deaths in children occur in sub-Saharan Africa.

Micronutrient deficiencies are common in HIV-infected children and have been associated with an increased risk of adverse health outcomes. The vicious cycle of malnutrition and infection is exacerbated in children, who are particularly susceptible to nutrient deficiencies, stunting, and impaired immunity (Ivers et al., 2009). Additionally, as advances in and expansion of prophylaxis for HIV-infected mothers reduce mother-to-child transmission, a growing population of HIV-exposed, uninfected children presents a unique immunological profile and nutritional needs (Evans et al., 2016). Emerging evidence suggests that children who are exposed to HIV *in utero*, even if not HIV-infected, are at higher risk for malnutrition, morbidity, and mortality compared to unexposed, uninfected children (Afran et al., 2014; Evans et al., 2016).

Micronutrient supplementation has been shown to reduce the risk of co-infections and improve nutritional status, growth, and development in HIV-infected children (Irlam et al., 2013); however, there is limited evidence regarding the safety and efficacy of micronutrient supplementation in the context of antiretroviral therapy or among HIV-exposed, uninfected children. Therefore, a comprehensive review of the literature is needed to examine the existing evidence and inform future research priorities along with clinical care and public health approaches for both HIV-infected and HIV-exposed children.

OBJECTIVES

The objective of this review is to examine the evidence that links micronutrients and HIV in pediatric populations with an emphasis on randomized clinical trials (RCTs). We examine the efficacy and safety of micronutrient supplementation on health outcomes in HIV-infected and HIV-exposed children, including HIV infection, disease progression, all-cause and AIDS-related mortality, micronutrient status, growth, morbidity, and development. We then discuss research gaps, the role of micronutrient supplementation as an adjunct to essential ART, and the implications of findings for clinical care and public health practice for HIV-infected and HIV-exposed, uninfected children with an emphasis on resource-limited settings.

METHODS

SEARCH STRATEGY AND SELECTION PROCESS

A structured literature search was conducted using MEDLINE® electronic databases. Relevant Medical Subject Heading (MeSH®) terms were used to identify published studies through October 4, 2015. The MeSH terms used and the search selection strategy are summarized in Figure 8.1. Initial inclusion criteria for this review were the availability of an abstract and inclusion of data on micronutrient supplementation, children, and HIV/AIDS.

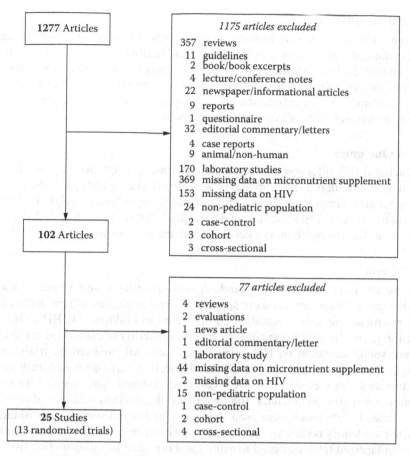

FIGURE 8.1 Study selection. Search terms: ((child[mh] OR infant[mh] OR adolescence[mh] OR pediatric OR paediatric OR child* OR newborn* OR adolescen* OR infan* OR preschool*[tw] OR teen*[tw] OR kindergarten*[tw] OR elementary school*[tw] OR nursery school*[tw] OR youth*[tw] OR baby* OR babies* OR schoolchild *[tw] OR toddler *[tw])) AND (((((((micronutrients OR micronutrient OR trace element OR trace elements OR vitamins OR vitamin OR carotenoids OR carotenoid OR carotenes OR carotene) OR ("24,25-dihydroxyvitamin D 3" OR "25-hydroxyvitamin D 2" OR "4- aminobenzoic acid" OR acetylcarnitine OR alpha-tocopherol OR aminobenzoic acids OR ascorbic acid OR beta carotene OR beta-tocopherol OR biotin OR boron OR cadmium OR calcifediol OR calcitriol OR carnitine OR cholecalciferol OR chromium OR cobalt OR cobamides OR cod liver oil OR calcium OR copper OR dehydroascorbic acid OR dihydrotachysterol OR dihydroxycholecalciferols OR ergocalciferols OR flavin OR folate OR mononucleotide OR folic acid OR formyltetrahydrofolates OR fursultiamin OR gamma-tocopherol OR hydroxocobalamin OR hydroxycholecalciferols OR inositol OR iodine OR iron OR leucovorin OR manganese OR magnesium OR molybdenum OR niacin OR niacinamide OR nickel OR nicorandil OR nicotinic acids OR palmitoylcarnitine OR pantothenic acid OR pteroylpolyglutamic acids OR pyridoxal OR pyridoxal phosphate OR pyridoxamine OR pyridoxine OR riboflavin OR selenium OR silicon OR tetrahydrofolates OR thiamine OR thiamine monophosphate OR thiamine pyrophosphate OR thiamine triphosphate OR thioctic acid OR tin OR tocopherols OR tocotrienols OR ubiquinone OR vanadium OR zinc)))) AND ((HIV Infections[MeSH] OR HIV[MeSH] OR hiv[tw] OR hiv-1*[tw] OR hiv-2*[tw] OR hiv1[tw] OR hiv2[tw] OR hiv infect*[tw] OR human immunodeficiency virus[tw] OR human immunedeficiency virus[tw] OR human immuno-deficiency virus[tw] OR human immune deficiency virus[tw] OR ((human immun*) AND (deficiency virus[tw])) OR acquired immunodeficiency syndrome[tw] OR acquired immunedeficiency syndrome[tw] OR acquired immunodeficiency syndrome[tw] OR acquired immune-deficiency syndrome[tw] OR ((acquired immun*) AND (deficiency syndrome[tw])) OR "sexually transmitted diseases, viral"[MESH:noexp]))))) NOT (animals[mh] NOT humans[mh]).

Micronutrient Supplementation

The following micronutrients were included in this review: vitamin A (retinol and carotenoids); vitamin C; vitamin B-complex, including vitamin B_1 (thiamine), vitamin B_2 (riboflavin), vitamin B_3 (niacin), vitamin B_5 (pantothenic acid), vitamin B_6 (pyridoxine), vitamin B_7 (biotin), vitamin B_9 (folic acid), and vitamin B_{12} (cobalamin); vitamin E; vitamin D; vitamin K; and the minerals boron, cadmium, calcium, chromium, cobalt, copper, iodine, iron, magnesium, manganese, molybdenum, nickel, selenium, silicon, vanadium, and zinc.

HIV-Related Outcomes

Outcomes included HIV infection; co-infections and clinical symptoms (i.e., measles, respiratory infections, diarrhea, malaria); anthropometry and growth (i.e., weight, length, head circumference, mid-upper arm circumference), including weight for age (WAZ), weight for length (WLZ), and length for age (LAZ) WHO z-scores (underweight, WAZ < –2; wasting, WLZ < –2; stunting, LAZ < –2); cognitive and psychomotor development; and anemia and micronutrient status.

Inclusion Criteria

Available abstracts of all studies were searched, full-text articles were extracted and reviewed, and the following inclusion criteria were applied: (1) human studies, (2) randomized trial study design, (3) micronutrient supplementation administered to children, (4) HIV-infected or HIV-exposed children from birth to 5 years of age, and (5) availability of data on the effects of pediatric micronutrient supplementation on HIV-related outcomes. All randomized trials and interventions, and quasi-randomized and uncontrolled trials meeting participant and methodological criteria were included. Sources were retrieved, collected, indexed, and assessed for micronutrient supplementation and HIV-related data. Bibliographies of published studies and manual searches of related articles in references were used to identify additional sources. An additional search was conducted to identify review articles, which were examined to cross-reference other relevant studies. A standardized table was used to extract and organize key information from the experimental studies that met the criteria noted here. Extracted data included publication date, authors, study design, setting, target population, micronutrient supplement type and composition, definitions of outcomes, main findings, and limitations.

LITERATURE REVIEW

The structured literature search yielded 1277 articles. Of these, 1175 studies were excluded based on abstracts: $n = 357$ reviews, $n = 11$ guidelines, $n = 2$ book chapters or excerpts, $n = 4$ conference proceedings, $n = 22$ newspaper or informational articles, $n = 9$ reports, $n = 4$ case reports, $n = 1$ questionnaire, $n = 32$ editorial commentary or letters, $n = 9$ non-human or animal studies, $n = 170$ in vitro/in vivo laboratory studies, $n = 369$ missing data on micronutrient supplementation, $n = 153$ missing data on HIV, $n = 24$ non-pediatric population, $n = 8$ not randomized trials (2 case-control, 3 cohort, and 3 cross-sectional). A total of 102 full-text articles were then extracted for further review; of these, 77 articles did not meet inclusion criteria: $n = 4$ reviews, $n = 2$ evaluations, $n = 1$ newspaper article, $n = 1$ commentary or letter, $n = 1$ laboratory study, $n = 44$ missing data on micronutrient supplementation, $n = 2$ missing data on HIV, $n = 15$ non-pediatric population, and $n = 7$ not randomized trials (1 case-control, 2 cohort, and 4 cross-sectional studies). Thus, a total of 25 papers from 13 randomized trials were included in this review. The structured literature search is summarized in Figure 8.1. Detailed findings from randomized trials are presented in Tables 8.1 to 8.4.

VITAMIN A

The World Health Organization (WHO) recommends high-dose vitamin A supplementation for children 6 to 59 months of age in settings where vitamin A deficiency is a public health problem, based on its demonstrated benefits on the risk of illness and death of infectious diseases, including measles and diarrhea (WHO, 2011). Vitamin A supplementation in both HIV-infected and HIV-uninfected children has been associated with reduced risk of lower respiratory tract infection and severe watery diarrhea, with similar protective effects against infectious disease morbidity and mortality. All-cause mortality and AIDS-related deaths have also been demonstrated to be lower in HIV-infected children supplemented with vitamin A. The effects of vitamin A supplementation on health outcomes in HIV-infected individuals have been previously reviewed in detail (Mehta and Fawzi, 2007) and are discussed in Chapter 1 of this volume.

Mortality

In a study of children hospitalized with pneumonia in Tanzania (687 total patients, 6 months to 5 years of age; 37 HIV-infected), children were randomized to receive either a vitamin A supplement (60 mg retinol or 30 mg retinol if $\leq$ 1 year old) or placebo at baseline, two days after enrollment, at four months, and at eight months after discharge (Fawzi et al., 1999). Among all children, vitamin A supplementation was associated with a 49% reduction in all-cause mortality (risk ratio [RR]: 0.51; 95% CI, 0.29–0.90; $p = 0.02$) and an even larger reduction in diarrhea-related mortality (RR, 0.07; 95% CI, 0.01–0.49; $p = 0.001$) during an average of 24.4 months of follow-up (standard deviation [SD] = 12.1 months; median = 27.8 months). In HIV-infected children, vitamin A supplementation was associated with a 63% reduction in all-cause mortality (RR, 0.37; 95% CI, 0.14–0.95; $p = 0.04$) and a 68% reduction in AIDS-related mortality (RR, 0.32; 95% CI, 0.10–0.99; $p < 0.05$).

A trial of vitamin A supplementation was conducted among HIV-infected children in Uganda ($n = 201$) who were supplemented from 15 to 36 months of age (Semba et al., 2005). Children were randomized to receive either a vitamin A supplement (60 mg retinol) or placebo every three months. Children who received vitamin A supplementation experienced a decrease in overall mortality over a 21-month follow-up period (RR, 0.54; 95% CI, 0.30–0.98; $p = 0.044$). Another randomized, placebo-controlled trial with vitamin A supplementation was conducted among HIV-infected mothers and their children ($n = 14,110$ mother–infant pairs) (Humphrey et al., 2006). The mother–infant pairs were randomized to one of four groups and supplemented with a single large dose shortly after birth as follows: (1) vitamin A supplementation for both mother (400,000 IU) and infant (50,000 IU) (MI); (2) supplementation for infant only (I); (3) supplementation for mother only (M); or (4) placebo for both mother and infant (P). In analyses among children who were HIV-infected in the first six weeks of life (i.e., whose HIV status changed from HIV-uninfected at baseline or at birth to HIV-infected by six weeks of age), as determined by polymerase chain reaction (PCR), vitamin A supplementation was associated with a 28% reduction in the risk of mortality in the first 24 months of life compared to placebo (hazard ratio [HR], 0.72; 95% CI, 0.57–0.92; $p = 0.01$) (Humphrey et al., 2006). However, HIV-exposed infants who were not HIV-infected by six weeks of age demonstrated a twofold increase in mortality by 24 months, although this was not statistically significant (Table 8.4) (HR, 1.41; 95% CI, 0.97–2.05; $p = 0.07$).

Morbidity

A randomized trial was conducted in South Africa to investigate the effects of vitamin A supplementation in HIV-exposed, full-term infants ($n = 118$) (Coutsoudis et al., 1995). The infants were randomly assigned to receive either vitamin A or placebo every three months (50,000 IU at one and three months, 100,000 IU at three and five months, and 200,000 IU at 12 and 15 months). HIV-infected children supplemented with vitamin A had lower odds of diarrhea (odds ratio [OR], 0.51;

TABLE 8.1

Micronutrient Supplementation in HIV-Infected and HIV-Exposed Children

Location and Ref.	Participants	Methods	Exposures	Outcomes	Main Findings
Dar es Salaam, Tanzania Kupka et al. (2013)	2387 infants born from HIV-infected mothers (≥32 weeks gestation)	Baseline interviews were conducted at time of enrollment for mothers and infants. All women received the same vitamins pre- and postnatally. Standard prenatal care included daily doses of 200 mg ferrous sulfate (60 mg ferrous Fe equivalent), folic acid (0.25 mg), and malaria prophylaxis. Prenatal and postnatal care also included vitamins B-complex, C, and E. Infants were randomized at 5–7 weeks of age to receive daily multivitamins or placebo until 104 weeks of age. At monthly visits, primary and secondary outcomes were measured. Supplements were provided to caretakers for the next month. HIV infection was evaluated 6 weeks and at 18 months of age. ART was administered only once to the mother and child at labor and at delivery to prevent transmission. As the study progressed, ART became available to all children and eligible mothers.	Placebo (n = 1194) Micronutrient supplementation: vitamins B-complex, C, and E (n = 1193) (60 mg vitamin C, 8 mg vitamin E, 0.5 mg B$_1$, 0.6 mg B$_2$, 4 mg B$_3$, 0.6 mg vitamin B$_6$, 130 µg folic acid, 1 mg vitamin B$_{12}$) Children under 6 months given 1 capsule and older children given 2 capsules per day	*Primary outcomes* Length-for-age z-score (LAZ) Weight-for-age z-score (WAZ) Weight-for-length z-score (WLZ) *Secondary outcomes* Stunting (LAZ <2) Underweight (WAZ <2) Wasting (WLZ <2)	No change in LAZ ($p = 0.94$), WAZ ($p = 0.97$), and WLZ ($p = 0.78$) between groups for HIV-infected and uninfected children No statistical difference in secondary outcomes Stunting (HR, 0.92; 95% CI, 0.79–1.08) Underweight (HR, 0.95; 95% CI, 0.81–1.10) Wasting (HR, 0.92; 95% CI, 0.79–1.07)

Dar es Salaam, Tanzania Duggan et al. (2012)	See above. Cohort of infants with mothers on ART (n = 429)	See above.	*Primary outcomes* Mortality *Secondary outcomes* Morbidity (diarrhea, cold, cough, fever, difficulty breathing, appetite, hospitalizations, vomiting, ear infections)	Lower risk of mortality with supplementation (HR, 1.13; 95% CI, 0.88–1.44; p = 0.3) Lower risk of fever (RR, 0.92; 95% CI, 0.85–0.99; p = 0.02) and vomiting (RR, 0.78; 95% CI, 0.65–0.93; p = 0.007) with micronutrient supplementation compared to placebo Lower incidences of hospitalizations (RR, 0.48; 95% CI, 0.24–0.95; p = 0.035), fever (RR, 0.7; 95% CI, 0.67–0.93; p = 0.005), and cough and fever (RR, 0.79; 95% CI, 0.65–0.96; p = 0.019)
Dar es Salaam, Tanzania Liu et al. (2013)	See above. Blood samples and hemoglobin (Hb) concentrations were measured at baseline and at 6, 12, 18, and 24 months follow-up. Only 10 children and 20% of mothers received ART.	See above. Placebo (n = 1006) Micronutrients (n = 1002)	*Primary outcomes* Anemia (Hb < 11 g/dL) Severe anemia (Hb < 8.5 g/dL) *Secondary outcomes* Mother-to-child transmission	Hb concentrations significantly higher in micronutrient group vs. placebo group at 12 months (9.77 vs. 9.64 g/dL; p = 0.03), at 18 months (9.76 vs. 9.57 g/dL; p = 0.004), and at 24 months (9.93 vs. 9.75 g/dL; p = 0.02) Risk of anemia 12% lower in micronutrient group vs. placebo group (HR, 0.88; 95% CI, 0.79– 0.99; p = 0.03) Risk of anemia 28% lower in micronutrient group children born to non-anemic mothers (HR, 0.72; 95% CI, 0.56–0.92; p = 0.008) No lower risk in micronutrient group of children born to anemic mothers (HR, 1.10; 95% CI, 0.79–1.54; p = 0.57) No association of mother-to-child-transmission with micronutrient supplementation (OR, 1.23; 95% CI, 0.77–1.95; p = 0.39)

(continued)

TABLE 8.1 (continued)
Micronutrient Supplementation in HIV-Infected and HIV-Exposed Children

Location and Ref.	Participants	Methods	Exposures	Outcomes	Main Findings
Dar es Salaam, Tanzania Manji et al. (2014)	See above.	See above. Bayley Scales cognition test was administered to 206 infants aged 15 months.	See above. Placebo ($n = 99$) Micronutrients ($n = 93$)	*Primary outcomes* Bayley Scales of Infant and Toddler Development—Third Edition test scores (cognitive functioning, receptive and language skills, fine and gross motor skills)	No significant improvement in fine motor skills with supplementation (mean difference = 0.38; 95% CI, −0.01–0.78; $p = 0.06$) No significant differences in cognitive (OR, 0.57; 95% CI, 0.29–1.14; $p = 0.11$), expressive language (OR, 1.10; 95% CI, 0.55–2.21; $p = 0.78$), receptive language (OR, 0.84; 95% CI, 0.37–1.91; $p = 0.67$), fine motor skills (OR, 0.49; 95% CI, 0.17–1.38; $p = 0.18$), or gross motor skills (OR, 1.10; 95% CI, 0.55–2.21; $p = 0.78$) scores
Durban, South Africa Coutsoudis et al. (1995)	118 HIV-infected and uninfected full-term infants born to HIV-infected mothers	HIV-infected mothers living within 10 miles of the hospital were included. Baseline characteristics were measured in mothers and infants. Children were randomized to the placebo or vitamin A group. Supplementation was provided every 3 months and follow-up at 2, 3, 6, 9, 12, 16, and 18 months. HIV testing in infants included positive HIV antibody test at 15 months. Outcomes were measured as incidence density (episodes per 100 months) ($n = 806$ child months). Serum vitamin A levels were measured in a subset of 36 infants at 1 and 9 months. Mothers were also administered vitamin A.	Placebo ($n = 416$ child months) Vitamin A (50,000 IU 1–3 months, 100,000 IU 6–9 months, 200,000 IU 12–15 months) ($n = 390$ child months)	*Primary outcomes* Morbidity associated with diarrhea (≥4 watery stools/day) Upper respiratory infections (rhinitis, throat or ear infection, cough) Lower respiratory infection (rapid breathing coughing, wheezing, crackling) Fever, thrush, rash *Secondary outcomes* Anthropometry Serum vitamin A levels	Lower morbidity in vitamin A group (OR, 0.69; 95% CI, 0.48–0.99) due to diarrhea, diarrhea lasting more than 7 days, hospitalization for diarrhea, thrush, lower respiratory tract infection (LRTI), hospitalization for LRTI, and upper respiratory tract infection Incidence of diarrhea lower in HIV-infected ($n = 28$) vitamin A-supplemented children (OR, 0.51; 95% CI, 0.27–0.99) Significantly higher mean serum vitamin A concentrations at 9 months in vitamin A vs. placebo group (38.4 µg/dL and 30.0 µg/dL, respectively; $p < 0.001$)

TABLE 8.2

Micronutrient Supplementation in HIV-Infected and HIV-Uninfected Children

Location and Ref.	Participants	Methods	Exposures	Outcomes	Main Findings
Kwa-Zulu Natal Province, South Africa Luabeya et al. (2007)	HIV-infected children ($n = 32$), HIV-uninfected children born to HIV-infected mothers ($n = 154$), HIV-uninfected children (6–24 months) born to HIV-uninfected mothers ($n = 187$)	Baseline anthropometry measures were documented. Three cohorts of children were randomized to one of three treatment groups. Exclusion criteria for children: diarrhea >7 days at enrollment; weight-for-age in 40th percentile of U.S. standards; supplementation received in last month. Supplementation from 6 to 24 months of age daily. Weekly visits conducted to provide tablet supplies and collect data on primary and secondary outcomes via questionnaires for caretakers. HIV testing conducted by HIV RNA assays	Vitamin A alone ($n = 124$) vs. vitamin A + zinc ($n = 123$) vs. vitamin A + zinc + multiple micronutrients ($n = 126$) Vitamin A (1250 IU) Zinc (10 mg) Micronutrients (0.5 mg of vitamin B_1, B_2, and B_6; 0.9 μg B_{12}; 35 mg C; 5 μg D; 6 mg E; 10 μg K; 0.6 mg copper, 50 μg I, 10 mg iron, 150 μg folic acid, 6 mg B_3)	*Primary outcomes* Percentage of days of diarrhea (frequent, looser, and/or bloody stools) *Secondary outcomes* Upper respiratory problems (cough, runny nose) Pneumonia (fast breathing or chest movements)	There were no significant differences between treatment groups for main outcomes: percent of days with diarrhea, upper respiratory problems, and pneumonia incidences in HIV exposed ($p = 0.852, 0.94, 0.084$), HIV-uninfected ($p = 0.857, 0.766, 0.397$), and HIV-infected ($p = 0.688, 0.222, 0.371$) children. Note: p = diarrhea, upper respiratory, pneumonia incidence

(continued)

TABLE 8.2 (continued)

Micronutrient Supplementation in HIV-Infected and HIV-Uninfected Children

Location and Ref.	Participants	Methods	Exposures	Outcomes	Main Findings
KwaZulu-Natal Province, South Africa Chhagan et al. (2010)	HIV-infected children (n = 32), HIV-uninfected but exposed children (n = 154), HIV-uninfected children (6–24 months) (n = 187)	See above. Anthropometry was measured at baseline and at 7, 8, 9, 12, 15, 18, 21, and 24 months. Hemoglobin was measured at baseline and at 12 months.	See above.	*Primary outcomes* Length-for-age z-score (LAZ) (stunting, z-score < 2 SD) Anemia (Hg < 11 g/dL) Effect of diarrhea (>6 episodes) on growth	There were no significant differences between treatment groups in LAZ score changes over 18 months among all children. Stunted children (LAZ < −2) in the multiple micronutrient (MM) group had significant improvement in LAZ over time (+0.7 z-score) compared to declines of 0.3 in vitamin A+ zinc (VAZ) and 0.2 in vitamin A (VA) (p = 0.029) groups. Among HIV-uninfected children experiencing diarrhea, those receiving MM showed no decline in LAZ compared to 0.5 and 0.6 z-score declines in the VAZ and VA groups, respectively (p = 0.006). At 12 months, there was a 24% decrease in the number of children with anemia in the MM group (p = 0.001), 11% decrease in the VAZ group (p = 0.131), and 18% decrease in the vitamin A group (p = 0.019) (between group differences p = 0.10).
KwaZulu-Natal Province, South Africa Chhagan et al. (2009)	HIV-infected children (n = 32), HIV-uninfected but exposed children (n = 154), HIV-uninfected children (6–24 months) (n = 187)	See above. Information about duration and episodes of diarrhea was extracted from daily records. HIV-uninfected children born to HIV-uninfected and infected mothers were clumped together in analyses due to similarity in diarrheal results.	See above.	*Primary outcomes* Incidence of diarrhea (defined as period of diarrhea separated by 2 or more days without diarrhea)	There were no significant differences in diarrhea incidence among treatment arms for HIV-infected (p = 0.76) and HIV-uninfected children (p = 0.69). Stunted HIV-uninfected children had lower diarrhea incidence with zinc supplementation (RR, 0.52; 95% CI, 0.45–0.60) (2.04 episodes/year) or multiple micronutrients (RR, 0.57; 95% CI, 0.49–0.67) (2.23 episodes/year) compared with just vitamin A (3.92 episodes/year (p = 0.024 comparing control vs. zinc and MM group combined).

Location / Author	Population	Intervention	Methods / Outcomes	Results
Kampala, Uganda, and surrounding areas Srinivasan et al. (2012)	352 children with severe pneumonia (6–59 months)	Zinc (10 mg if <12 months; 20 mg if ≥12 months) vs. placebo	Children were randomly assigned to the two treatment groups. Supplementation occurred daily for 7 days with water-soluble tablets. Outcomes were measured every 6 hours for 7 days or until death or discharge. Antibiotics were administered to treat pneumonia. *Primary outcomes* Low oxygen saturation (<92%) Rapid breathing rate (>50 breaths/min children younger than 1 year; >40 breaths/min children older than 1 year) Fever Time to normalization of above outcomes was measured. *Secondary outcomes* Case fatality/mortality due to disease	Among HIV-infected children, supplementation with vitamin A plus zinc or multiple micronutrients had a higher risk of persistent diarrhea ($p = 0.02$) and severe diarrhea ($p = 0.01$), compared to vitamin A alone. Case fatality was lower in the zinc group than the placebo group for HIV-infected (RR, 0.1; 95% CI, 0.0–1.0) and HIV-uninfected children (RR, 0.7; 95% CI, (0.2–2.2). Case fatality was lower in the zinc group than the control group among all children combined (mixed HIV status) (RR, 0.33; 95% CI, 0.15–0.76; $p <$ 0.05). Oxygen saturation (HR, 1.04; 95% CI, 0.74–1.46; $p = 0.823$), breathing rate (HR, 0. 88; 95% CI, 0.69–1.13; $p = 0.306$), and fever (HR, 1.016; 95% CI, 0.79–1.30; $p = 0.897$) times to normalization were not significant between treatment groups ($p >$ 0.05).
Dar es Salaam, Tanzania Fawzi et al. (2000)	687 children (6–60 months) with pneumonia (HIV-infected, $n =$ 37; HIV-uninfected, $n =$ 363)	Vitamin A (60 mg retinol) vs. placebo	Children were supplemented and blood samples were taken at baseline (at the hospital) and 4 and 8 months after discharge. Children were supplemented with enhanced corn oil which also contained 0.24 mg/mL of vitamin E for both groups. Children older than 1 year received 1 mL of the dosage; children younger received 0.5 mL	*Primary outcomes* Diarrhea (acute, 1–14 days; persistent, >14 days) Respiratory symptoms (cough, rapid breathing, fever) Hospitalizations Morbidity	There were no significant differences among treatment groups for HIV-infected children for acute diarrhea (RR, 1.55; 95% CI, 0.75–3.17; $p =$ 0.23) and for respiratory symptoms (RR, 0. 54; 95% CI, 0.24–1.20; $p = 0.13$) compared to placebo. HIV-uninfected children supplemented with vitamin A had an increased risk of cough and rapid respiratory rate (RR, 1.47; 95% CI, 1.16–1.86; $p =$ 0.001) compared to HIV-uninfected children given placebo. The odds of severe watery diarrhea (watery stools for ≥14 days) were reduced (OR, 0.56; 95% CI, 0.32–0.99; $p = 0.04$) compared to placebo in all children.

(continued)

TABLE 8.2 (continued)
Micronutrient Supplementation in HIV-Infected and HIV-Uninfected Children

Location and Ref.	Participants	Methods	Exposures	Outcomes	Main Findings
		Morbidity was measured up to 1 year after being discharged. HIV testing was carried out by immunoassay and western blot.			Higher odds of cough and rapid respiratory rate were associated with supplementation (OR, 1.67; 95% CI, 1.17–2.36; $p = 0.004$) in all children.
Dar es Salaam, Tanzania Fawzi et al. (1999)	See above.	See above. Mortality was monitored during monthly visits and clinic visits. The mean duration of follow-up was 24.4 ± 12.1 months (median = 27.8).	See above.	*Primary outcome* Mortality	Mortality was higher in HIV-infected children than in HIV-uninfected children (RR, 5.0; 95% CI, 3.0–8.4; $p < 0.0001$). In HIV-infected children, vitamin A supplementation reduced all-cause mortality by 63% (RR, 0.37; 95% CI, 0.14–0.95; $p = 0.04$) and was associated with a 68% reduction in AIDS-related deaths ($p = 0.05$). In HIV-uninfected children, vitamin A supplementation reduced all-cause mortality by 42% (RR, 0.58; 95% CI, 0.28–1.19; $p = 0.14$). In all children, vitamin A supplementation reduced mortality from diarrhea by 93% (RR, 0.07; 95% CI, 0.00–0.49; $p = 0.001$) and reduced all-cause mortality by 49% (RR, 0.51; 95% CI, 0.29, 0.90; $p = 0.02$).

Dar es Salaam, Tanzania Villamor et al. (2002)	See above.	See above. Morbidity data were collected at biweekly visits. Participants were followed-up for 1 year.	See above. Vitamin A (100,000 IU for children < 1 yr; 200,000 IU for older children)	*Primary outcomes* Morbidity (diarrhea, respiratory infections) Anthropometry (stunting, HAZ < −2; wasting, WHZ < −2) *Secondary outcomes* HIV disease progression Malaria	*HIV-infected children* There was a significant increase in height in the vitamin A group (2.8 cm; 95% CI, 1.0–4.6 cm; $p = 0.003$) for children 6–18 months. No risk of stunting was associated with persistent diarrhea in the vitamin A group (controlled for HIV infection status) (RR, 1.0; 95% CI, 0.3–1.3). *Mixed HIV status* There was a non-significant 23% (95% CI, −4%–44%; $p = 0.09$) decrease in the risk of stunting (AHR, 0.78; 95% CI, 0.57–1.06; $p = 0.11$) with vitamin A. Supplementation led to a non-significant 50% (95% CI, 2–74%; $p = 0.08$, test for interaction) decrease in risk of stunting in children exclusively breastfed 4–6 months. There was a non-significant reduced risk of wasting in supplemented children with malaria (RR, 0.28; 95% CI, 0.07–1.02; $p = 0.04$, test for interaction) and low arm circumference (<25th percentile) (RR, 0.55; 95% CI, 0.27–1.10; $p = 0.06$, test for interaction).

TABLE 8.3

Micronutrient Supplementation in HIV-Infected Children

Location and Ref.	Participants	Methods	Exposures	Outcomes	Main Findings
Kampala, Uganda, and surrounding areas Ndeezi et al. (2011)	847 HIV-infected children only (ages 1–5 years) included in trial 214 participants analyzed in study	847 children were enrolled in a micronutrient supplementation study. HAART was administered after enrollment. Children were randomized to receive 2× RDA or SOC doses at the 4-year old level. Blood samples were collected at baseline and at 6 months and analyzed for serum vitamin B_{12} and folate levels for 214 children.	Twice recommended dietary allowance (RDA) vs. standard of care (SOC) SOC: Children received SOC doses of 6 micronutrients (n = 114) (400 µg vitamin A, 0.6 mg vitamin B_1, 0.6 mg vitamin B_2, 8 mg niacin, 25 mg vitamin C, 200 IU vitamin D). Twice RDA: Children received 2× the RDA for 14 micronutrients (n = 104) (800 µg vitamin A, 1.2 mg vitamin B_1, 1.2 mg vitamin B_2, 16 mg niacin, 1.2 mg vitamin B_6, 2.4 µg vitamin B_{12}, 50 mg vitamin C, 400 IU vitamin D, 14 mg vitamin E, 40 µg folate, 60 µg selenium, 10 mg zinc, 800 µg copper, 180 µg iodine). Children received daily 4 g of supplementation powder mixed in milk or water.	*Primary outcomes* Low serum vitamin B_{12} levels (<221 pmols/L) Low serum folate levels (<13.4 nmols/L) *Secondary outcomes* Low CD4+ cell counts (<25%) Hemoglobin levels	At baseline for all total children, 28% had low serum vitamin B_{12} and 29% had low folate levels. In the 2× RDA group, there was a significant increase in vitamin B_{12} (median [IQR], 285.5 [216.5–371.8] to 401.5 [264.3–518.8] pmol/L; p < 0.001) and folic acid levels (median [IQR], 17.3 [13.5–26.6) to 27.7 [21.1–33.4] nmol/L; p < 0.001). In the SOC group, there was no significant difference in vitamin B_{12} (median [IQR]: 280 [211.5–386.3] to 288.5 [198.8–391.0; p = 0.78) and folic acid (median [IQR]: 15.7 [11.9–22.1] to 16.5 [11.7–22.1]; p = 0.44) levels before and after supplementation. Children on HAART (n = 44) experienced a significant increase in vitamin B_{12} levels (median [IQR]: 262.0 [215.0–342.0] to 453.0 [261.0–594.0] pmol/L; p = 0.002) and folate levels (median [IQR]: 18.6 [13.8–23.9] to 25.0 [21.3–32.9; p = 0.040). Hemoglobin levels increased in 2× RDA group (p = 0.04) and in the SOC group (p < 0.001). CD4 levels did not significantly change in 2× RDA (p = 0.16) nor in the SOC group (p = 0.52). Of the children on HAART, 32.5% had CD4% <25 compared to 63.5% of HAART-naïve children (p = 0.001).

Location	Population	Methods	Sample	Outcomes	Results
Kampala, Uganda, and surrounding areas Ndeezi et al. (2010)	847 HIV-infected children (ages 1–5 years)	See above. Clinic follow-ups occurred at baseline and at 6, 9, and 12 months. Anthropometry, morbidity, and mortality were recorded. After 6 months, both treatment groups received SOC doses.	See above. ART strata: 2× RDA (n = 43), SOC (n = 42) ART-naïve strata: 2× RDA (n = 383), SOC (n = 379)	*Primary outcome* Mortality *Secondary outcomes* Morbidity Anthropometry (WAZ, WHZ) HIV disease progression (CD4 cell count)	There was no significant difference in mortality at 12 months between treatment groups (RR, 0.9; 95% CI, 0.5–1.5). There was no significant difference in mortality between ART groups (RR, 1.0; 95% CI, 0.6–1.6). Fever (HR, 2.1; 95% CI, 1.1–3.9; $p = 0.02$), cough (HR, 1.8; 95% CI, 0.9–3.5; $p = 0.08$), recurrent hospitalization (HR, 2.6; 95% CI, 1.2–5.7; $p = 0.02$), WAZ < –2 (HR, 2.6; 95% CI, 1.2–5.8; $p = 0.02$), and HIV stages 3 and 4 (HR, 2.9; 95% CI, 1.5–5.6; $p < 0.01$) were all associated with higher mortality. Cotrimoxazole regimen decreased mortality risk (RR, 0.4; 95% CI, 0.2–0.9; $p = 0.03$). There was no significant difference in CD4 cell counts between treatment groups (OR, 0.74; 95% CI, 0.74–1.17).
Kampala, Uganda, and surrounding areas Ndeezi et al. (2012)	847 HIV-infected children (ages 1–5 years)	See above. Diarrhea episodes were recorded at baseline and during monthly clinic visits up to 6 months.	See above. HAART strata: 2× RDA) (n = 43), SOC (n = 42) HAART-naïve strata: 2× RDA (n = 383), SOC (n = 379)	*Primary outcome* Diarrhea incidence (3+ watery or loose stools in the past 24 hr)	Diarrhea incidence ratio was not significantly different between treatment groups. *Overall* 2× RDA SOC (RR, 1.1; 95% CI, 0.9–1.3; $p = 0.43$) HAART-naïve 2× RDA SOC (RR, 1.1; 95% CI, (0.9–1.2), $p = 0.44$) HAART (RR, 1.1; 95% CI, 0.5–2.3; $p = 0.94$) Children on HAART had a lower incidence of diarrhea compared to HAART-naïve children (OR, 0.6; 95% CI, 0.3–0.9; $p = 0.03$). *(continued)*

TABLE 8.3 (continued)

Micronutrient Supplementation in HIV-Infected Children

Location and Ref.	Participants	Methods	Exposures	Outcomes	Main Findings
Pretoria, South Africa Mda et al. (2013)	201 HIV-infected, ART-naïve children (4–24 months)	In a 6-month study, children were randomly assigned to receive daily tablets of micronutrient supplementation or placebo. Children at HIV stages 3 or 4 and at CD4 counts <15% received ART. Blood samples were collected at baseline and at 3 and 6 months. Participants were visited twice per week.	Placebo (n = 97) Micronutrients (300 μg A, 0.6 mg B₁, 0.6 mg B₂, 8 mg B₃, 0.6 mg B₆, 1 μg B₁₂, 70 μg folic acid, 25 mg C, 5 μg D, 7 mg E, 700 μg copper, 8 mg iron, 30 μg selenium, and 8 mg zinc) (n = 104)	*Primary outcomes* Mortality Diarrhea (3+ watery or loose stools) Respiratory infections (cough and/or fever, ≥50 breaths/min) Anthropometry CD4 cell count	There was no significant difference in mortality between groups (n = 27 vs. 16; p = 0.12). Weight-for-height z-scores significantly increased in the micronutrient group compared to placebo (0.40; 95% CI, 0.09–0.71 vs. −0.04; 95% CI, −0.39–0.31; p < 0.05) There was a lower incidence of diarrhea in the micronutrient group (0.25; 95% CI, 0.17–0.33) than in the placebo group (0.36; 95% CI, 0.26–0.33; p = 0.09). There was a lower incidence of respiratory symptoms in the micronutrient group (0.66; 95% CI, 0.52–0.80) than in the placebo group (1.01; 95% CI, 0.83–1.79; p < 0.05) There were no significant differences in CD4 cell counts: change in 6 months, placebo (−1.44; 95% CI, −3.71–0.83) vs. micronutrients (−0.64; 95% CI, −3.39–2.11).
Pretoria, South Africa Mda et al. (2010a)	201 HIV-infected, ART-naïve children (4–24 months)	See above.	See above. Placebo (n = 52) Micronutrients (n = 54)	*Primary outcome* Hospitalization duration for diarrhea and respiratory infections	Hospitalization duration, independent of admission diagnosis (diarrhea or pneumonia), was significantly shorter for the micronutrient group (7.3 ± 3.9 days) than for the placebo group (9.0 ± 4.9) (p < 0.05). Duration for diarrhea was shorter for the micronutrient group by 1.6 days and 1.9 days for pneumonia (p > 0.05).

| Pretoria, South Africa Mda et al. (2010b) | 201 HIV-infected ART-naïve children (6–24 months) | Children were randomly assigned to daily micronutrient supplementation or placebo for 6 months. Anthropometric measures were recorded at monthly clinic visits. Appetite tests were conducted at baseline, 3 months, and 6 months. To test appetite, children fasted from dinner until the test. Without encouragement, caretakers fed 75 g of warm porridge to the child, and the amount consumed was measured. | Placebo ($n = 65$) Micronutrients (300 mg vitamin A, 0.6 mg vitamin B_1, 0.6 mg vitamin B_2, 8 mg vitamin B_3, 0.6 mg vitamin B_6, 1 mg vitamin B_{12}, 70 mg folic acid, 25 mg vitamin C, 5 mg vitamin D, 7 mg vitamin E, 700 mg copper; 8 mg iron, 30 mg selenium, 8 mg zinc) ($n = 75$) | *Primary outcomes* Appetite (change in amount eaten per kilogram body weight) Anthropometry *Secondary outcomes* Serum zinc, iron, and ferritin | After 3 months, log ferritin was significantly higher in the micronutrient supplementation group ($p < 0.05$). Change in amount eaten was significantly higher in the micronutrient group vs. placebo group (mean ± SD: 108 ± 112 vs. 57 ± 130 g) ($p < 0.05$). Change in eating rate was higher in the micronutrient group compared to placebo (mean ± SD: 4.7 ± 14.7 vs. 1.4 ± 15.1 g/min) ($p < 0.05$). |
| Kampala, Uganda, and surrounding areas Semba et al. (2005) | 201 HIV-infected children (6–36 months) | Children, enrolled at 6 months old, were randomly assigned to receive either vitamin A supplementation or placebo once every 3 months at a clinic from ages 15–36 months. Trimethoprim–sulfsmethoxazole was also supplemented daily. Morbidity data for the last 7 days (last 30 days for hospitalizations) and other outcome data were collected every 3 months. | Vitamin A (60 mg retinol) ($n = 83$) Placebo ($n = 85$) | *Primary outcomes* Mortality Morbidity (diarrhea, cough, fast breathing, fever, ear discharge, bloody stools) Hospitalizations Anthropometry Clinical presentations of vitamin A deficiency (night blindness, Bitot's spots, corneal xerosis, and/or ulceration) | Mortality was lower in the vitamin A group (20.6%) compared to the placebo group (20.6%) (RR, 0.54; 95% CI, 0.30–0.98; $p = 0.044$). Children in the vitamin A group experienced lower incidences of cough (OR, 0.47; 95% CI, 0.23–0.96; $p = 0.038$), diarrhea (OR, 0.48; 95% CI, 0.19–1.18; $p = 0.11$), and durations of ear infections ($p = 0.03$) compared to the placebo group. |

(continued)

TABLE 8.3 (continued)

Micronutrient Supplementation in HIV-Infected Children

Location and Ref.	Participants	Methods	Exposures	Outcomes	Main Findings
Malawi Esan et al. (2013)	209 HIV-infected children (6–59 months) with moderate anemia (7.0–9.9 Hg g/dL)	Children were randomly assigned to each treatment arm. Children were supplemented daily for 3 months and observed for a total of 6 months. Children were followed up at 1, 2, 3, and 6 months and outcomes were measured.	Multivitamin (1500 IU/mL vitamin A, 35 mg/mL vitamin C, 400 IU/mL vitamin D) vs. multivitamin + iron (3 mg/kg/day)	*Primary outcomes* Hemoglobin concentrations (anemia, Hb < 11 g/dL) Iron deficiency (serum ferritin < 30 µg/dL with CRP ≥ 5.0 mg/L, or serum ferritin < 12 µg/dL with CRP < 5.0 mg/L) Respiratory infections (>40–50 breaths/min, cough, respiratory distress, etc.) Low CD4 cell counts (<20%) Malaria incidence (presence of parasites)	Multivitamin + iron group was associated with increased hemoglobin concentration (adjusted mean difference: 0.60; 95% CI, 0.06–1.13; $p = 0.03$), lower prevalence in anemia (PR, 0.59; 95% CI, 0.38–0.92; $p = 0.02$), and higher incidence of malaria (adjusted IRR, 1.81; 95% CI, 1.04–3.16; $p = 0.04$) compared to placebo at 6 months. There were higher CD4 counts in the multivitamin + iron group (MD, 6.00; 95% CI, 1.84–10.16; $p = 0.005$) and lower risk of iron deficiency (adjusted prevalence ratio [APR], 0.28; 95% CI, 0.15–0.49; $p < 0.001$) only after 3 months. After 3–6 months/post-intervention, iron supplementation led to a lower incidence of respiratory infections (IR, 0.28; 95% CI, 0.09–0.91; $p = 0.04$), higher risk of malaria in children less than 2 years (IR, 3.30; 95% CI, 1.28–8.49; $p = 0.01$), and, in iron-deficient children, lower risk of HIV disease progression to AIDS (IR, 0.25; 95% CI, 0.08–0.83; $p = 0.02$).
Pietermaritzburg, South Africa Bobat et al. (2005)	96 HIV-infected children (6–60 months)	Children were randomly assigned daily supplementation of zinc or placebo. HIV viral load and CD4 cell counts were measured at baseline and at 3, 6, and 9 months.	Placebo vs. zinc (10 mg zinc sulfate)	*Primary outcomes* Plasma HIV viral load CD4 cell count *Secondary outcomes* Mortality Hemoglobin concentrations Diarrhea	There were no significant differences between treatment groups for CD4 cell counts (−0.8; 95% CI, −4–3), hemoglobin concentrations ($p = 0.20$), HIV viral load (linear regression coefficient, −0.026; 95% CI, −0.250–0.197; $p = 0.82$), or mortality ($p = 0.10$). Zinc supplementation was associated with a lower incidence of watery diarrhea ($p = $

| Agra, India Gautam et al. (2014) | 127 HIV-infected children (≤15 yr) | Children on ART ($n = 58$) were randomly assigned to micronutrient supplementation or placebo; children not on ART were assigned to each treatment group. Micronutrients were administered for 6 months daily (5 mL syrup form) and probiotics for 3 months twice daily (2.5×10^{10} CFU/5 g, 10 g). CD4 cell counts were measured at baseline and at 6 months. Other outcomes were measured at baseline and every month after up to 6 months for the micronutrient group and up to 3 months for the probiotic group. | Micronutrients and/or probiotics vs. placebo Micronutrients (25 µg copper, 5 mg zinc, 10 µg selenium, 38 µg iodine, 1250 IU vitamin A, 0.75 mg vitamin B_1, 0.75 mg vitamin B_2, 0.5 mg vitamin B_6, 1.25 mg vitamin B_5, 0.5 µg vitamin B_{12}, 100 IU vitamin D, 2.5 IU vitamin E) Probiotics (2.5×10^{10} CFU/5 g) | *Primary outcome* HIV disease progression (WHO clinical and immunological stages, CD4 cell count) Body mass index (BMI) | 0.001) and a reduced number of illness visits compared to the placebo group (0.11 vs. 0.16 visits/month; $p = 0.05$). *Not on ART: supplemented with micronutrients* Significant improvement from clinical stage 2 to 1 (+8 [30.8%] to clinical stage 1 at follow-up) ($p = 0.01$; $p = 0.049$ when compared to controls) Significant improvement in BMI (+8 [30.8%] to "normal" BMI at follow-up) ($p = 0.04$; $p = 0.8$ compared to controls) Significant improvement in immunological status (+9 [34.6%] to "not significant") ($p = 0.02$; $p = 0.20$ compared to controls) *On ART: placebo; ≤5 years* Significant decrease in CD4 cell count at follow-up compared to baseline (−65.3 ± 33.5 change in CD4 cells/mm³) ($p = 0.005$; $p = 0.92$ compared to controls) |

(continued)

TABLE 8.3 (continued)
Micronutrient Supplementation in HIV-Infected Children

Location and Ref.	Participants	Methods	Exposures	Outcomes	Main Findings
New Delhi, India Lodha et al. (2014)	52 HIV-infected children (≥6 months) on ART	Placebo or zinc supplementation occurred daily for 24 weeks. Follow-up visits occurred every 4 weeks and outcomes were measured at baseline and at 12 and 24 weeks.	Placebo vs. zinc (20 mg)	*Primary outcomes* CD4% value and cell count *Secondary outcomes* Anthropometry Viral load Morbidity Serum zinc levels	There were no significant differences between treatment groups in percentage increase in CD4+ T-cell counts at 24 weeks ($p = 0.30$). CD4 absolute cell count increased in the zinc group compared to placebo (416; 95% CI, 263–560 cells/mm^3 vs. 250; 95% CI, 102–314 cells/mm^3; $p = 0.30$). Viral load (log reduction) also decreased in both groups (3.2; 95% CI, 2.2–4.2 vs. 2.89; 95% CI, 1.6–3.85; $p = 0.43$). Serum zinc was higher but not significant in the zinc group (median [IQR]: 59.97 [45.2–69.69] vs. 52.98 [44.4–61.81] µg/dL; $p = 0.25$). There were no significant differences in diarrheal episodes between treatment groups after 24 weeks ($p = 0.17$).

Note: APR, adjusted prevalence ratio; ART, antiretroviral therapy; BMI, body mass index; CI, confidence interval; HAART, highly active antiretroviral therapy; HR, hazard ratio; IQR, inter-quartile range; IRR, incidence rate ratio; OR, odds ratio; PR, prevalence ratio; RDA, recommended dietary allowance; RR, risk ratio; SOC, standard of care; WAZ, weight-for-age z-score; WHZ, weight-for-height z-score.

TABLE 8.4
Micronutrient Supplementation in HIV-Infected Mothers and Their Children

Location and Ref.	Participants	Methods	Exposure	Outcomes	Main Findings
Zimbabwe Miller et al. (2006)	2854 infants (analyzed 999 HIV-uninfected and 273 HIV-infected children) Measurements taken for 1592 infants total	After delivery, maternal and infant baseline characteristics, anthropometry, and HIV status were evaluated. Infants were randomly assigned to one of four treatment groups. Follow-up visits occurred at 6 weeks and 3, 6, 9, and 12 months of age. Infant morbidity and anthropometric measures were evaluated at all follow-up visits. HIV testing was conducted by assays. Iron status was tested at birth and at 6 months.	One of four treatment groups: (1) Mothers and infants received vitamin A; (2) mothers received vitamin A, and infants received placebo; (3) mothers received placebo, and infants received vitamin A; (4) mothers and infants both received placebo Vitamin A supplementation: 400,000 IU in mothers; 50,000 IU in infants	*Primary outcome* Anemia (Hb < 10.5 g/dL) *Secondary outcomes* HIV status Low total body iron at birth (<12 μg/L) Maternal HIV status Morbidity (diarrhea, fever, cough, timing of infection)	Vitamin A supplementation in either the mother or infant had no effect on anemia among treatment arms regardless of the HIV status of infants ($p > 0.05$). HIV-infected children had a >5× increased risk of anemia (odds ratio [OR], 4.46; 95% CI, 3.32– 5.99) independent of vitamin A supplementation. Male gender ($p < 0.001$ HIV-uninfected; $p = 0.012$ HIV-infected), total body iron ($p < 0.001$ HIV-uninfected; $p = 0.007$ HIV-infected at birth only), frequent morbidity ($p = 0.003$ HIV-infected), early timing of infection ($p < 0.001$ HIV-infected), and low maternal CD4 counts ($p = 0.002$ HIV-infected) were predictors for anemia in infants.
Zimbabwe Humphrey et al. (2006)	14,110 mother–infant pairs (4495 HIV-exposed infants)	See above. Change in HIV-status was taken into account for analyses.	MI: Supplementation for both mother and infant M: Mother received vitamin A, and infant received placebo I: Mother received placebo, infant received vitamin A) P: placebo for both mother and infant	*Primary outcomes* Mother-to-child transmission Mortality	At 12 months, infection-or-death rates were higher in infants born to HIV-infected mothers in the M and I groups ($p < 0.05$). At 24 months, there was a 28% reduction in 2-year mortality in HIV-infected infants supplemented at 6 weeks (infants infected during the late intrauterine/intrapartum/early postnatal period) (hazard ratio [HR], 0.72; 95% CI, 0.57–0.92; $p = 0.01$). Infants who were HIV-uninfected at 6 weeks and vitamin A supplemented showed a 2× increase in mortality (HR, 1.41; 95% CI, 0.97–2.05; $p = 0.07$). However, after analyzing the infants who were HIV-uninfected at 6 weeks ($n = 116$), some of the infants became HIV-infected before death ($n = 46$) and, after assigning an HIV-infection likelihood score, $n = 25$ infants were likely to have been HIV-infected before death.

95% CI, 0.27–0.99; $p < 0.05$) compared to placebo. Vitamin A supplementation also decreased the odds of a combined endpoint of morbidity (i.e., diarrhea, respiratory infections, thrush, and rash) compared to placebo (OR, 0.69; 95% CI, 0.48–0.99; $p < 0.05$).

In the previously described trial in Tanzania, although vitamin A-supplemented children with pneumonia had reduced odds of severe watery diarrhea (watery stools for ≥14 days) (OR, 0.56; 95% CI, 0.32–0.99; $p = 0.04$) compared to placebo in overall analyses, supplementation was associated with higher odds of a combined endpoint of cough and rapid respiratory rate (OR, 1.67; 95% CI, 1.17–2.36; $p = 0.004$) (Fawzi et al., 2000). In analyses among HIV-infected children with pneumonia, there were no significant differences in the incidences of diarrhea (RR, 1.55; 95% CI, 0.75–3.17; $p = 0.23$) and respiratory symptoms (i.e., cough and rapid respiratory rate) (RR, 0.54; 95% CI, 0.24–1.20; $p = 0.13$) between the treatment and placebo groups. However, in analyses among HIV-uninfected children (HIV-exposed children were not explicitly identified within this group), vitamin A was associated with an increased risk of cough and rapid respiratory rate (RR, 1.47; 95% CI, 1.16–1.86; $p = 0.001$) compared to placebo.

In the aforementioned Ugandan trial in HIV-infected children, vitamin A supplementation was associated with lower odds of cough (OR, 0.47; 95% CI, 0.23–0.96; $p = 0.038$) and significantly shorter duration of ear infections ($p = 0.03$) compared to placebo (Semba et al., 2005). The previously mentioned trial in Zimbabwe, which supplemented HIV-infected mothers and/or their HIV-exposed and HIV-infected children with vitamin A, found that there was no significant difference in the risk of anemia (defined as hemoglobin [Hb] levels < 10.5 g/dL) ($p > 0.05$) compared to placebo, regardless of child HIV status (Miller et al., 2006).

Growth and Development

In the previously described Tanzanian trial, vitamin A supplementation of HIV-infected children with pneumonia did not have a significant effect on the risk of stunting (LAZ < –2; HR, 0.60; 95% CI, 0.21–1.67; $p > 0.05$) or wasting (WAZ < –2; HR, 0.31; 95% CI, 0.06–1.52; $p > 0.05$) (Villamor et al., 2002). In analyses among HIV-infected infants ages 6 to 18 months, vitamin A supplementation was associated with a significant increase in length (mean difference [MD], 2.8 cm; 95% CI, 1.0–4.6; $p = 0.003$) compared to placebo.

Vitamins B-Complex, C, and E

B-vitamin deficiencies are common in HIV-infected individuals and have been associated with increased HIV infection progression and adverse health outcomes in observational studies (Friis, 2001). Vitamin B_{12} and folate are required for *de novo* nucleotide biosynthesis, DNA methylation, and cellular division and proliferation, including immune cells (Finkelstein et al., 2015). Randomized trials of B-complex vitamins at single and multiple RDA levels have reduced HIV infection progression and increased CD4, CD3, and CD8 T-cells in HIV-infected individuals (Friis, 2001). Other chapters in this volume review in detail the evidence regarding the efficacy and safety of B vitamins (see Chapter 2) and antioxidants (see Chapter 5) for HIV-infected individuals.

Morbidity

HIV-exposed infants ($n = 2387$) in Tanzania were randomized to receive either a daily dose of multiple micronutrients comprised of vitamins B_1, B_2, B_3, B_6, B_{12}, folic acid, C, and E at 133 to 800% RDA level (1 capsule daily from 6 weeks to <6 months of age; 2 capsules at ≥6 months of age) or a placebo from 6 weeks to 2 years of age (Liu et al., 2013). There was no effect of multivitamins on the odds of mother-to-child transmission of HIV during breastfeeding (OR, 1.23; 95% CI, 0.77–1.95; $p = 0.39$) at the end of 24 months of follow-up compared to placebo. Multivitamin supplementation significantly increased Hb concentrations in children at 12 months (9.77 vs. 9.64 g/dL; $p = 0.03$), 18 months (9.76 vs. 9.57 g/dL; $p = 0.004$), and 24 months (9.93 vs. 9.75 g/dL; $p = 0.02$) compared to placebo. Multivitamin supplementation was also associated with a 12% lower risk of anemia (defined as Hb < 11.0 g/dL) (HR, 0.88; 95% CI, 0.79–0.99; p = 0.03) and a 28% lower risk of severe anemia (defined as Hb < 8.5 g/dL) (HR, 0.72; 95% CI, 0.56–0.92; p = 0.008), compared to placebo, among children born to mothers without anemia. Supplementation also led to a lower risk of fever (RR, 0.92; 95% CI, 0.85–0.99; p = 0.02) and vomiting (RR, 0.78; 95% CI, 0.65–0.93; p = 0.007) compared to placebo (Duggan et al., 2012). In subgroup analyses among children whose mothers were on ART (n = 429), multivitamin supplementation was associated with a lower risk of hospitalizations (RR, 0.48; 95% CI, 0.24–0.95; p = 0.035), fever (RR, 0.7; 95% CI, 0.67–0.93; p = 0.005), and a combined endpoint of cough and fever (RR, 0.79; 95% CI, 0.65–0.96; p = 0.019) compared to placebo.

Growth and Development

In the previously mentioned Tanzanian study among HIV-exposed children, multivitamin supplementation had no overall effects on the incidence of stunting (HR, 0.92; 95% CI, 0.79–1.08; p = 0.30), wasting (HR, 0.92; 95% CI, 0.79–1.07; p = 0.29), or being underweight (HR, 0.95; 95% CI, 0.81–1.10; p = 0.48) compared to placebo (Kupka et al., 2013). The Bayley Scales of Infant and Toddler Development, Third Edition, was administered to a subset of 206 HIV-exposed children who participated in the Tanzanian trial at 15 months of age. Between treatment groups, there were no significant differences in the odds of scoring below the 25th percentile in the following components: cognitive development (OR, 0.57; 95% CI, 0.29–1.14; p = 0.11), expressive language (OR, 1.10; 95% CI, 0.55–2.21; p = 0.78), receptive language (OR, 0.84; 95% CI, 0.37–1.91; p = 0.67), fine motor skills (OR, 0.49; 95% CI, 0.17–1.38; p = 0.18), or gross motor skills (OR, 1.10; 95% CI, 0.55–2.21; p = 0.78) (Manji et al., 2014).

ZINC

Mortality

In a Ugandan trial, both HIV-infected (highly active ART [HAART]-naïve) and HIV-uninfected children (ages 6 months to 5 years) who had been diagnosed with severe pneumonia (i.e., cough, rapid breathing, chest indrawing) were randomly assigned to receive a daily zinc supplement (10 mg zinc if < 12 months; 20 mg zinc if > 12 months) or placebo in addition to standard antibiotics (Srinivasan et al., 2012). Supplementation was administered for seven days, and the risk of mortality was assessed during this time period. In analyses among all children (i.e., HIV-infected and HIV-uninfected), there was a lower risk of case fatality in children who received zinc supplementation compared to placebo (RR, 0.33; 95% CI, 0.15–0.76; p < 0.05). However, in analyses within HIV strata, zinc supplementation was not associated with significantly lower risk of case fatality among HIV-infected children not on HAART (p > 0.05) or in HIV-uninfected children (p > 0.05) compared to placebo.

Morbidity

In the aforementioned Ugandan trial of daily zinc supplementation for HIV-infected and HIV-uninfected children, there were no significant differences in hazards of fever (HR, 1.02; 95% CI, 0.79–1.30; p = 0.897), normalization of low oxygen saturation (defined as <92%) (HR, 1.04; 95% CI, 0.74–1.46; p = 0.823), or low breathing rate (HR, 0.88; 95% CI, 0.69–1.13; p = 0.306) between the two treatment groups (Srinivasan et al., 2012). In a randomized trial in South Africa, ART-naïve HIV-infected children were supplemented with either zinc (10 mg zinc sulfate) or a placebo daily for six months (Bobat et al., 2005). There were no differences in Hb concentrations, HIV-1 RNA viral load, or CD4 T-cell counts (p > 0.05) between the treatment groups after nine months of supplementation. There was a significantly lower rate of watery diarrhea among children receiving zinc supplements vs. placebo (7.4 vs. 14.5% watery diarrhea diagnosis during follow-up; p = 0.001). However, there were no significant differences in the number of visits for illness between treatment groups (0.11 vs. 0.16 visits/month; p = 0.05).

Another trial was conducted in India among HIV-infected children on ART: two nucleoside reverse transcriptase inhibitors (NRTIs) + nevirapine for children < 3 years; two NRTIs + efavirenz for children ≥ 3 years. HIV-infected children (n = 52) were randomized to a zinc (20 mg) or placebo supplement daily for 24 weeks (Lodha et al., 2014). Zinc supplementation exhibited no significant effects on serum zinc levels (median [IQR]: 59.97 [45.2–69.69] vs. 52.98 [44.46–61.81] µg/dL; p = 0.25) or log reduction in HIV-1 RNA viral load (3.2 [2.2–4.2] vs. 2.89 [1.6–3.85] log copies/mL; p = 0.43) compared to placebo at the end of follow-up (i.e., after 24 weeks). However, zinc supplementation did result in an increase in absolute CD4 T-cell counts (416 [263–560] vs. 250 [102–314] cells/mm^3; p = 0.0035) compared to the placebo group at 24 weeks of follow-up. There was no significant difference in percentage increase in CD4+ T-cell counts between treatment groups at 24 weeks (p = 0.30). In terms of diarrheal episodes, there were no significant differences between treatment groups after 24 weeks (p = 0.17).

MULTIPLE MICRONUTRIENTS

Mortality

A recent randomized trial in Uganda enrolled 847 HIV-infected children under 5 (1–5 years) stratified by ART (10% ART vs. 90% no ART). Children were randomly assigned to receive either twice the recommended dietary allowance (RDA) of multiple micronutrients (vitamins A, B_1, B_2, B_3, B_6, B_{12}, folic acid, C, D, and E; selenium; zinc; copper; and iodine) or the single RDA level (vitamins A, B_1, B_2, B_3, C, and D) (Ndeezi et al., 2010). There was no significant difference between treatment groups in the risk of mortality after 12 months of follow-up (RR, 0.90; 95% CI, 0.50–1.50; p > 0.05). There were also no significant differences in average weight-for-length (WLZ) or weight-for-height (WHZ) z-scores (0.70 ± 1.43; 95% CI, 0.52–0.88 vs. 0.59 ± 1.15; 95% CI, 0.45–0.75; p > 0.05) or average CD4+ T-cell counts (1024 ± 592; 95% CI, 942–1107 vs. 1060 ± 553; 95% CI, 985–1136 cells/µL; p > 0.05) over 12 months between the multiple-RDA group and the single-RDA group. In analyses among children receiving ART, there were no significant effects of the higher dose regimen on mortality (RR, 1.00; 95% CI, 0.60–1.60; p > 0.05). In analyses of predictors of mortality in HIV-infected children, the following baseline characteristics were associated with increased risk in mortality: fever (adjusted hazard ratio [AHR], 2.10; 95% CI, 1.10–3.90; p = 0.02), recurrent hospitalization (AHR, 2.60; 95% CI, 1.20–5.70; p = 0.02), WAZ < –2 (AHR, 2.60; 95% CI, 1.20– 5.80; p = 0.02), and WHO HIV disease stage 3 or 4 (AHR, 2.90; 95% CI, 1.50–5.60; p < 0.01) at baseline. Treatment with cotrimoxazole was associated with lower mortality (AHR, 0.40; 95% CI, 0.20–0.90; p = 0.03) in both treatment arms as well.

In a randomized trial in South Africa, ART-naïve, HIV-infected children (n = 201) were randomly assigned to receive a multiple micronutrient (vitamins B_1, B_2, B_3, B_6, B_{12}, folic acid, C, D, and E; copper; iron; selenium; and zinc) or placebo as a daily supplement for six months (Mda et al., 2013). There was no significant difference in the number of deaths that occurred in the micronutrient supplementation and placebo groups (n = 27 vs. 16; p = 0.12).

Morbidity

In a South African trial, 373 children (ages 6 to 24 months) with mixed HIV status (Group 1, 32 HIV-infected children; Group 2, 154 HIV-exposed children [HIV-uninfected children born to HIV-infected mothers]; Group 3, 187 HIV-uninfected children [born to HIV-uninfected mothers]) were randomly assigned daily supplements of (1) vitamin A (1250 IU), (2) vitamin A and zinc (10 mg), or (3) vitamin A, zinc, and other micronutrients (vitamins B_1, B_2, B_3, B_6, B_{12}, folic acid, C, D, E, and K; copper; iodine; iron) (Luabeya et al., 2007). There were no significant differences between multivitamin treatments in the incidence of diarrhea and no differences in findings by HIV status (p > 0.05) (Chhagan et al., 2009). In analyses among HIV-infected children, vitamin A plus zinc supplementation (0.27; 95% CI, 0.10–0.71) and multiple micronutrient supplementation (0.39; 95% CI, 0.19–0.78) were associated with higher incidence of persistent diarrhea compared to vitamin A supplementation alone (0.05; 95% CI, n/a; p = 0.02). In analyses among HIV-infected children, vitamin A plus zinc supplementation (0.27; 95% CI, 0.11–0.66) and multiple micronutrient supplementation (0.39; 95% CI, 0.21–0.74) were associated with higher incidences of severe diarrhea compared to vitamin A supplementation alone (0.05; 95% CI, n/a; p = 0.01). In a subgroup of children who were stunted and HIV-uninfected, there were lower incidences of diarrhea in the vitamin A and zinc group (2.04 episodes/year; RR, 0.52; 95% CI, 0.45–0.60; p < 0.05) and multiple micronutrient group (2.23 episodes/year; RR, 0.57; 95% CI, 0.49–0.67; p < 0.05) compared to vitamin A alone (3.92 episodes/year; p = 0.024 comparing control vs. zinc and multiple micronutrient groups' incidences combined). No significant differences between treatment arms were found with respect to the percent of days with diarrhea, upper respiratory infection (URI) symptoms, or pneumonia among HIV-infected children (p > 0.05), HIV-exposed children (p > 0.05), and HIV-uninfected children (p > 0.05) (Luabeya et al., 2007). At the end of 12 months of follow-up in the overall sample (combining HIV-infected, HIV-exposed, and HIV-uninfected children), the prevalence of anemia was significantly reduced by 24% with multiple micronutrient supplementation (p = 0.001) and 18% with vitamin A supplementation (p = 0.02) but was not significantly reduced with vitamin A and zinc supplementation (11%; p = 0.13) (Chhagan et al., 2010). In analyses among HIV-exposed and HIV-uninfected children, multiple micronutrient supplementation (p = 0.002) and vitamin A supplementation alone (p = 0.03) were associated with a significantly reduced prevalence of anemia at the end of 12 months of follow-up compared to baseline.

In a Ugandan study supplementing HIV-infected children (10% on HAART; 90% not on HAART) with either twice the RDA of multiple micronutrients (vitamins A, B_1, B_2, B_3, B_6, B_{12}, folic acid, C, D, and E; selenium; zinc; copper; and iodine) or single-RDA multivitamins (vitamins A, B_1, B_2, B_3, C, and D), serum vitamin B_{12} (p < 0.001) and folate (p < 0.001) concentrations significantly increased in the multiple-RDA group compared to the single-RDA group (Ndeezi et al., 2011). Hemoglobin levels significantly increased in both the multiple-RDA regimen (p = 0.04) and the single-RDA regimen (p < 0.001) compared to baseline measurements. There were no significant changes in CD4 T-cell counts in either group (p > 0.05) compared to baseline. There were no significant effects of regimen on the incidence of diarrhea (p > 0.05); however, children in both treatment groups who were on HAART had lower incidences of diarrhea when compared to HAART-naïve children (OR, 0.60; 95% CI, 0.30– 0.90; p = 0.03) (Ndeezi et al., 2012).

In the South African trial described previously among HIV-infected children, the multiple micronutrient group had significantly lower hospitalization duration, independent of hospital admission diagnosis (diarrhea or pneumonia) (mean ± SD: 7.3 ± 3.9 vs. 9.0 ± 4.9 days; p < 0.05) compared to the placebo (Mda et al., 2010a). When individually analyzed, duration of pneumonia was reduced by 1.9 days (20% reduction), and diarrheal episodes were reduced by 1.6 days (19% reduction), although these reductions were not significant (p > 0.05). The number of respiratory infections per month was lower in the group receiving micronutrients vs. the placebo: 0.66 episodes/month (95% CI, 0.52–0.80) vs. 1.01 episodes/month (95% CI, 0.83–1.19) (p < 0.05), but there were no differences in the occurrence of diarrhea between groups (p = 0.09) (Mda et al., 2013). There were no significant differences in changes in CD4 T-cell counts between treatment groups at three or six months of follow-up (p > 0.05).

In a randomized trial in India, 127 HIV-infected children less than 15 years of age were randomized to receive daily supplements of (1) multiple micronutrients (vitamins A, B_1, B_2, B_5, B_6, B_{12}, D, and E; copper; selenium; iodine; and zinc) for six months; (2) probiotics for three months; or (3) placebo supplements for six months (Gautam et al., 2014). The ART-naïve children (≤15) supplemented with micronutrients showed significant improvement in HIV disease progression from WHO HIV stage 2 to 1 (p = 0.01) and from "mild" to "not significant" WHO classifications (p = 0.02) during follow-up compared to the placebo group.

Growth and Development

In the South African trial among 373 children with mixed HIV status (Group 1, 32 HIV-infected children; Group 2, 154 HIV-exposed children; Group 3, 187 HIV-uninfected children born to HIV-uninfected mothers), in analyses among stunted (LAZ < –2) children, multiple micronutrient supplementation was associated with significant increases in LAZ compared to supplementation with vitamin A alone or vitamin A plus zinc ($p = 0.029$) (Chhagan et al., 2010). In another trial in South Africa among HIV-infected children, multiple micronutrient supplementation led to a larger increase in the amount of food eaten over six months (mean ± SD: 108 ± 112 vs. 57 ± 130 g) and in eating rate (4.7 ± 14.7 vs. –1.4 ± 15.1 g/min) compared to the placebo (Mda et al., 2010b). Children receiving micronutrient supplements also had a significant increase in weight-for-height z-scores compared to the placebo group: 0.40 (95% CI, 0.09–0.71) vs. –0.04 (95% CI, –0.39–0.31) ($p < 0.05$) (Mda et al., 2013). Finally, in a trial among HIV-infected children (<15 years of age) in India, there were significant increases in body mass index (BMI) with micronutrient supplementation ($p = 0.04$) after six months of follow-up compared to baseline measurements in children who were not on ART (Gautam et al., 2014).

IRON

Morbidity

In Malawi, 209 HIV-infected children with mild anemia (Hb, 7.0–9.9 g/dL) were randomized to receive either (1) daily iron (3 mg/kg/day) and multivitamins (vitamins A, C, and D), or (2) daily multivitamins alone for three months (Esan et al., 2013). Children were followed up for a total of six months: three months during the intervention and an additional three months post-intervention. Combined iron and multivitamin supplementation were associated with significantly higher CD4 T-cell counts (adjusted mean difference [AMD], 6.00, 59% CI, 1.84–10.16; $p = 0.005$) and a lower risk of iron deficiency (adjusted prevalence ratio [APR], 0.28; 95% CI, 0.15–0.49; $p < 0.001$) after three months compared to multivitamins alone, after adjusting for baseline Hb concentrations, HAART use, CD4 T-cell percentages, bed net use, and history of blood transfusions. However, these differences were no longer significant after six months of follow-up ($p > 0.05$). Iron and multivitamin supplementation resulted in increased Hb concentrations (AMD, 0.60; 95% CI, 0.06–1.13; $p = 0.03$) and lower prevalence of anemia (APR, 0.59; 95% CI, 0.38–0.92; $p = 0.02$) but a higher incidence of malaria (incidence ratio [IR], 1.81; 95% CI, 1.04–3.16; $p = 0.04$) after six months of follow-up compared to multivitamins alone. During the post-intervention phase, children who had received iron and multivitamin supplementation had a lower risk of respiratory infections (IR, 0.28; 95% CI, 0.09–0.91; $p = 0.04$) compared to multivitamins alone. In subgroup analyses among iron-deficient children, iron and multivitamin supplementation was associated with a lower risk of HIV infection progression during the post-intervention period compared to multiple micronutrients alone (IR, 0.25; 95% CI, 0.08–0.83; $p = 0.02$).

DISCUSSION

Micronutrient deficiencies are common in HIV-infected children and have been associated with adverse health outcomes. This chapter reviewed data from 13 randomized clinical trials involving micronutrient supplementation in HIV-exposed and HIV-infected infants and children in papers from 25 publications (Tables 8.1 to 8.4). In general, among HIV-infected children, multiple micronutrient supplementation has been shown to decrease co-infection risk and improve child nutritional status, growth, and development. Our review examines the literature on existing gaps in terms of the safety and efficacy of specific micronutrients, as well as supplementation in the context of ART and among HIV-exposed children.

Overview of Findings

Vitamin A

Overall, randomized trials to date on vitamin A supplementation indicate significant decrease in risk of mortality in HIV-infected children, including infants who were infected with HIV in the late intrauterine, intrapartum, or early postnatal period (Fawzi et al., 1999; Semba et al., 2005; Humphrey et al., 2006). Studies have suggested that the effect of vitamin supplementation may vary with timing of HIV infection. In one study, although vitamin A supplementation reduced two-year mortality in HIV-infected infants, supplementation in HIV-exposed, uninfected infants actually doubled the risk of mortality (Humphrey et al., 2006). *In vitro* studies indicate that human monocytes, pretreated with retinoic acid prior to infection with HIV, produced increased amounts of virus (Kitano et al., 1990; Poli et al., 1992; Turpin et al., 1992; Humphrey et al., 2006). A more recent study examining the effects of *in vivo* vitamin A supplementation of pregnant and lactating HIV-infected women found no increase in mortality of infants and children from six weeks to five years, but a doubling of the two- to five-year mortality among the HIV-infected children of the supplemented mothers ($p = 0.04$ unadjusted; $p = 0.06$ when adjusted for baseline maternal characteristics) (Khavari et al., 2014). The variation in effects of timing of both HIV infection and vitamin A administration on health outcomes highlight a need for future trials to evaluate safety and efficacy of supplementation for HIV-exposed and HIV-infected children.

Zinc

Studies on zinc supplementation offer conflicting results. Although in some trials zinc supplementation reduced case fatality among HIV-infected children (Srinivasan et al., 2012) and risk of diarrhea in ART-naïve children (Bobat et al., 2005), other studies indicate no significant effect on diarrheal episodes in HIV-infected children on ART (Lodha et al., 2014). Further investigation is needed to determine the effect of zinc supplementation on morbidity among HIV-exposed children, especially in the context of ART. Future studies should also evaluate the effect of zinc supplementation on anthropometric outcomes, as zinc supplementation has been known to improve growth and development and reduce the risk of stunting in children less than 5 years of age (Imdad and Bhutta, 2011).

Iron

Trials to date indicate that iron supplementation with micronutrients in HIV-infected children may improve HIV infection outcomes and lower risk of anemia, but they also indicate an increased risk of malaria (Esan et al., 2013). Although a recent Cochrane Review found that iron supplementation does not increase risk of malaria where malaria prevention services are available (Neuberger et al., 2016), there is limited evidence on the effects of iron supplementation on health outcomes in children co-infected with HIV and malaria.

Multiple Micronutrients

Multiple micronutrient supplementation has been shown to reduce morbidity in HIV-infected children (Mda et al., 2010a; Chhagan et al., 2009, 2010) and to improve hemoglobin concentrations and reduce risk of anemia in HIV-exposed children (Liu et al., 2013). Multiple micronutrient supplementation has also been shown to improve most anthropometric outcomes and appetite in ART-naïve, HIV-infected children (Mda et al., 2010b, 2013; Gautam et al., 2014). Further trials are needed to elucidate the role of multiple micronutrient supplementation in HIV-exposed, uninfected children to inform standard of care for this vulnerable population.

RESEARCH GAPS

Study Design

Variations across trials in dosage, timing (e.g., intermittent vs. daily), and administration (e.g., pill, capsule, powder) limit the ability to draw definitive conclusions on the effects of supplementation on HIV-related outcomes in children. Additionally, multiple micronutrient supplementation and variations in regimens constrain causal inference of the effects of specific micronutrients on outcomes and the ability to compare findings across studies.

Generalizability

All of the trials were conducted in resource-limited, developing areas, limiting generalizability beyond these settings. Additionally, some trials included children co-infected with pneumonia or malaria (Fawzi et al., 1999; Srinivasan et al., 2012; Mda et al., 2010a; Esan et al., 2013), hindering comparison with other studies and populations.

HIV Status in Children

Categorization of HIV status varied across trials. Although some studies explicitly identified HIV-exposed, uninfected children, other trials included this subgroup within a more broadly defined group of HIV-uninfected children. However, current evidence confirms that uninfected children exposed to HIV *in utero* present a distinct risk profile for HIV-associated and other health outcomes (Afran et al., 2014). Future studies should record and report the HIV status of the participating children and the timing of its change in case of occurrence of seroconversion.

As mother-to-child transmission declines, the population of HIV-exposed, uninfected children is increasing. Studies have reported higher rates of mortality in HIV-exposed infants compared to HIV-unexposed infants (Brahmbhatt et al., 2006; Marinda et al., 2007; Sutcliffe et al., 2008), and evidence suggests that this group presents higher risks of infection, malnutrition, diarrhea, and adverse health outcomes (Evans et al., 2013). There is limited evidence on the effect of micronutrient supplementation on health outcomes in HIV-exposed infants and children. Further research and long-term longitudinal studies are needed to assess the health needs of this population, taking into account variations in maternal ART regimen, infant feeding modality, and confirmation of HIV status with follow-up.

Micronutrient Supplementation in the Context of Antiretroviral Therapy

Trials employed varying study designs in the context of ART, a critical factor in evaluating health outcomes of HIV-infected populations. Although some trials administered HAART to all participants at enrollment (Ndeezi et al., 2011), other trials only included ART-naïve participants (Mda et al., 2013). Some trials stratified participants by ART status to take into account the associations among medications, micronutrient status, and health outcomes (Ndeezi et al., 2010). In other trials, ART status changed throughout the course of the trials as medication became available, which constrains the ability to attribute improved health outcomes to micronutrient supplementation as opposed to ART (Kupka et al., 2013). The variability in ART status limits the ability to compare results across trials.

Additionally, HAART itself may adversely affect micronutrient status, as studies have reported various side effects that diminish dietary intake and nutrient absorption, including diminished appetite, nausea, and diarrhea (Ivers et al., 2009; Sicotte et al., 2014). Where resources permit, guidelines recommend individualized therapy regimens based on side effects, expected adherence, individual health profiles, co-infections, stage of disease, drug resistance, and other risk factors (Van den Eynde and Podzamczer, 2014; WHO, 2016). Because individual receptivity to each treatment regimen varies, it is difficult to identify optimal treatment strategies in adjunct to ART. Health outcomes also depend enormously on ART adherence, and in studies that did not measure adherence it is difficult to draw conclusions on the efficacy of micronutrient supplementation interventions in the context of ART. Overall, in trials employing micronutrient supplementation in adjunct to ART, it is difficult to identify causality of improved health outcomes, particularly across studies including a range of medications.

IMPLICATIONS OF FINDINGS FOR CLINICAL CARE AND PUBLIC HEALTH PRACTICE IN HIV-INFECTED AND HIV-EXPOSED CHILDREN

Supplementation with vitamin A is recommended for HIV-infected and HIV-exposed children, consistent with both WHO recommendations for uninfected and unexposed children ages 6 to 59 months (WHO, 2011) and with a previous Cochrane Review conducted on this topic (Irlam et al., 2013). Further investigation, however, is required to elucidate the effect of vitamin A supplementation in children younger than 6 months, particularly HIV-exposed infants. Additionally, although zinc supplementation appears to reduce the risk of diarrhea in HIV-infected children, further investigation is required concerning dosage and its effect on HIV-exposed children. Randomized trials have also suggested that multiple micronutrient supplementation reduces morbidity and improves growth and development in both HIV-infected and HIV-exposed children. Overall, micronutrient supplementation is likely to benefit both HIV-infected and HIV-exposed children. However, further research is needed to evaluate recommendations, particularly in the context of antiretroviral therapy and for HIV-exposed, uninfected children.

REFERENCES

Afran, L., M. Garcia Knight, E. Nduati, B. C. Urban, R. S. Heyderman, and S. L. Rowland-Jones. (2014). HIV-exposed uninfected children: a growing population with a vulnerable immune system? *Clinical & Experimental Immunology* 176(1): 11–22.

Bobat, R., H. Coovadia, C. Stephen, K. L. Naidoo et al. (2005). Safety and efficacy of zinc supplementation for children with HIV-1 infection in South Africa: a randomised double-blind placebo-controlled trial. *The Lancet* 366(9500): 1862–67.

Brahmbhatt, H., G. Kogozi, and F. Wabwire-Mangen et al. (2006). Mortality in HIV-infected and uninfected children of HIV-infected and uninfected mothers in rural Uganda. *Journal of Acquired Immune Defiency Syndrome* 41(4): 504–8.

Chhagan, M. K., J. Van den Broeck, K. K. Luabeya, N. Mpontshane, K. L. Tucker, and M. L. Bennish. (2009). Effect of micronutrient supplementation on diarrhoeal disease among stunted children in rural South Africa. *European Journal of Clinical Nutrition* 63(7): 850–57.

Chhagan, M. K., J. Van den Broeck, K. K. Luabeya, N. Mpontshane, A. Tomkins, and M. L. Bennish. (2010). Effect on longitudinal growth and anemia of zinc or multiple micronutrients added to vitamin A: a randomized controlled trial in children aged 6–24 months. *BMC Public Health* 10: 145.

Coutsoudis, A., R. A. Bobat, H. M. Coovadia, L. Kuhn, W. Y. Tsai, and Z. A. Stein. (1995). The effects of vitamin A supplementation on the morbidity of children born to HIV-infected women. *American Journal of Public Health* 85(8, Pt. 1): 1076–81.

Duggan, C., K. P. Manji, R. Kupka et al. (2012). Multiple micronutrient supplementation in Tanzanian infants born to HIV-infected mothers: a randomized, double-blind, placebo-controlled clinical trial. *American Journal of Clinical Nutrition* 96(6): 1437–46.

Esan, M. O., M. B. van Hensbroek, E. Nkhoma et al. (2013). Iron supplementation in HIV-infected Malawian children with anemia: a double-blind, randomized, controlled trial. *Clinical Infectious Diseases* 57(11): 1626–34.

Evans, C., C. E. Jones, and A. J. Prendergast. (2016). HIV-exposed, uninfected infants: new global challenges in the era of paediatric HIV elimination. *The Lancet Infectious Diseases* 16(6): e92–e107.

Fawzi, W. W., R. L. Mbise, E. Hertzmark et al. (1999). A randomized trial of vitamin A supplements in relation to mortality among human immunodeficiency virus-infected and uninfected children in Tanzania. *Pediatric Infectious Disease Journal* 18(2): 127–33.

Fawzi, W. W., R. Mbise, D. Spiegelman, M. Fataki, E. Hertzmark, and G. Ndossi. (2000). Vitamin A supplements and diarrheal and respiratory tract infections among children in Dar es Salaam, Tanzania. *Journal of Pediatrics* 137(5): 660–7.

Finkelstein, J. L., A. J. Layden, and P. J. Stover. (2015). Vitamin B-12 and perinatal health. *Advances in Nutrition* 6(5): 552–63.

Friis, H., Ed. (2001). *Micronutrients and HIV Infection*. Boca Raton, FL: CRC Press.

Gautam, N., R. Dayal, D. Agarwal et al. (2014). Role of multivitamins, micronutrients and probiotics supplementation in management of HIV infected children. *Indian Journal of Pediatrics* 81(12): 1315–20.

Humphrey, J. H., P. J. Iliff, E. T. Marinda et al.; ZVITAMBO Study Group. (2006). Effects of a single large dose of vitamin A, given during the postpartum period to HIV-positive women and their infants, on child HIV infection, HIV-free survival, and mortality. *Journal of Infectious Diseases* 193(6): 860–71.

Imdad, A. and Z. A. Bhutta. (2011). Effect of preventive zinc supplementation on linear growth in children under 5 years of age in developing countries: a meta-analysis of studies for input to the lives saved tool. *BMC Public Health* 11(Suppl. 3): S22.

Irlam, J. H., N. Siegfried, M. E. Visser, and N. C. Rollins. (2013). Micronutrient supplementation for children with HIV infection. *Cochrane Database Systematic Reviews* 10: CD010666.

Ivers, L. C., K. A. Cullen, K. A. Freedberg, S. Block, J. Coates, and P. Webb. (2009). HIV/AIDS, undernutrition and food insecurity. *Clinical Infectious Diseases* 49(7): 1096–102.

Khavari, N., H. Jiang, K. Manji et al. (2014). Maternal multivitamin supplementation reduces the risk of diarrhoea among HIV-exposed children through age 5 years. *International Health* 6(4): 298–305.

Kitano, K., G. C. Baldwin, M. A. Raines, and D. W. Golde. (1990). Differentiating agents facilitate infection of myeloid leukemia cell lines by monocytotropic HIV-1 strains. *Blood* 76(10): 1980–8.

Kupka, R., K. P. Manji, R. J. Bosch et al. (2013). Multivitamin supplements have no effect on growth of Tanzanian children born to HIV-infected mothers. *Journal of Nutrtion* 143(5): 722–7.

Liu, E., C. Duggan, K. P. Manji et al. (2013). Multivitamin supplementation improves haematologic status in children born to HIV-positive women in Tanzania. *Journal of the International AIDS Society* 16(1): 18022.

Lodha, R., N. Shah, N. Mohari et al. (2014). Immunologic effect of zinc supplementation in HIV-infected children receiving highly active antiretroviral therapy: a randomized, double-blind, placebo-controlled trial. *Journal of Acquired Immune Deficiency Syndromes* 66(4): 386–92.

Luabeya, K. K., N. Mpontshane, M. Mackay et al. (2007). Zinc or multiple micronutrient supplementation to reduce diarrhea and respiratory disease in South African children: a randomized controlled trial. *PLoS One* 2(6): e541.

Manji, K. P., C. M. McDonald, R. Kupka et al. (2014). Effect of multivitamin supplementation on the neurodevelopment of HIV-exposed Tanzanian infants: a randomized, double-blind, placebo-controlled clinical trial. *Journal of Tropical Pediatrics* 60(4): 279–86.

Marinda, E., J. H. Humphrey, and P. J. Iliff et al. (2007). Child mortality according to maternal and infant HIV status in Zimbabwe. ZVITAMBO Study Group. *Pediatric Infectious Disease Journal* 26(6): 519–26.

Mda, S., J. M. van Raaij, F. P. de Villiers, U. E. MacIntyre, and F. J. Kok. (2010a). Short-term micronutrient supplementation reduces the duration of pneumonia and diarrheal episodes in HIV-infected children. *Journal of Nutrition* 140(5): 969–74.

Mda, S., J. M. van Raaij, U. E. Macintyre, F. P. de Villiers, and F. J. Kok. (2010b). Improved appetite after multi-micronutrient supplementation for six months in HIV-infected South African children. *Appetite* 54(1): 150–5.

Mda, S., J. M. van Raaij, F. P. de Villiers, and F. J. Kok. (2013). Impact of multi-micronutrient supplementation on growth and morbidity of HIV-infected South African children. *Nutrients* 5(10): 4079–92.

Mehta, S. and W. W. Fawzi. (2007). Effects of vitamins, including vitamin A, on HIV/AIDS patients. *Vitamins and Hormones*. 75: 355–83.

Miller, M. F., R. J. Stoltzfus, P. J. Iliff, L. C. Malaba, N. V. Mbuya, and J. H. Humphrey; Zimbabwe Vitamin A for Mothers and Babies Project (ZVITAMBO) Study Group. (2006). Effect of maternal and neonatal vitamin A supplementation and other postnatal factors on anemia in Zimbabwean infants: a prospective, randomized study. *American Journal of Clinical Nutrition* 84(1): 212–22.

Ndeezi, G., T. Tylleskär, C. M. Ndugwa, and J. K. Tumwine. (2010). Effect of multiple micronutrient supplementation on survival of HIV-infected children in Uganda: a randomized, controlled trial. *Journal of the International AIDS Society* 13: 18.

Ndeezi, G., J. K. Tumwine, C. M. Ndugwa, B. J. Bolann, and T. Tylleskär. (2011). Multiple micronutrient supplementation improves vitamin B(1)(2) and folate concentrations of HIV infected children in Uganda: a randomized controlled trial. *Nutrition Journal* 10: 56.

Ndeezi, G., T. Tylleskär, C. M. Ndugwa, and J. K. Tumwine. (2012). Multiple micronutrient supplementation does not reduce diarrhoea morbidity in Ugandan HIV-infected children: a randomised controlled trial. *Paediatrics and International Child Health* 32(1): 14–21.

Neuberger, A., J. Okebe, D. Yahav, and M. Paul. (2016). Oral iron supplements for children in malaria-endemic areas. *Cochrane Database of Systematic Reviews* 2: CD006589.

Poli, G., A. L. Kinter, J. S. Justement, P. Bressler, J. H. Kehrl, and A. S. Fauci. (1992). Retinoic acid mimics transforming growth factor β in the regulation of human immunodeficiency virus expression in monocytic cells. *Proceedings of the National Academy of Sciences (USA)* 89(7): 2689–93.

Semba, R. D., C. Ndugwa, R. T. Perry et al. (2005). Effect of periodic vitamin A supplementation on mortality and morbidity of human immunodeficiency virus-infected children in Uganda: a controlled clinical trial. *Nutrition* 21(1): 25–31.

Sicotte, M., É. V. Langlois, J. Aho, D. Ziegler, and M. V. Zunzunegui. (2014). Association between nutritional status and the immune response in HIV+ patients under HAART: protocol for a systematic review. *Systematic Reviews* 3: 9.

Srinivasan, M. G., G. Ndeezi, C. K. Mboijana et al. (2012). Zinc adjunct therapy reduces case fatality in severe childhood pneumonia: a randomized double blind placebo-controlled trial. *BMC Medicine* 10: 14.

Sutcliffe, C. G., S. Scott, N. Mugala et al. (2008). Survival from 9 months of age among HIV-infected and uninfected Zambian children prior to the availability of antiretroviral therapy. *Clinical Infectious Diseases* 47(6): 837–44.

Turpin, J. A., M. Vargo, and M. S. Meltzer. (1992). Enhanced HIV-1 replication in retinoid-treated monocytes: retinoid effects mediated through mechanisms related to cell differentiation and to a direct transcriptional action on viral gene expression. *Journal of Immunology* 148(8): 2539–46.

UNAIDS (Joint United Nations Programme on HIV/AIDS). (2016). *AIDS Data*. Geneva: Joint United Nations Programme on HIV/AIDS (http://www.unaids.org/sites/default/files/media_asset/2016-AIDS-data_en.pdf).

Van den Eynde, E. and D. Podzamczer. (2014). Switch strategies in antiretroviral therapy regimens. *Expert Review of Anti-Infectective Therapy* 12(9): 1055–74.

Villamor, E., R. Mbise, D. Spiegelman et al. (2002). Vitamin A supplements ameliorate the adverse effect of HIV-1, malaria, and diarrheal infections on child growth. *Pediatrics* 109(1): E6.

WHO. (2011). *Guideline: Vitamin A Supplementation in Infants and Children 6–59 Months of Age*. Geneva: World Health Organization.

WHO. (2016). *Consolidated Guidelines on the Use of Antiretroviral Drugs for Treating and Preventing HIV Infection: Recommendations for a Public Health Approach*, 2nd ed. Geneva: World Health Organization.

9 Macronutrient Supplementation to HIV and TB Patients during Treatment

Henrik Friis, Mette Frahm Olsen, and Suzanne Filteau

CONTENTS

INTRODUCTION

In low-income countries, undernutrition and infectious diseases are major health problems. Their coexistence is partly due to poverty being an important determinant of both problems, but also due to the two-way causal interactions between nutritional deficiencies and infections, whereby infections exacerbate nutritional deficiencies, which in turn increase infectious disease morbidity and mortality. Most research has been conducted on the relationship between generalized malnutrition or micronutrient deficiencies and childhood infections. Control of infectious diseases is now considered important in prevention of undernutrition, and evidence-based nutritional interventions have been established to reduce childhood morbidity and mortality.

In contrast, not much research has been done to develop effective nutritional interventions that target two of the major infectious diseases in adults: tuberculosis (TB) and HIV infection. Despite obvious differences between HIV and TB, both are characterized by wasting and often affect underprivileged individuals. Furthermore, HIV is a strong determinant of TB, so co-infections are common. In some settings, more than half of the TB patients starting anti-TB treatment are HIV co-infected (Range et al., 2001). Similarly, a large proportion of HIV-patients starting ART treatment will also have TB, partly because newly diagnosed TB patients are tested for HIV and referred for treatment and because HIV patients are screened for TB.

Some studies have shown that micronutrient supplementation may affect progression and transmission of HIV (Fawzi et al., 2002, 2004), and micronutrients may be of importance for primary TB infection or actual TB disease (van Lettow and Whalen, 2008). As such, there might be a role for micronutrient interventions that target individuals at risk of HIV and TB infections or in the early stages of these infections. Patients with advanced HIV infection and clinical TB disease often live in food-insecure settings, and their habitual diet does not contain enough energy and nutrients to meet their requirements. There is, therefore, a need for effective nutritional interventions that target HIV and TB patients as part of comprehensive medical and social care packages. In addition to ameliorating food security and nutritional status, such interventions may also have a beneficial impact on disease and treatment outcomes.

HISTORY, CURRENT PRACTICES, AND RECOMMENDATIONS

TUBERCULOSIS

Tuberculosis is an ancient disease for which effective drugs have only become available over the last half-century. Because the cardinal manifestation of TB is wasting or cachexia, the potential role of nutrition in its prevention and treatment was recognized early. Initially based on anecdotal evidence and layman wisdom, but later supported by research, nutrition became the backbone of TB treatment for centuries. The history of TB and the early research on the effect of nutrition and diet have been reviewed elsewhere (van Lettow and Whalen, 2008).

After the discovery of the first effective anti-TB drugs—streptomycin in 1948 and rifampicin in 1952 (Whalen and Semba, 2001)—nutrition was no longer the main TB therapy and apparently did not find its place as auxiliary therapy, not even in low-income settings. A seminal study that reflected and contributed to this paradigm shift was conducted in the late 1950s in Madras City, now Chennai, India, and published in the paper, "The Role of Diet in the Treatment of Pulmonary Tuberculosis: An Evaluation in a Controlled Chemotherapy Study in Home and Sanatorium Patients in South India" (Ramakrishnan et al., 1961). In brief, patients with TB from a poverty-stricken community in Madras City were randomized to treatment at home or at a sanitarium. Both groups received the same treatment, but those treated at home had a markedly poorer diet while also being physically more active, as compared to those treated at the sanatorium. The paper concluded that, "initial chemotherapy of patients at home can be successful even if the dietary intake is low throughout the period of treatment," although sputum conversion seemed to occur earlier and weight was considerably greater in those treated at the sanatorium (Ramakrishnan et al., 1961) (Figure 9.1).

Since then, TB patients have usually been treated at home, through the Directly Observed Treatment Short-Course (DOTS) program, and do not usually receive nutritional support when coming for drugs. The seriously sick patient, requiring initial inpatient treatment, may receive hospital food, although in many settings no food at all is provided. In TB programs where nutritional support is given, as actual food supplements, food vouchers, or cash, it has often not been specifically for nutritional reasons, but as an incentive to improve adherence, as poor adherence can be a cause of treatment failure and transmission.

In 2013, the World Health Organization (WHO) published *Guideline: Nutritional Care and Support for Patients with Tuberculosis* (WHO, 2013), which represented the first nutritional recommendations in this area. The guideline recommended that individuals with TB disease should receive an assessment of their nutritional status and appropriate counseling. TB patients with moderate undernutrition who fail to regain normal body mass index (BMI) after two months of TB

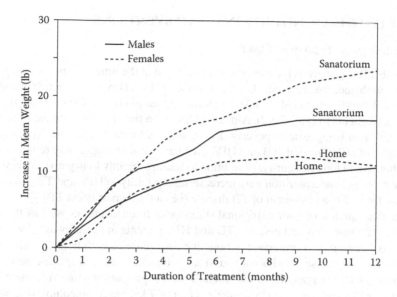

FIGURE 9.1 Weight changes over a 12-month period, according to sex of patients and place of treatment. (From Ramakrishnan, C.V. et al., *Bulletin of the World Health Organization*, 25(3), 339–359, 1961.)

treatment should be evaluated for adherence and comorbidity, receive nutrition assessment and counseling, and, if indicated, be provided with locally available nutrient-rich or fortified supplementary foods. Furthermore, it is recommended that TB patients with severe acute malnutrition should be treated in accordance with WHO guidelines for treatment of malnutrition.

HIV INFECTION

HIV is a more recent disease, first reported in 1980 among homosexual men in the United States (CDC, 1981) and in Africa in 1983 (Clumeck et al., 1983). These case reports were followed by studies showing a huge prevalence in a number of sub-Saharan countries (Melbye et al., 1986). The early research agenda focused on drugs and vaccines, given the success from the field of TB and other infections. The first drug, zidovudine, became available in 1987, less than a decade after the first case reports, and effective treatment was developed within 15 years (highly active antiretroviral treatment in the early 1990s) (Sepkowitz, 2001). Nutritional research, on the other hand, was slow to get underway, and for many years focused on micronutrient supplementation only.

In 2003, WHO published a report from a technical consultation titled *Nutrient Requirements for People Living with HIV/AIDS* (WHO, 2004), which concluded that energy requirements are likely to increase by 10% in asymptomatic and 20% to 30% in symptomatic HIV-infected adults. However, to date, there are no recommendations for patients with HIV, as there are for TB patients. Currently, governments and non-governmental organizations (NGOs) are distributing various food supplements, through either community organizations or health facilities, to HIV patients and their families. These include food baskets, fortified blended foods, and lipid-based nutrient supplements (LNS). Supplementation may target HIV patients with different stages of HIV infection (pre-ART or ART) and may be based on different inclusion criteria or simply judgment. The objectives also differ among supplementation programs. The aim may be to ameliorate household food insecurity, often considerably exacerbated by HIV infection, or to increase adherence to ART programs, or supplementation may be given in the hope that it will affect HIV progression, treatment outcomes, and survival. The effects of such programs are rarely evaluated, and in some settings several programs are running simultaneously without proper coordination.

POTENTIAL EFFECTS OF NUTRITIONAL INTERVENTIONS

Nutritional Status at Treatment Start

Individuals with TB are likely to have been undernourished at the time of exposure, as poverty is not only associated with undernutrition but also with risk factors for TB exposure, which include crowding, alcohol, and smoking (Frieden et al., 2003). The same applies to HIV, as food insecurity is associated with unsafe sex (Kalichman et al., 2012). Although HIV often thrives in the context of socioeconomic inequality rather than being strictly poverty driven, poor individuals are much more vulnerable to the consequences of HIV. For both TB and HIV, even early disease stages may reduce work capacity and result in household food insecurity, in addition to leading directly to negative energy and nutrient balances. Furthermore, undernutrition may increase susceptibility to HIV and TB infection, and it is certainly a risk factor for development of TB disease (i.e., a flare-up of latent TB).

Thus, as a consequence of poor nutritional status prior to exposure, as well as the indirect and direct effects of the infection and disease, TB and HIV patients are often wasted when diagnosed and treatment is initiated. It is important to note that even patients with normal and high BMI may have lost lean mass (i.e., muscle and organ mass), as well as fat mass and specific nutrients. A study among TB patients in Mwanza, Tanzania, found that TB patients starting treatment had a mean weight deficit of 10 kg and a mean grip strength deficit of 7 kg, based on comparison with age- and sex-matched neighborhood controls (PrayGod et al., 2011b). HIV co-infection was not associated with increased deficits, probably reflecting that the risk of TB disease occurs early in the course of HIV infection, as compared to other opportunistic infections (Fertel and Pitchenik, 1989). Deficits of weight and muscle strength are likely to be smaller among HIV patients when starting ART but depend on ART eligibility criteria, treatment lag time, and the proportion of patients with TB and other opportunistic infections.

General and Disease-Specific Outcomes

Nutritional deficiencies are known to have effects on a wide range of general health outcomes, which may translate into effects on human capital. In addition, nutritional deficiencies may affect a range of disease-specific outcomes among individuals who are exposed to TB or HIV, who have latent or symptomatic infection, or who are receiving treatment for these infections, as shown in Table 9.1. During treatment of either TB or HIV, nutritional deficiencies—or lack of food to go with the medicine—may affect adherence, absorption, and metabolism of the drugs. These factors may result in too high or too low drug concentrations, which may result in toxicities or impair efficacy and lead to treatment failure and resistance. Nutritional deficiencies may also directly affect immune functions and the infectious agent. As proof of principle, low intake of zinc results in what amounts to a dietary thymectomy—that is, disappearance of the thymus, a key immunological organ in both young animals (Fraker et al., 2000) and children (Schonland, 1972). Additionally, host selenium deficiency has been shown to turn avirulent coxsackie virus virulent in a laboratory animal model (Beck et al., 1995).

The effects of a nutritional intervention do not necessarily negate the effects of the deficiencies it targets. Even if a deficiency is considered harmful, the nutritional intervention aimed to correct it may paradoxically also be harmful. This has mainly been a concern in relation to micronutrient supplementation, where iron supplementation has been shown to increase infectious disease morbidity in children living in areas with a high incidence of malaria (Sazawal et al., 2006). Harmful effects of nutrients given in a food matrix may be less likely, unless very high amounts are given, but the possibility cannot be precluded. Similarly, giving energy to starved individuals may also be harmful, as it may lead to the potentially fatal refeeding syndrome (Heimburger et al., 2010; Koethe et al., 2013). A nutritional intervention, therefore, cannot simply be assumed to be beneficial or even harmless but should be tested in rigorously conducted trials before being implemented.

TABLE 9.1

Potential General and Disease-Specific Effects of Nutritional Deficiencies

General	Health	Reproduction, including fertility and pregnancy outcome
		Child growth and development
		Risk of infections
		Risk of chronic diseases
	Human capital	Working capacity
		Intelligence and educational achievement
		Quality of life
		Survival
HIV-specific	Natural history	Sexual transmission
	Treatment outcomes	Mother-to-child transmission
		Progression of HIV infection
		Opportunistic infections
		Drug absorption, metabolism, efficacy, toxicity, resistance
		Adherence to HIV treatment
		Risk of metabolic syndrome
		Mortality
TB-specific	Natural history	Primary, latent infection
		Overt TB disease
		Progression of disease
	Treatment outcomes	Drug absorption, metabolism, efficacy, toxicity, resistance
		Resolution of lesions
		Sputum conversion, cure, recurrence, and relapse
		Mortality

WHY NUTRITIONAL SUPPORT DURING TREATMENT?

Among TB patients starting treatment, both low BMI and poor early weight gain have been associated with increased mortality (Zachariah et al., 2002; Hanrahan et al., 2010) and other adverse treatment outcomes (Khan et al., 2006; Krapp et al., 2008). Similarly, among HIV patients, low BMI at the start of ART is a predictor of mortality (Lawn et al., 2008; May et al., 2010; Gupta et al., 2011), as is low weight gain during the early stage of treatment (Madec et al., 2009; Koethe et al., 2010; Sudfield et al., 2013). For example, among 40,000 adult HIV patients starting ART in Lusaka, Zambia, a very clear inverse relationship was seen between initial BMI and mortality (Koethe et al., 2010). Compared to those with BMI above 18.5 kg/m^2, mortality was roughly two, three, and five times higher in those with BMI of 17 to 18.5, 16 to 17, or below 16 kg/m^2, respectively. Although such findings from observational studies certainly suggest a role for nutrition, it is important to note that the low BMI and poor weight gain could reflect disease severity and treatment failure, although attempts have been made to adjust for these factors. Yet, although possible effects on mortality spur an interest in nutrition, there are many other important potential outcomes to be considered.

Most TB and HIV patients will gain weight when put on treatment. Unfortunately, this often leads clinicians to wrongly conclude that the drugs are effective in solving the nutritional problem that the patient may have had, and they consequently see no need for nutritional support. In fact, such a judgment accords with the WHO recommendations for TB patients, as long as weight is not declining and BMI is above 18.5 after the first two months of treatment (WHO, 2013). For example, if an adult TB patient with moderate undernutrition gains 2 kg of weight during the first two months of TB treatment, after which the BMI is 19, then the patient is considered to have nutritionally recovered. If this patient, however, had originally lost 10 kg, then the aim would obviously be to regain not just the weight lost but also the lean mass (i.e., muscles and organ tissues, which are essential to a range of body functions). If the regain of weight is inadequate, or if the lean mass that was lost is replaced by fat, then the patient will not recover the body functions lost and may be further at risk of diabetes and other chronic diseases.

It is therefore not correct to argue that treatment of the infection, which initially caused the weight loss, and a subsequent weight gain will solve the nutritional problems of the patient. In fact, in the short term it will actually increase the requirement for energy and nutrients as the patient tries to regain the lost lean and fat mass.

CURRENT EVIDENCE

TUBERCULOSIS

Only few trials on the effect of food supplementation among TB patients at the initiation of treatment have been conducted. A Cochrane Review from 2011 identified six trials assessing the effects of macronutrient supplements (Sinclair et al., 2011). In Singapore, 36 TB patients were randomized to receive either a high-energy commercial nutritional supplement for six weeks with counseling or counseling alone (Paton et al., 2004). The supplementation resulted in a greater weight gain and, importantly, greater gains in lean mass and grip strength. Recruitment and supplementation began up to two weeks after the start of TB treatment. The patients were initially given 600 kcal/day, which increased to 900 kcal/day after one week, if tolerated. In Timor-Leste, 270 new TB patients were randomized to receive nutritional support or nutritional advice only for 32 weeks (Martins et al., 2009). For the first eight weeks, a daily bowl of feijuada—a local stew with meat, red kidney beans, and vegetables that provided 430 kcal/day—was served at the clinic. In the remaining 24 weeks, a food parcel containing unprepared red kidney beans, rice, and oil was given. The intervention had no effect on treatment completion or adherence but resulted in a modestly higher weight gain (10.1% vs. 7.5% of baseline weight).

In Andhra Pradesh, India, 100 TB patients, who had started treatment within two weeks were randomized to receive nutritional supplementation or nutritional advice only for three months (Jahnavi and Sudha, 2010). The supplement was locally produced sweet balls made from wheat flour, caramel, groundnuts, and vegetable ghee, which provided 6 g protein and 600 kcal energy, as well as 100 g of sprouted grains and nuts for vitamins and minerals, provided daily. The intervention group had greater weight gain after three months (3.4 kg vs. 1.1 kg, or 8.6% vs. 2.6%). In Tamil Nadu, India, a pilot study was carried out among 103 TB patients, of whom 22 were HIV co-infected (Sudarsanam et al., 2011). The patients were randomized to either a local cereal–lentil mixture that provided 930 kcal and a micronutrient supplement or no supplementation. There was no effect on compliance to or completion of treatment or on body composition after one year.

In Mwanza, Tanzania, two trials were carried out among 1250 TB patients, of which 50% were HIV co-infected (PrayGod et al., 2011a, 2012). Those with culture-positive TB and HIV co-infection were randomized to receive either one (150 kcal/d) or six (880 kcal/day) biscuits daily for the first two months of treatment (PrayGod et al., 2012). The higher energy supplement had no overall effects on body weight or grip strength after two months but was associated with 1.3 kg greater grip strength after five months. However, subgroup analysis showed that, among those with CD4 counts above 350 cells/μL, the intervention increased weight by 1.9 kg at two months and grip strength by 2.3 kg at five months, whereas there was no effect among those with low CD4 counts.

HIV INFECTION

In Malawi, 491 adult HIV patients starting ART were randomized to supplementation with LNS or a corn–soy blend that provided 1360 kcal/day for three months (Ndekha et al., 2009). Only patients with BMI below 18.5 were included. At the end of the three-month supplementation period, those receiving LNS had 0.5 greater increase in BMI and 0.7 kg greater increase in lean mass, measured using bioimpedance. There was no difference between the groups in mortality (27% vs. 26%) or other secondary outcomes, such as CD4 count, HIV viral load, adherence to ART, or quality of life. A Cochrane Review of macronutrient intervention trials among HIV patients included only trials using unsupplemented control groups (Grobler et al., 2013). No published trial data among adults were included from HIV-prevalent, food-insecure settings; however, unpublished data from a trial in Kenya of malnourished HIV patients starting ART were described. In this trial, 1057 HIV patients, stratified according to ART status (pre-ART patients and patients initiating ART within five weeks of recruitment), were randomized to receive a supplement of 300 g/day of fortified, blended food or no supplement for six months; both groups received nutrition counseling for 12 months. The fortified, blended food was based on maize and soy, with whey protein concentrate, and provided 1320 kcal/day. The trial found that, after the first three months, supplementation increased weight gain by 1.22 kg in pre-ART patients and 1.12 kg in ART patients compared to no supplementation.

In Ethiopia, 318 HIV patients starting ART were included in the ARTFood trial, which compared the effect of LNS with whey and soy protein for the first three months of ART or the subsequent three months (Olsen et al., 2014). HIV patients eligible for ART were included if BMI was above 16, yet those with BMI between 16 and 17 were randomized to the early supplementation group only. Thus, it was possible to compare the effect of LNS with whey or soy to no supplementation for the first three months among patients with BMI above 17. After three months, those receiving LNS had increased their weight by 2.05 kg in addition to the 0.87-kg weight gain seen among participants receiving only ART. Furthermore, those on early supplementation gained 0.90 kg of lean body mass, assessed by the deuterium dilution technique, compared to individuals in the control group, who in effect did not gain lean mass at all. After six months, when all groups had completed three months of supplementation, those receiving the delayed intervention had a 1.2-kg greater weight gain compared to those receiving supplementation early. This secondary comparison was complicated by the fact that those receiving early supplementation actually lost weight during the subsequent three months; however, this weight loss was accounted for by loss of fat mass, whereas lean mass accretion continued. Actually, consumption of the supplement was reduced during the first few weeks after the start of ART (Olsen et al., 2013); hence, intake was greater in those with delayed supplementation, but this only partially explained the difference in weight gain. At six months, there was no difference in lean mass, but grip strength and physical activity were higher in the early supplemented group. In addition, at three months, those receiving the LNS with whey had a significant increase in CD3 and CD8 and a marginally significant increase in CD4 when compared with the delayed supplementation group. The differences between the LNS with whey or soy, however, were not significant. In contrast to other studies, this trial did not exclude patients with BMI above a certain cut-off and found that the effects of nutritional supplementation were not modified by BMI.

In Tanzania and Zambia, the NUSTART trial assessed the effects of not only macro- and micronutrients but also bulk minerals, such as phosphorus, potassium, and magnesium, given in LNS. Patients starting ART with BMI below 18.5 were randomized to receive 30 g of LNS from recruitment until two weeks after the start of ART and then 250 g of LNS from weeks 2 to 6 of ART, with additional macro- and microminerals, as well as vitamins. The control group received similar amounts of LNS, with no added vitamins and minerals. This trial was based on the paradoxically high early mortality among HIV patients starting ART, despite indications that the drugs are effective in reducing viral load, and the observation that mortality is predicted by low serum phosphate, a common metabolic abnormality associated with malnutrition. This led to the hypothesis that mortality was due to ART-related hypophosphatemia, similar to refeeding hypophosphatemia, seen when starved individuals receive too much energy too early. Both groups gained about 5 kg between referral for ART and 12 weeks of ART, and high-energy supplements were associated with greater increases in anthropometric measures in the group with high vitamins and minerals (Rehman et al., 2015). However, there was no difference in mortality rate, which was high in both groups (NUSTART Study Team et al., 2015).

RESEARCH GAPS

SUPPLEMENTATION PRODUCTS AND APPROACHES

A wide variety of intervention products have been used with few direct comparisons between them. In the trial in Malawi (Ndekha et al., 2009), LNS improved anthropometry more than a corn–soy blend. In the NUSTART trial, LNS with high levels of vitamins and minerals had modest benefits for anthropometry over and above unfortified LNS (Rehman et al., 2015). In the ARTFood trial, there were no significant differences between LNS that contained whey or soy protein. Overall, it appears that high-nutrient, energy-dense LNS are a good choice in the short term for patients who begin ART in a malnourished state. However, long-term supplementation with these products is unlikely to be sustainable, so they are suitable only for acute care. Longer term nutritional interventions will require other foods or other approaches, such as food vouchers or livelihood support.

INCLUSION CRITERIA—ALL OR LOW BMI?

Nutritional intervention studies for HIV or TB usually target patients with low BMI or food insecurity, or some combination of the two. The inclusion criteria should depend, in part, on what type of intervention is planned. BMI is easier to measure precisely as a trial or programmatic outcome compared with food insecurity. It is important if nutritional interventions for HIV or TB are to be included in policies and scaled up that there is a strong evidence base from trials with clear aims and inclusion criteria and evaluations that clearly address the aims, something that has not always been the case in the past.

TIMING OF SUPPLEMENTATION

Both the ARTFood (Olsen et al., 2013, 2014) and NUSTART trials (Rehman et al., 2014) found that appetite was depressed in the first couple of weeks after starting ART, presumably in response to the drugs themselves. This appetite depression likely reduces the potential benefits of nutritional supplements started at the time of starting ART, which is the most frequent approach in current controlled studies. Findings from the ARTFood trial, described above, also suggested some benefits of delaying supplementation until after viral load has declined. From a nutritional standpoint, it might seem sensible to delay the nutritional support until several weeks after starting ART. Research is needed to determine the optimal timing of supplementation. However, this may not always be feasible in practice, as clinic visits, during which supplements and associated counseling could be provided, are not scheduled within the first few weeks after starting ART in all ART programs. An alternative approach, which needs to be investigated, would involve slowly increasing the amount of supplementation after initiating ART.

INFLAMMATION

The NUSTART trial found that increases in anthropometric measures and lean mass were associated with decreases in systemic inflammation, as measured by C-reactive protein (CRP) (NUSTART Study Team et al., 2015; Rehman et al., 2015; PrayGod et al., 2016). Fat mass deposition, in contrast, was not associated with changes in CRP. This is similar to a finding of the ARTFood trial in which lean mass deposition at three months of ART was greater in patients who had obtained an undetectable HIV viral load. In both cases, it appears that ongoing infection and inflammation inhibit lean tissue deposition and, perhaps, result in fat deposition instead. In view of the need for lean mass in the short term and the potential adverse effects of fat deposition in the long term, it is important to investigate the reasons for ongoing inflammation and its effects on tissue deposition in patients being treated for HIV or TB.

RISK OF CHRONIC DISEASES

Interventions for HIV and TB in low-income countries have focused on acute care and nutritional deficiencies; however, HIV is now becoming a chronic disease, and there is evidence that long-term ART can increase the risks of lipid abnormalities, diabetes, hypertension, and cardiovascular disease (Narayan et al., 2014). There is also evidence that severe infections themselves (i.e., not just the treatments) can have similar long-term risks. Currently, not much is known about the development of such risks in patients from low-income countries who have been treated for HIV or TB or about how to manage these risks. However, these chronic diseases in other situations can be mitigated by nutritional interventions, so there is a need to determine what interventions may work and be acceptable in low-income settings.

PERCEPTIONS, ACCEPTABILITY, AND PROGRAMMATIC ISSUES

Although the ARTFood and NUSTART trials both found good adherence to LNS products, several nutritional programs have reported problems with low adherence to supplementation among HIV patients. It is therefore important to consider how supplementation can be scaled up so that it can be implemented through the normal HIV care facilities. There is a continued need to determine the optimal duration and amount of supplementation. The ARTFood trial showed beneficial effects of three months of supplementation with 200 g/day of LNS, although other experiences from supplementation programs suggest that larger amounts of LNS for extended periods may not be feasible (Kebede and Haidar, 2014). Other barriers to adherence have been identified as patients' concerns about the risk of HIV disclosure and, in some settings, patients' dislike of the taste of LNS, which is often very different from their usual foods. On the other hand, the fact that LNS products are distinct from household foods and provided with medical treatment can facilitate patient adherence and reduce the risk of supplements being shared among household members (Olsen et al., 2013). It is crucial to consider acceptability issues in the specific context of supplementation programs. In settings where patients are affected by general food insecurity, other types of programs are needed to complement the time-limited nutritional support at the initiation of treatment.

CONCLUSION

Nutritional support to TB and HIV patients is important. The first few months may be particularly critical, as the energy and nutrient requirements are very high. If these are not met, then patients may not regain lost tissues and functions and may even be at risk of chronic diseases. However, a number of research questions remain to be addressed in order to inform revisions to policies and programs aimed at promoting good nutrition among people with HIV and TB infections.

REFERENCES

Beck, M. A., Q. Shi, V. C. Morris, and O. A. Levander. (1995). Rapid genomic evolution of a non-virulent coxsackievirus B3 in selenium-deficient mice results in selection of identical virulent isolates. *Nature Medicine* 1(5): 433–6.

CDC. (1981). Pneumocystis pneumonia—Los Angeles. *Morbidity and Mortality Weekly Report (MMWR)* 30(21): 250–2.

Clumeck, N., F. Mascart-Lemone, J. de Maubeuge, D. Brenez, and L. Marcelis. (1983). Acquired immune deficiency syndrome in Black Africans. *Lancet* 1(8325): 642.

Fawzi, W. W., G. I. Msamanga, D. Hunter et al. (2002). Randomized trial of vitamin supplements in relation to transmission of HIV-1 through breastfeeding and early child mortality. *AIDS* 16(14): 1935–44.

Fawzi, W. W., G. I. Msamanga, D. Spiegelman et al. (2004). A randomized trial of multivitamin supplements and HIV disease progression and mortality. *New England Journal of Medicine* 351(1): 23–32.

Fertel, D. and A. E. Pitchenik. (1989). Tuberculosis in acquired immune deficiency syndrome. *Seminars in Respiratory Infections* 4(3): 198–205.

Fraker, P. J., L. E. King, T. Laakko, and T. L. Vollmer. (2000). The dynamic link between the integrity of the immune system and zinc status. *Journal of Nutrition* 130(5S, Suppl.): 1399S–1406S.

Frieden, T. R., T. R. Sterling, S. S. Munsiff, C. J. Watt, and C. Dye. (2003). Tuberculosis. *Lancet* 362(9387): 887–99.

Grobler, L., N. Siegfried, M. E. Visser, S. S. N. Mahlungulu, and J. Volmink. (2013). Nutritional interventions for reducing morbidity and mortality in people with HIV. *Cochrane Database of Systematic Reviews* 2: CD004536.

Gupta, A., G. Nadkarni, W.-T. Yang et al. (2011). Early mortality in adults initiating antiretroviral therapy (ART) in low- and middle-income countries (LMIC): a systematic review and meta-analysis. *PLoS One* 6(12): e28691.

Hanrahan, C. F., J. E. Golub, L. Mohapi et al. (2010). Body mass index and risk of tuberculosis and death. *AIDS* 24(10): 1501–8.

Heimburger, D. C., J. R. Koethe, C. Nyirenda et al. (2010). Serum phosphate predicts early mortality in adults starting antiretroviral therapy in Lusaka, Zambia: a prospective cohort study. *PLoS One* 5(5): e10687.

Jahnavi, G., and C. H. Sudha. (2010). Randomised controlled trial of food supplements in patients with newly diagnosed tuberculosis and wasting. *Singapore Medical Journal* 51(12): 957–62.

Kalichman, S. C., M. Watt, K. Sikkema, D. Skinner, and D. Pieterse. (2012). Food insufficiency, substance use, and sexual risks for HIV/AIDS in informal drinking establishments, Cape Town, South Africa. *Journal of Urban Health* 89(6): 939–51.

Kebede, M. A. and J. Haidar. (2014). Factors influencing adherence to the food by prescription program among adult HIV positive patients in Addis Ababa, Ethiopia: a facility-based, cross-sectional study. *Infectious Diseases of Poverty* 3(1): 20.

Khan, A., T. R. Sterling, R. Reves, A.Vernon, and C. R. Horsburgh. (2006). Lack of weight gain and relapse risk in a large tuberculosis treatment trial. *American Journal of Respiratory and Critical Care Medicine* 174(3): 344–8.

Koethe, J. R., A. Lukusa, M. J. Giganti et al. (2010). Association between weight gain and clinical outcomes among malnourished adults initiating antiretroviral therapy in Lusaka, Zambia. *Journal of Acquired Immune Deficiency Syndromes* 53(4): 507–13.

Koethe, J. R., M. Blevins, C. K. Nyirenda et al. (2013). Serum phosphate predicts early mortality among underweight adults starting ART in Zambia: a novel context for refeeding syndrome? *Journal of Nutrition and Metabolism* 2013(4): 545439.

Krapp, F., J. C. Véliz, E. Cornejo, E. Gotuzzo, and C. Seas. (2008). Bodyweight gain to predict treatment outcome in patients with pulmonary tuberculosis in Peru. *International Journal of Tuberculosis and Lung Disease* 12(10): 1153–9.

Lawn, S. D., A. D. Harries, X. Anglaret, L. Myer, and R. Wood. (2008). Early mortality among adults accessing antiretroviral treatment programmes in sub-Saharan Africa. *AIDS* 22(15): 1897–908.

Madec, Y., E. Szumilin, C. Genevier et al. (2009). Weight gain at 3 months of antiretroviral therapy is strongly associated with survival: evidence from two developing countries. *AIDS* 23(7): 853–61.

Martins, N., P. Morris, and P. M. Kelly. (2009). Food incentives to improve completion of tuberculosis treatment: randomised controlled trial in Dili, Timor-Leste. *BMJ* 339: b4248.

May, M., A. Boulle, S. Phiri et al.; IeDEA Southern Africa and West Africa. (2010). Prognosis of patients with HIV-1 infection starting antiretroviral therapy in sub-Saharan Africa: a collaborative analysis of scale-up programmes. *Lancet* 376(9739): 449–57.

Melbye, M., A. Bayley, E. K. Njelesani et al. (1986). Evidence for heterosexual transmission and clinical manifestations of human immunodeficiency virus infection and related conditions in Lusaka, Zambia. *Lancet* 328(8516): 1113–5.

Narayan, K. M., P. G. Miotti, N. P. Anand et al. (2014). HIV and noncommunicable disease comorbidities in the era of antiretroviral therapy: a vital agenda for research in low- and middle-income country settings. *Journal of Acquired Immune Deficiency Syndromes* 67(Suppl. 1): S2–7.

Ndekha, M. J., J. J. G. van Oosterhout, E. E. Zijlstra et al. (2009). Supplementary feeding with either ready-to-use fortified spread or corn-soy blend in wasted adults starting antiretroviral therapy in Malawi: randomised, investigator blinded, controlled trial. *BMJ* 338(7706): 1309–12.

NUSTART Study Team, S. Filteau, G. PrayGod, L. Kasonka et al. (2015). Effects on mortality of a nutritional intervention for malnourished HIV-infected adults referred for antiretroviral therapy: a randomised controlled trial. *BMC Medicine* 13: 17.

Olsen, M. F., M. Tesfaye, P. Kæstel, H. Friis, and L. Holm. (2013). Use, perceptions, and acceptability of a ready-to-use supplementary food among adult HIV patients initiating antiretroviral treatment: a qualitative study in Ethiopia. *Patient Preference and Adherence* 7: 481–8.

Olsen, M. F., A. Abdissa, P. Kæstel et al. (2014). Effects of nutritional supplementation for HIV patients starting antiretroviral treatment: randomised controlled trial in Ethiopia. *BMJ* 348: g3187.

Paton, N. I., Y.-K. Chua, A. Earnest, and C. B. Chee. (2004). Randomized controlled trial of nutritional supplementation in patients with newly diagnosed tuberculosis and wasting. *American Journal of Clinical Nutrition* 80(2): 460–5.

PrayGod, G., N. Range, D. Faurholt-Jepsen et al. (2011a). Daily multi-micronutrient supplementation during tuberculosis treatment increases weight and grip strength among HIV-uninfected but not HIV-infected patients in Mwanza, Tanzania. *Journal of Nutrition* 141(4): 685–91.

PrayGod, G., N. Range, D. Faurholt-Jepsen et al. (2011b). Weight, body composition and handgrip strength among pulmonary tuberculosis patients: a matched cross-sectional study in Mwanza, Tanzania. *Transactions of the Royal Society of Tropical Medicine and Hygiene* 105(3): 140–7.

PrayGod, G., N. Range, D. Faurholt-Jepsen et al. (2012). The effect of energy-protein supplementation on weight, body composition and handgrip strength among pulmonary tuberculosis HIV-co-infected patients: randomised controlled trial in Mwanza, Tanzania. *British Journal of Nutrition* 107(2): 263–71.

PrayGod, G., M. Blevins, S. Woodd et al. (2016). A longitudinal study of systemic inflammation and recovery of lean body mass among malnourished HIV-infected adults starting antiretroviral therapy in Tanzania and Zambia. *European Journal of Clinical Nutrition* 70(4): 499–504.

Ramakrishnan, C. V., K. Rajendran, P. G. Jacob, W. Fox, and S. Radhakrishna. (1961). The role of diet in the treatment of pulmonary tuberculosis: an evaluation in a controlled chemotherapy study in home and sanatorium patients in South India. *Bulletin of the World Health Organization* 25(3): 339–59.

Range, N., Y. A. Ipuge, R. J. O'Brien et al. (2001). Trend in HIV prevalence among tuberculosis patients in Tanzania, 1991–1998. *International Journal of Tuberculosis and Lung Disease* 5(5): 405–12.

Rehman, A. M., S. Woodd, M. Chisenga et al. (2014). Appetite testing in HIV-infected African adults recovering from malnutrition and given antiretroviral therapy. *Public Health Nutrition* 18(4): 742–51.

Rehman, A. M., S. Woodd, G. PrayGod et al. (2015). Effects on anthropometry and appetite of vitamins and minerals given in lipid nutritional supplements for malnourished HIV-infected adults referred for antiretroviral therapy: results from the NUSTART Randomized Controlled Trial. *Journal of Acquired Immune Deficiency Syndromes* 68(4): 405–12.

Sazawal, S., R. E. Black, M. Ramsan et al. (2006). Effects of routine prophylactic supplementation with iron and folic acid on admission to hospital and mortality in preschool children in a high malaria transmission setting: community-based, randomised, placebo-controlled trial. *Lancet* 367(9505): 133–43.

Schonland, M. (1972). Depression of immunity in protein-calorie malnutrition: a post-mortem study. *Journal of Tropical Pediatrics and Environmental Child Health* 18(3): 217–24.

Sepkowitz, K. A. (2001). AIDS—the first 20 years. *New England Journal of Medicine* 344(23): 1764–72.

Sinclair, D., K. Abba, L. Grobler, and T. D. Sudarsanam. (2011). Nutritional supplements for people being treated for active tuberculosis. *Cochrane Database of Systematic Reviews* (11): CD006086.

Sudarsanam, T. D., J. John, G. Kang et al. (2011). Pilot randomized trial of nutritional supplementation in patients with tuberculosis and HIV-tuberculosis coinfection receiving directly observed short-course chemotherapy for tuberculosis. *Tropical Medicine & International Health* 16(6): 699–706.

Sudfeld, C. R., S. Isanaka, F. M. Mugusi et al. (2013). Weight change at 1 mo of antiretroviral therapy and its association with subsequent mortality, morbidity, and CD4 T cell reconstitution in a Tanzanian HIV-infected adult cohort. *American Journal of Clinical Nutrition* 97(6): 1278–87.

Van Lettow, M. and C. Whalen. (2008). Tuberculosis. In: *Nutrition and Health in Developing Countries*, 2nd ed. (Semba, R.D. and Bloem, M.W., Eds.), pp. 275–306. Totowa, NJ: Humana Press.

Whalen, C. and R. D. Semba. (2001). Tuberculosis. In: *Nutrition and Health in Developing Countries* (Semba, R.D. and Bloem, M.W., Eds.), pp. 209–235. Totowa, NJ: Humana Press.

WHO. (2004). *Nutrient Requirements for People Living with HIV/AIDS: Report of a Technical Consultation, 13–15 May, 2003, Geneva, Switzerland.* Geneva: World Health Organization (http://www.who.int/nutrition/publications/hivaids/9241591196/en/).

WHO. (2013). *Guideline: Nutritional Care and Support for Patients with Tuberculosis.* Geneva: World Health Organization (http://www.who.int/nutrition/publications/guidelines/nutcare_support_patients_with_tb/en/).

Zachariah, R., M. P. Spielmann, A. D. Harries, and F. M. L. Salaniponi. (2002). Moderate to severe malnutrition in patients with tuberculosis is a risk factor associated with early death. *Transactions of the Royal Society of Tropical Medicine and Hygiene* 96(3): 291–4.

Index

endothelial damage, selenium and, 200
env gene, 8
ergocalciferol, 176
erythrocyte sedimentation rate, 163
Escherichia coli, 13, 259
esophageal candidiasis, 4
exclusive breastfeeding (EBF), 247–248, 252, 262, 263, 265, 266
exclusive formula feeding (EFF), 247
extended-release niacin, 68–72, 79–80, 81, 83

F

fat deposition, 314
febrile proteinuria, 4
ferritin, *see* serum ferritin
ferrous sulfate, 193, 238
fetal death
　multivitamins, and, 13, 75, 237, 238
　selenium supplementation, and, 200, 235, 237
　vitamin A supplementation, and, 236
　zinc supplementation, and 236
fever, 3–4
　vitamin B supplementation, and, 77
　multivitamin supplementation, and 297, 298
　zinc supplementation, and, 297
fibroblast growth factor 23 (FGF-23), 176
flow-mediated dilatation (FMD), 80, 164, 177, 178
flow-mediated vasodilation, 80
folate, 28, 29, 30, 76, 82, 193, 296; *see also* vitamin B$_9$
　antagonists, 79
　biomarkers for, 31
　deficiency, 234
　highly active antiretroviral therapy (HAART), and, 29
folic acid, 32, 34–36, 53–65, 67, 78–79, 81, 83, 98, 101, 127, 211, 222, 223, 230, 231, 232, 278, 280, 283, 288, 290, 291, 298, 299
　anemia, and, 134, 137, 140, 142, 143, 208, 236
　anthropometry and growth, and, 77
　birthweight, and, 236, 238
　cardiovascular outcomes, and, 79
　cognitive and psychomotor development, and, 78
　hematologic status, and, 78
　HIV disease progression, and, 33, 237
　HIV transmission, and, 76, 296
　HIV viral load, and, 73, 236
　immune function, and, 28, 73
　pregnancy, and, 75
　supplementation with iron, 142, 143, 208, 236, 239
　tuberculosis, and, 74
folinic acid, 78
formula feeding, 253–266
　exclusive, 247, 264

G

galactopoesis, 249
gestational age at delivery
　iron, and, 93, 134, 142
　micronutrient supplementation, and, 208
　vitamin B supplementation, and, 31, 75
glutathione peroxidase, 200
grip strength, 312, 313
gynecological infections, 9, 11

H

HAART, *see* highly active antiretroviral therapy
height for age (HAZ)
　iron supplementation, and, 137, 140, 141
　vitamin B supplementation, and 62, 77
　zinc supplementation, and 202
hemoglobin
　ART, and, 143
　HAART, and, 141
　HIV viral load, and, 138
　iron, and, 90, 91, 93, 134, 135, 138
　multivitamins, and, 238
　selenium, and, 237
　stavudine, and, 140
　vitamin A, and, 296
　vitamin D, and, 164
　zidovudine, and, 142, 234
　zinc, and, 193, 199, 236, 297
hepatitis C virus (HCV), vitamin D and, 165
hepcidin, 93, 135, 137, 138, 139, 144–145
highly active antiretroviral therapy (HAART), 14–18, 21, 33, 73, 79, 80, 82
　iron, and, 91, 136, 140–143, 145–146
　lipid-based nutrient supplements, and, 143
　micronutrient supplementation, and, 239, 299, 302–303
　selenium, and, 199–200, 237
　vitamin B, and, 29
　zinc supplementation, and, 199, 297
HIV-1-LTR reporter gene activity, 156
HIV-1 transactivator factor (Tat), 3
HIV Epidemiology Research Study (HERS), 11
HIV viral load, *see* viral load
HL-60 promyelocytic cell line, 155–156
homeostatic model assessment of insulin resistance (HOMA-IR), 80, 177, 202
human immunodeficiency virus (HIV)
　antioxidants, and, 191–203
　as chronic disease, 315
　deaths due to, 1
　in utero exposure to, 140, 235, 245, 276, 302
　infant feeding, and, 243–267
　iron, and, 89–146
　macronutrients, and, 307–315
　micronutrients, and, 207–239, 275–303
　prevalence, 191, 276
　vitamin A, and, 1–21
　vitamin B, and, 27–83
　vitamin D, and, 153–180
　weight and muscle strength deficits, 310
human papillomavirus (HPV), 11
hypertension
　antiretroviral therapy, and, 315
　multivitamin supplementation, and, 75
　prenatal multivitamins, and, 238
　vitamin D, and, 164
hypochromasia, 135, 139, 142, 164
hypophosphatemia, 313

I

immune function, 3, 12, 13
　iron, and, 90
　nutritional deficiencies, and, 310

Printed in the United States
by Baker & Taylor Publisher Services

Printed in the United States
by Baker & Taylor Publisher Services